Anticancer Inhibitors

Anticancer Inhibitors

Editors

Marialuigia Fantacuzzi
Alessandra Ammazzalorso

MDPI • Basel • Beijing • Wuhan • Barcelona • Belgrade • Manchester • Tokyo • Cluj • Tianjin

Editors
Marialuigia Fantacuzzi
Pharmacy
"G. d'Annunzio" University
of Chieti-Pescara
Chieti
Italy

Alessandra Ammazzalorso
Pharmacy
"G. d'Annunzio" University
of Chieti-Pescara
Chieti
Italy

Editorial Office
MDPI
St. Alban-Anlage 66
4052 Basel, Switzerland

This is a reprint of articles from the Special Issue published online in the open access journal *Molecules* (ISSN 1420-3049) (available at: www.mdpi.com/journal/molecules/special_issues/anticancer_inhibitor).

For citation purposes, cite each article independently as indicated on the article page online and as indicated below:

LastName, A.A.; LastName, B.B.; LastName, C.C. Article Title. *Journal Name* **Year**, *Volume Number*, Page Range.

ISBN 978-3-0365-4920-0 (Hbk)
ISBN 978-3-0365-4919-4 (PDF)

Contents

About the Editors vii

Alessandra Ammazzalorso and Marialuigia Fantacuzzi
Anticancer Inhibitors
Reprinted from: *Molecules* **2022**, *27*, 4650, doi:10.3390/molecules27144650 1

Alessandra Ammazzalorso, Mariangela Agamennone, Barbara De Filippis and Marialuigia Fantacuzzi
Development of CDK4/6 Inhibitors: A Five Years Update
Reprinted from: *Molecules* **2021**, *26*, 1488, doi:10.3390/molecules26051488 5

Huda S. Al-Salem, Md Arifuzzaman, Hamad M. Alkahtani, Ashraf N. Abdalla, Iman S. Issa and Aljawharah Alqathama et al.
A Series of Isatin-Hydrazones with Cytotoxic Activity and CDK2 Kinase Inhibitory Activity: A Potential Type II ATP Competitive Inhibitor
Reprinted from: *Molecules* **2020**, *25*, 4400, doi:10.3390/molecules25194400 27

Mohamed E. Abdallah, Mahmoud Zaki El-Readi, Mohammad Ahmad Althubiti, Riyad Adnan Almaimani, Amar Mohamed Ismail and Shakir Idris et al.
Tamoxifen and the PI3K Inhibitor: LY294002 Synergistically Induce Apoptosis and Cell Cycle Arrest in Breast Cancer MCF-7 Cells
Reprinted from: *Molecules* **2020**, *25*, 3355, doi:10.3390/molecules25153355 43

Eva Konkoľová, Monika Hudáčová, Slávka Hamuľaková, Rastislav Jendželovský, Jana Vargová and Juraj Ševc et al.
Tacrine-Coumarin Derivatives as Topoisomerase Inhibitors with Antitumor Effects on A549 Human Lung Carcinoma Cancer Cell Lines
Reprinted from: *Molecules* **2021**, *26*, 1133, doi:10.3390/molecules26041133 59

Sei-ichi Tanuma, Kiyotaka Katsuragi, Takahiro Oyama, Atsushi Yoshimori, Yuri Shibasaki and Yasunobu Asawa et al.
Structural Basis of Beneficial Design for Effective Nicotinamide Phosphoribosyltransferase Inhibitors
Reprinted from: *Molecules* **2020**, *25*, 3633, doi:10.3390/molecules25163633 73

Tal Tilayov, Tal Hingaly, Yariv Greenshpan, Shira Cohen, Barak Akabayov and Roi Gazit et al.
Engineering Stem Cell Factor Ligands with Different c-Kit Agonistic Potencies
Reprinted from: *Molecules* **2020**, *25*, 4850, doi:10.3390/molecules25204850 89

Hui Yang, Jasmine Heyer, Hui Zhao, Shengxian Liang, Rui Guo and Li Zhong
The Potential Role of Cathepsin K in Non-Small Cell Lung Cancer
Reprinted from: *Molecules* **2020**, *25*, 4136, doi:10.3390/molecules25184136 107

Yun Chen, Ya-Hui Tsai and Sheng-Hong Tseng
Regulation of ZMYND8 to Treat Cancer
Reprinted from: *Molecules* **2021**, *26*, 1083, doi:10.3390/molecules26041083 119

Silvie Rimpelová, Michal Kolář, Hynek Strnad, Tomáš Ruml, Libor Vítek and Helena Gbelcová
Comparison of Transcriptomic Profiles of MiaPaCa-2 Pancreatic Cancer Cells Treated with Different Statins
Reprinted from: *Molecules* **2021**, *26*, 3528, doi:10.3390/molecules26123528 131

Yaomin Wang, Chen Xia, Lianfu Chen, Yi Charlie Chen and Youying Tu
Saponins Extracted from Tea (*Camellia Sinensis*) Flowers Induces Autophagy in Ovarian Cancer Cells
Reprinted from: *Molecules* **2020**, *25*, 5254, doi:10.3390/molecules25225254 . . . . **153**

Youying Tu, Lianfu Chen, Ning Ren, Bo Li, Yuanyuan Wu and Gary O. Rankin et al.
Standardized Saponin Extract from Baiye No.1 Tea (*Camellia sinensis*) Flowers Induced S Phase Cell Cycle Arrest and Apoptosis via AKT-MDM2-p53 Signaling Pathway in Ovarian Cancer Cells
Reprinted from: *Molecules* **2020**, *25*, 3515, doi:10.3390/molecules25153515 . . . . **165**

Henrik Franzyk and Søren Brøgger Christensen
Targeting Toxins toward Tumors
Reprinted from: *Molecules* **2021**, *26*, 1292, doi:10.3390/molecules26051292 . . . . **183**

About the Editors

Marialuigia Fantacuzzi

Marialuigia Fantacuzzi is an Assistant Professor in Medicinal Chemistry at the Department of Pharmacy, "G. d'Annunzio"University of Chieti-Pescara (Italy). She received a degree in Pharmaceutical Chemistry and Technology and a Ph.D. in Pharmaceutical Sciences from the same university. Her research interests are mainly focused on design, synthesis, biological evaluation, and docking study of compounds of pharmaceutical interest useful for the treatment of inflammatory pathology, metabolic syndrome, neurodegenerative diseases, and cancer.

Her scientific activity is certified by 61 papers in international peer reviewed journals and different communications in scientific meetings. Her commitment to pharmaceutical chemistry is rounded out by her role as a reviewer for major international medicinal chemistry journals, as well as her participation as an editorial board member and as a Special Issue guest editor.

Alessandra Ammazzalorso

Alessandra Ammazzalorso is an Assistant Professor in Medicinal Chemistry at the Department of Pharmacy, "G. d'Annunzio"University of Chieti-Pescara (Italy). She obtained her degree in Pharmaceutical Chemistry and Technology and Ph.D. in Pharmaceutical Sciences. Her research activity is devoted to the synthesis of small molecules endowed with biological activity. In detail, her studies are focused on compounds targeting Peroxisome Proliferator-Activated Receptors, with special attention to the antitumor potential of their agonists and antagonists. She is also involved in the identification of novel inhibitors of nitric oxide synthase and aromatase as anticancer agents. Her research activity is documented by 74 peer reviewed papers, several contributions to scientific meetings, and participation in international and national research projects. She is also a reviewer for several high-ranked medicinal chemistry journals, and she serves as an editorial board member for different international journals.

molecules MDPI

Editorial

Anticancer Inhibitors

Alessandra Ammazzalorso * and Marialuigia Fantacuzzi *

Department of Pharmacy, "G. d'Annunzio" University of Chieti-Pescara, Via dei Vestini 31, 66100 Chieti, Italy
* Correspondence: alessandra.ammazzalorso@unich.it (A.A.); marialuigia.fantacuzzi@unich.it (M.F.); Tel.: +39-08713554682 (A.A.); +39-08713554684 (M.F.)

Citation: Ammazzalorso, A.; Fantacuzzi, M. Anticancer Inhibitors. *Molecules* **2022**, *27*, 4650. https://doi.org/10.3390/molecules27144650

Received: 1 July 2022
Accepted: 16 July 2022
Published: 21 July 2022

1. Introduction

Cancer is a multifactorial disorder caused by several aberrations in gene expression that generate a homeostatic imbalance between cell division and death. Because of the worldwide increasing burden and the complexity of the mechanisms involved, considerable efforts have been devoted to cancer management. Many chemotherapeutics have been developed, but most of them have failed in cancer treatment. Antitumor drugs can be divided in non-specific (cytotoxic) drugs and specific drugs (targeted). Due to the inability of non-specific drugs to selectively target tumor cells, targeted therapy has grown more in recent years, allowing researchers to identify drugs characterized by a high specificity towards receptors and enzymes involved in cancer proliferation [1–7]. Since multiple pathogenetic mechanisms are involved in the development of cancer, the characterization of different types of cancers, which distinguishes them from healthy cells and other cancers, allows for the identification of specific targets for each individual tumor.

The Special Issue "Anticancer Inhibitors" covers twelve contributes (nine original research papers and three reviews). As guest editors, we briefly report an overview of these contributions.

2. Results

The roles of cyclin-dependent kinases (CDKs) in different cancers allows for targeting specific kinases to obtain a selective action in the cell cycle and gene transcription. In the last years, CDK4/6 inhibitors revealed a therapeutic role for the treatment of breast cancer. Structural modifications of the three FDA-approved CDK4/6 inhibitors furnished novel molecules currently under clinical investigation as antitumor drugs. The novel generation of PROTACs (proteolysis targeting chimeras) has also been reviewed, allowing for a selective degradation of CDK4 or CDK6 by varying the chemical structures of inhibitors and linkers [8].

Al-Salem et al. synthesized a series of isatin-hydrazones with cytotoxic effects against MCF-7 and A2780 cell lines. Structure–activity relationship studies highlighted the structural modifications mainly responsible for the CDK2 IC_{50s} nanomolar range activity. In silico ADME demonstrated the recommended drug likeness properties, while computational predictions of the binding mode confirmed type II ATP competitive inhibition [9].

Phosphatidylinositide-3-kinase (PI3K)/Akt signaling pathway inhibitors have undergone pre-clinical evaluation as a promising therapy for cancer treatment; the combination use of LY294002 and tamoxifen in breast cancer MCF-7 cells was indagated by Abdallah and coworkers. A synergistic cytotoxic effect of the combination, achieved by the induction of apoptosis and cell cycle arrest through cyclin D1, pAKT, caspases, and Bcl-2 signaling pathways, was found helpful to develop novel and effective therapeutic combination against breast cancer and reduce the toxicity and resistance of LY294002 and tamoxifen [10].

Konkol'ová et al. synthesized novel tacrine–coumarin hybrids as inhibitors of topoisomerase, and enzyme involved in DNA metabolism. Novel compounds inhibit the metabolic activity of A549 cell line in a time- and dose-dependent manner, increase the accumulation of cells in the G0/G1 phase, and topoisomerase I inhibition was confirmed as the mechanism of action of this class of hybrids [11].

Tanuma et al. synthesized novel azaindole–piperidine or azaindole–piperazine to develop effective and safer (no gastrointestinal symptoms and thrombocytopenia) anticancer nicotinamide phosphoribosyltransferase (NAMPT) inhibitors [12].

Tilayov et al. combined rational and combinatorial engineering approaches for transforming dimeric stem cell factor (SCF) into ligands with different agonistic potencies by engineering variants with a reduced dimerization potential and an increased affinity for c-Kit. The combinatorial site-directed engineering of both ligand–ligand and ligand–receptor interactions provides the means to generate improved therapeutic mediators and to gain insights into the dynamics of receptor tyrosine kinases (RTK)–ligand interactions [13].

The involvement of Cathepsin K in non-small-cell lung cancer has been investigated by Yang et al. through in vitro experiments of cell proliferation, migration, and invasion in human cell line A549. The results showed that Cathepsin K was overexpressed, promoting the proliferation, migration, invasion, and activation of the mammalian target of the rapamycin (mTOR) signaling pathway [14].

The review by Chen collects the literature evidence about both pro-oncogenic and tumor-suppressive effects of ZMYND8 (zinc finger myeloid, nervy, and deformed epidermal autoregulatory factor 1-type containing 8) in various types of cancer [15].

Rimpelová et al. studied the effect of statins on the expression of genes, whose products are implicated in cancer inhibition. The study on MiaPaCa-2 pancreatic cancer cells analyzes the genes involved in the metabolism of lipids and steroids that were affected by statin treatment [16].

The pivotal role played by natural products in the discovery and development of novel anticancer agents is well known [17]. The anticancer effect of saponins from tea (*Camellia sinensis*) was investigated by Wang et al. The extracted saponins decreased cell viability and induced morphological changes in OVCAR-3 cells. The autophagic effect occurred independently from Akt/mTOR/p70S6K pathway signaling, but it is linked to ERK activation and ROS generation [18]. A further evaluation on a high purity standardized saponin extract, namely, Baiye No.1 tea flower saponin, demonstrated its potential to be used as a nutraceutical for the prevention and treatment of ovarian cancer [19].

Franzyk and Christensen reviewed the recent literature reports on advanced prodrug concepts targeting toxins to cancer tissues. These strategies include antibody-directed enzyme prodrug therapy (ADEPT), gene-directed enzyme prodrug therapy (GDEPT), lectin-directed enzyme-activated prodrug therapy (LEAPT), and antibody-drug conjugated therapy (ADC). In addition, recent examples of protease-targeting chimeras (PROTACs) were also analyzed and discussed; these methods involve ubiquitination enzyme complexes that undergo proteolytic degradation to release the drug. Overall, these innovative strategies of tumor targeting may lead to future new anticancer drugs that are urgently needed for. However, many of these recently developed targeting principles remain to result in approved drugs, which emphasizes the need for further research [20].

3. Conclusions

This collection contributes to improving the knowledge on anticancer inhibitors, focusing on the synthesis and evaluation of novel compounds able to inhibit enzymes involved in tumorigenesis and proliferation, the role of transcription factors, the use of natural molecules as lead compounds for anti-cancer drug development, and, finally, the search for innovative strategies to overcome pharmacokinetic limitations.

Funding: This research received no external funding.

Acknowledgments: The Guest Editors wishes to thank all the authors for their contributions to this Special Issue, all the reviewers for their work in evaluating the submitted articles, and the editorial staff of *Molecules* for their kind assistance.

Conflicts of Interest: The authors declare no conflict of interest.

References

1. Guo, T.; Ma, S. Recent Advances in the Discovery of Multitargeted Tyrosine Kinase Inhibitors as Anticancer Agents. *ChemMedChem* **2021**, *16*, 600–620. [CrossRef] [PubMed]
2. Højfeldt, J.W.; Agger, K.; Helin, K. Histone lysine demethylases as targets for anticancer therapy. *Nat. Rev. Drug. Discov.*. **2013**, *12*, 917–930. [CrossRef] [PubMed]
3. Fantacuzzi, M.; Gallorini, M.; Gambacorta, N.; Ammazzalorso, A.; Aturki, Z.; Balaha, M.; Carradori, S.; Giampietro, L.; Maccallini, C.; Cataldi, A.; et al. Design, Synthesis and Biological Evaluation of Aromatase Inhibitors Based on Sulfonates and Sulfonamides of Resveratrol. *Pharmaceuticals* **2021**, *14*, 984. [CrossRef] [PubMed]
4. Ammazzalorso, A.; Gallorini, M.; Fantacuzzi, M.; Gambacorta, N.; De Filippis, B.; Giampietro, L.; Maccallini, C.; Nicolotti, O.; Cataldi, A.; Amoroso, R. Design, synthesis and biological evaluation of imidazole and triazole-based carbamates as novel aromatase inhibitors. *Eur. J. Med. Chem.* **2021**, *211*, 113115. [CrossRef] [PubMed]
5. Giampietro, L.; Gallorini, M.; Gambacorta, N.; Ammazzalorso, A.; De Filippis, B.; Della Valle, A.; Fantacuzzi, M.; Maccallini, C.; Mollica, A.; Cataldi, A.; et al. Synthesis, structure-activity relationships and molecular docking studies of phenyldiazenyl sulfonamides as aromatase inhibitors. *Eur. J. Med. Chem.* **2021**, *224*, 113737. [CrossRef] [PubMed]
6. Ammazzalorso, A.; Bruno, I.; Florio, R.; De Lellis, L.; Laghezza, A.; Cerchia, C.; De Filippis, B.; Fantacuzzi, M.; Giampietro, L.; Maccallini, C.; et al. Sulfonimide and Amide Derivatives as Novel PPARα Antagonists: Synthesis, Antiproliferative Activity, and Docking Studies. *ACS Med. Chem. Lett.* **2020**, *11*, 624–632. [CrossRef] [PubMed]
7. Maccallini, C.; Di Matteo, M.; Gallorini, M.; Montagnani, M.; Graziani, V.; Ammazzalorso, A.; Amoia, P.; De Filippis, B.; Di Silvestre, S.; Fantacuzzi, M.; et al. Discovery of N-{3-[(ethanimidoylamino)methyl]benzyl}-l-prolinamide dihydrochloride: A new potent and selective inhibitor of the inducible nitric oxide synthase as a promising agent for the therapy of malignant glioma. *Eur. J. Med. Chem.* **2018**, *152*, 53–64. [CrossRef] [PubMed]
8. Ammazzalorso, A.; Agamennone, M.; De Filippis, B.; Fantacuzzi, M. Development of CDK4/6 Inhibitors: A Five Years Update. *Molecules* **2021**, *26*, 1488. [CrossRef] [PubMed]
9. Al-Salem, H.S.; Arifuzzaman, M.; Alkahtani, H.M.; Abdalla, A.N.; Issa, I.S.; Alqathama, A.; Albalawi, F.S.; Rahman, A.F.M.M. A Series of Isatin-Hydrazones with Cytotoxic Activity and CDK2 Kinase Inhibitory Activity: A Potential Type II ATP Competitive Inhibitor. *Molecules* **2020**, *25*, 4400. [CrossRef] [PubMed]
10. Abdallah, M.E.; El-Readi, M.Z.; Althubiti, M.A.; Almaimani, R.A.; Ismail, A.M.; Idris, S.; Refaat, B.; Almalki, W.H.; Babakr, A.T.; Mukhtar, M.H.; et al. Tamoxifen and the PI3K Inhibitor: LY294002 Synergistically Induce Apoptosis and Cell Cycle Arrest in Breast Cancer MCF-7 Cells. *Molecules* **2020**, *25*, 3355. [CrossRef] [PubMed]
11. Konkoľová, E.; Hudáčová, M.; Hamuľaková, S.; Jendželovský, R.; Vargová, J.; Ševc, J.; Fedoročko, P.; Kožurková, M. Tacrine-Coumarin Derivatives as Topoisomerase Inhibitors with Antitumor Effects on A549 Human Lung Carcinoma Cancer Cell Lines. *Molecules* **2021**, *26*, 1133. [CrossRef] [PubMed]
12. Tanuma, S.-I.; Katsuragi, K.; Oyama, T.; Yoshimori, A.; Shibasaki, Y.; Asawa, Y.; Yamazaki, H.; Makino, K.; Okazawa, M.; Ogino, Y.; et al. Structural Basis of Beneficial Design for Effective Nicotinamide Phosphoribosyltransferase Inhibitors. *Molecules* **2020**, *25*, 3633. [CrossRef] [PubMed]
13. Tilayov, T.; Hingaly, T.; Greenshpan, Y.; Cohen, S.; Akabayov, B.; Gazit, R.; Papo, N. Engineering Stem Cell Factor Ligands with Different c-Kit Agonistic Potencies. *Molecules* **2020**, *25*, 4850. [CrossRef] [PubMed]
14. Yang, H.; Heyer, J.; Zhao, H.; Liang, S.; Guo, R.; Zhong, L. The Potential Role of Cathepsin K in Non-Small Cell Lung Cancer. *Molecules* **2020**, *25*, 4136. [CrossRef] [PubMed]
15. Chen, Y.; Tsai, Y.-H.; Tseng, S.-H. Regulation of ZMYND8 to Treat Cancer. *Molecules* **2021**, *26*, 1083. [CrossRef] [PubMed]
16. Rimpelová, S.; Kolář, M.; Strnad, H.; Ruml, T.; Vítek, L.; Gbelcová, H. Comparison of Transcriptomic Profiles of MiaPaCa-2 Pancreatic Cancer Cells Treated with Different Statins. *Molecules* **2021**, *26*, 3528. [CrossRef] [PubMed]
17. De Filippis, B.; De Lellis, L.; Florio, R.; Ammazzalorso, A.; Amoia, P.; Fantacuzzi, M.; Giampietro, L.; Maccallini, C.; Amoroso, R.; Veschi, S.; et al. Synthesis and cytotoxic effects on pancreatic cancer cells of resveratrol analogs. *Med. Chem. Res.* **2019**, *28*, 984–991. [CrossRef]
18. Wang, Y.; Xia, C.; Chen, L.; Chen, Y.C.; Tu, Y. Saponins Extracted from Tea (*Camellia sinensis*) Flowers Induces Autophagy in Ovarian Cancer Cells. *Molecules* **2020**, *25*, 5254. [CrossRef] [PubMed]
19. Tu, Y.; Chen, L.; Ren, N.; Li, B.; Wu, Y.; Rankin, G.O.; Rojanasakul, Y.; Wang, Y.; Chen, Y.C. Standardized Saponin Extract from Baiye No.1 Tea (*Camellia sinensis*) Flowers Induced S Phase Cell Cycle Arrest and Apoptosis via AKT-MDM2-p53 Signaling Pathway in Ovarian Cancer Cells. *Molecules* **2020**, *25*, 3515. [CrossRef] [PubMed]
20. Franzyk, H.; Christensen, S.B. Targeting Toxins toward Tumors. *Molecules* **2021**, *26*, 1292. [CrossRef] [PubMed]

molecules

Review

Development of CDK4/6 Inhibitors: A Five Years Update

Alessandra Ammazzalorso, Mariangela Agamennone, Barbara De Filippis and Marialuigia Fantacuzzi *

Unit of Medicinal Chemistry, Department of Pharmacy, "G. d'Annunzio" University, 66100 Chieti, Italy; alessandra.ammazzalorso@unich.it (A.A.); mariangela.agamennone@unich.it (M.A.); barbara.defilippis@unich.it (B.D.F.)
* Correspondence: marialuigia.fantacuzzi@unich.it; Tel.: +39-0871-3554684

Abstract: The inhibition of cyclin dependent kinases 4 and 6 plays a role in aromatase inhibitor resistant metastatic breast cancer. Three dual CDK4/6 inhibitors have been approved for the breast cancer treatment that, in combination with the endocrine therapy, dramatically improved the survival outcomes both in first and later line settings. The developments of the last five years in the search for new selective CDK4/6 inhibitors with increased selectivity, treatment efficacy, and reduced adverse effects are reviewed, considering the small-molecule inhibitors and proteolysis-targeting chimeras (PROTACs) approaches, mainly pointing at structure-activity relationships, selectivity against different kinases and antiproliferative activity.

Keywords: cyclin-dependent kinase; cancer; resistance; small molecule inhibitors; PROTACs

Citation: Ammazzalorso, A.; Agamennone, M.; De Filippis, B.; Fantacuzzi, M. Development of CDK4/6 Inhibitors: A Five Years Update. *Molecules* **2021**, *26*, 1488. https://doi.org/10.3390/molecules26051488

Academic Editor: Margherita Brindisi

Received: 13 February 2021
Accepted: 6 March 2021
Published: 9 March 2021

Publisher's Note: MDPI stays neutral with regard to jurisdictional claims in published maps and institutional affiliations.

1. Introduction

Breast cancer (BC) is the most recurrent cancer in women worldwide, impacting 2.1 million women each year according to World Health Organization [1]. BC is a heterogeneous disease due to genetic factors that are reflected in different phenotypes. BC can be divided into different subtypes: luminal, in which estrogen receptors (ER) and/or progesterone receptors (PR) are expressed, further divided into luminal A and luminal B subtypes depending on the expression of Ki67 (low levels in A and high in B); HER2+, in which the human epidermal growth factor receptor 2 (HER2) is overexpressed and ER and PR are lacking; triple negative BC (TN), in which the previous targets are not expressed. The estrogen-receptor positive (ER+) BC is the most common type, with the prevalence of about 60% of cases in pre-menopausal women and 75% in post-menopausal women [2–5].

The anti-hormonal treatment involves the suppression or reduction of the estrogen effects and can be carried out using drugs that limit the production of these hormones, such as aromatase inhibitors (AIs), or act on the ER receptor, such as selective ER modulators (SERM) or down-regulators (SERD) [6–8]. The adjuvant therapy consists of 5–10 years of ER-directed endocrine therapy that result in a reduction of mortality in ER+ BC of more than 40%. Resistance to endocrine therapy leading to early-stage ER+ BC is common and decisive in the setting of advanced disease [9,10].

The aromatization reaction in the final step of estrogen biosynthesis is unique, therefore this reaction becomes an excellent target for inhibiting the synthesis of estrogens without affecting the production of other steroids. In recent decades, several aromatase inhibitors have been developed to adequately suppress estrogen production and have been used in the treatment of estrogen-dependent BC [11–16].

Given the high percentage of resistance to aromatase inhibitor treatment, new therapeutic strategies have been identified to make the treatment of ER+ BC more effective. One of the mechanisms involved in the resistance concerns the activation of cyclin-dependent kinases (CDKs) as an ER-independent growth signal, that involves the important protein kinase signaling pathway (PI3K/AKT/mTOR) (Figure 1) [17,18].

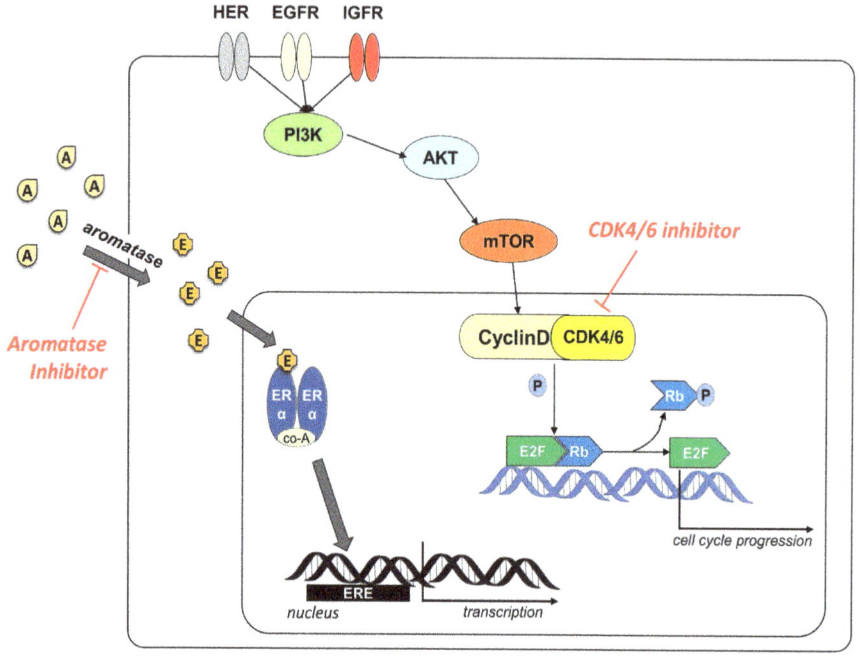

Figure 1. Schematic representation of the cyclinD/CDK4/6 involvement in overpassing resistance to aromatase inhibitors. Aromatase converts androgens (A) in estrogens (E) that bind to ER receptor. The recruitment of co-activators (co-A) allows the binding to ERE element on the target genes and the activation of the transcription. AIs block the production of estrogen inhibiting the ER-driven activation of cell cycle progression. The activation of cyclinD/CDK4/6 complex, mediated by the protein kinase signaling pathway (PI3K/AKT/mTOR), stimulates cell proliferation independently from aromatase. The use of CDK4/6 inhibitor blocks this alternative activation pathway.

CDKs, a family of serine/threonine kinases, regulate cell cycle progression into the four distinct phases G1, S (DNA synthesis), G2 and M, and are crucially involved in the regulation of cell division and proliferation. CDK stability, activation and downstream phosphorylation is controlled by cyclin counterpart and endogenous inhibitors. To date, 21 CDKs are known and their role in different types of cancer has been reported by many research groups [19–21]. In particular, CDK1, 2 and 4 regulate the transition of the cell cycle steps, CDK 7, 8, 9 and 11 regulate the gene transcription, while CDK 6 regulates both [22–24].

Mitogenic, hormonal, and growth factors allow the cyclin D to bind CDK4/6, forming the complex that regulates the phosphorylation status of retinoblastoma protein (Rb). The phosphorylated-Rb determines the dissociation of the transcription factor E2F that binds to DNA and promotes the expression of different genes, regulates DNA replication and cell division, with the transition from G1 to S phase (Figure 1). Several endogenous factors control cell proliferation, including INK4 family proteins (p16, p15, p18, p19), cyclin inhibitory proteins and kinase inhibitory proteins (KIPs, p21, p27) [25,26].

The dysregulation of cell cycle caused by the overexpression or gain-of-function mutations in the CDKs and cyclins or the loss of endogenous inhibitors expression and function, is recurrent in many cancer diseases. In BC, but also in other type of cancer, a dysregulation of this process leads to a proliferative stimulus, and a significant role in this mechanism is played by the overexpression of cyclin D. Inhibition of cell cycle using CDK4/6 inhibitor has emerged as antitumor treatment in BC in association to the hormonal therapy to overpass resistance to AIs and avoiding relapses [27–32].

Over the years several CDK inhibitors have been developed and tested in different types of cancer [33–37]. First generation inhibitors (flavopiridol and roscovitine) demonstrated an inadequate balance between efficacy and toxicity, due to their action on several kinases (pan-inhibitors) [38–40]. Second generation inhibitors (dinaciclib) were developed with the aim to increase selectivity and potency, but demonstrated limited efficacy and considerable toxicity in clinical studies. The toxicity of these compounds is associated with the multi-target activity against isoforms fundamental for the proliferation (CDK1) and survival (CDK9) of normal cells [41–44]. However, in recent years, the interest in identifying inhibitors of specific kinases with targeted action on tumor cells and with less toxic effects, has led to the discovery of selective CDK4/6 inhibitors [30,45]. Third generation CDK inhibitors selectively inhibit CDK4/6 with potent efficacy and reduced toxicity, such as the FDA approved palbociclib (**1**), ribociclib (**2**), and abemaciclib (**3**) (Figure 2) [46–49].

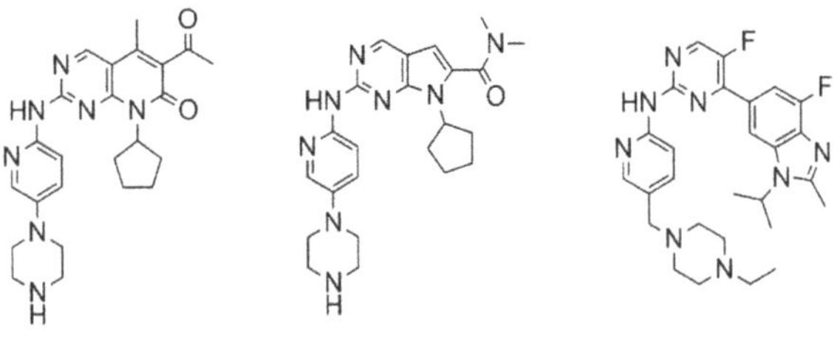

1 palbociclib (Ibrance®) Pfizer Inc. February 2015

2 ribociclib (Kisqali®) Novartis Pharmaceuticals Corp. March 2017

3 abemaciclib (VerzenioTM) Eli Lilly and Company September 2017

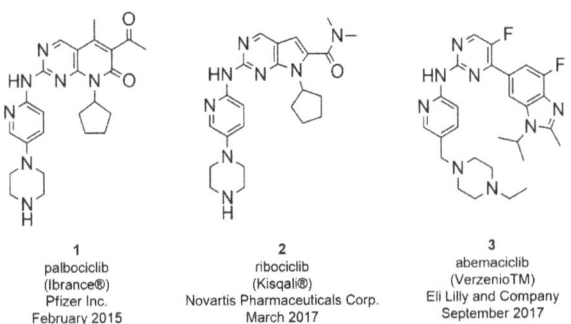

Figure 2. FDA approved CDK4/6 inhibitors palbociclib, ribociclib, and abemaciclib.

The search for even more selective CDK4/6 inhibitors is still a challenge in the development of novel anticancer therapies. To date, three ATP-competitive CDK 4/6 selective inhibitors (trilaciclib, lerociclib and SHR-6390) are under advanced clinical trials. Trilaciclib (G1T28, **4**, Figure 3) is currently ongoing phase II trials in patients with small cell lung cancer (NCT02514447, NTC02499770) and with hormone receptor negative BC (NCT02978716), while entered in phase III for metastatic colorectal cancer (NCT04607668) [50–53]. Phase II (NCT02983071) trial of lerocliclib (G1T38, **5**, Figure 3) examined the effect in combination with fulvestrant in hormone receptor-positive, HER2-negative locally advanced metastatic BC while another phase II study combined lerociclib with osimertinib in EGFR-mutant non-small cell lung cancer (NCT03455829) [54,55]. SHR-6390 (**6**, Figure 3) is currently ongoing phase II trial in patients with hormone receptor positive, ErbB2 negative BC (NCT03966898) [56,57]. Moreover, an abemaciclib related compound, BPI-16350 (**7**, Figure 3), recently entered phase I clinical trial (NCT03791112) in patients with advanced solid tumor and the estimated study completion date is in December 2021 [58].

Based on their mode of action, kinase inhibitors can be divided into two types: ATP-competitive and non-competitive inhibitors. The reported CDK4/6 small molecule inhibitors abemaciclib, palbociclib and ribociclib are ATP-competitive inhibitors, forming hydrogen bonds in the ATP binding site with the kinase "hinge" residues (Val101 in CDK6) and hydrophobic interactions in the region normally occupied by the ATP adenine ring (Figure 4A,C,D) [59–61].

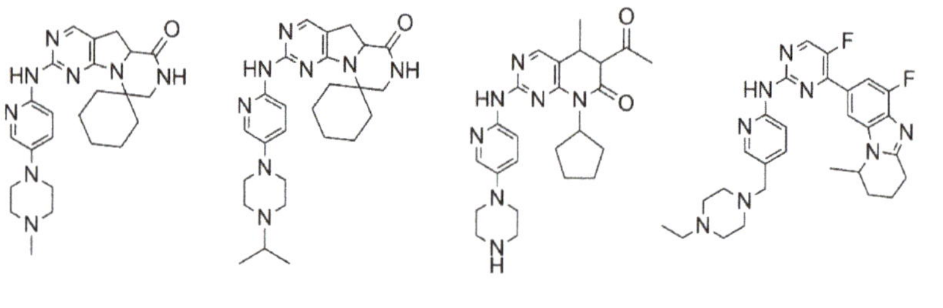

4
trilaciclib
(G1T28)

5
lerociclib
(G1T38)

6
SHR-6390

7
BPI-16350

Figure 3. Chemical structure of ATP-competitive CDK 4/6 selective inhibitors in clinical trials.

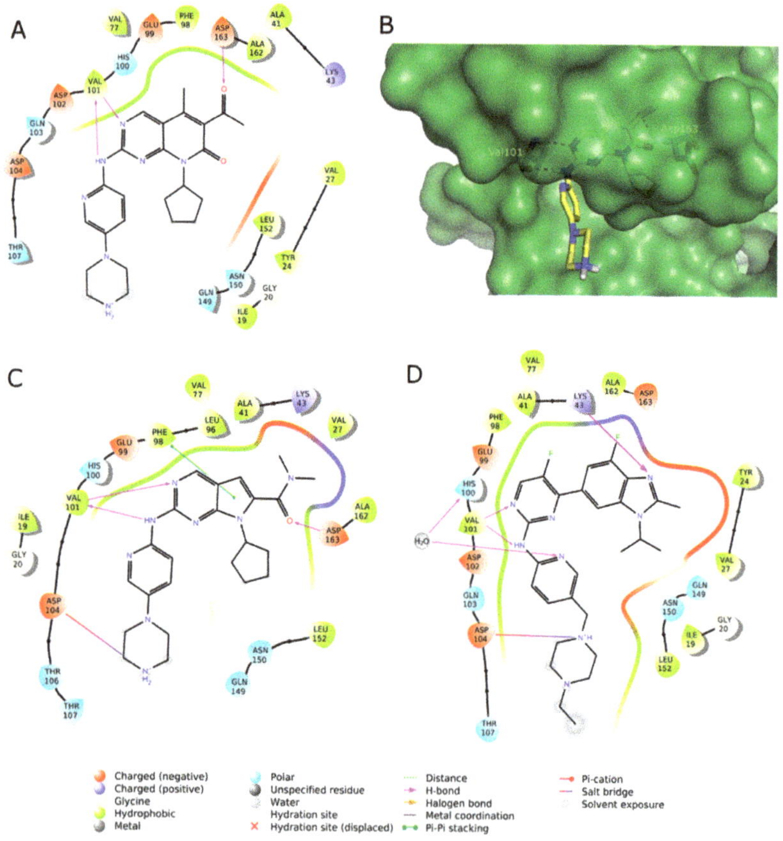

Figure 4. (**A**,**C**,**D**) 2D interaction diagram of the three approved CDK4/6 selective inhibitors as observed in their X-ray complexes into CDK6: (**A**) palbociclib (PDB ID: 5L2I); (**C**) ribociclib (PDB ID: 5L2T); (**D**) abemaciclib (PDB ID: 5L2S). (**B**) 3D representation of the X-ray binding geometry of palbociclib (stick, yellow C atoms) into the CDK6 binding site (dark green solid surface). Protein residues involved in key H-bond interactions are represented as stick; H-bonds are depicted as magenta dashed lines.

According to the study of Chen et al., the interactions enhancing the CDK inhibition and selectivity over other kinases are the H-bonds with the sidechains of His100 and

Lys43, as shown for abemaciclib (Figure 4B) and a solvent-mediated interaction of a positively charged atom of the ligand and a solvent-exposed ridge consisting of Asp104 and Thr107 [62].

Given the great similarity in the structure of the approved compounds, several research groups have tried to identify different compounds with increased CDK4/6 selectivity, reduced adverse effects while maintaining or improving treatment efficacy. In this review we focused the attention on the last five years progress in the optimization of clinically approved CDK4/6 inhibitors, primarily tested for their BC anti-tumor activity. The main works, considering both the small-molecule inhibitors and the PROteolysis-TArgeting Chimeras (PROTACs) are summarized.

2. Small-Molecule Inhibitors

Small molecule inhibitors (SMIs) are compounds of $\leq$500 Da size, often administered orally, useful in cancer diseases. The traditional chemotherapy includes single or combination-therapy of drug targeting dividing tumor cells. The principal drawback of this non-targeted approach is the non-selective action on both normal and cancer cells. SMIs bind to specific molecular targets (targeted therapy) and selectively eliminate malignant cells [63,64]. The small size allows to use these molecules towards extracellular, surface, or intracellular proteins, including anti-apoptotic proteins that play a key role in cell growth and promotion of metastases. The most interesting targets in the antitumor field are mainly kinases such as serine/threonine/tyrosine kinases, matrix metalloproteinases (MMP), and CDKs [63–68].

The following SMIs are classified based on their chemical scaffold.

2.1. *Thiazolyl-Pyrimidine Derivatives*

Starting from the structure of abemaciclib and considering the fundamental interactions with the hinge region of CDK4/6, Tadesse et al. synthesized three series of compounds keeping constant pyrimidine, pyridine, and the amino linker to maintain the coplanarity of the two rings for ATP-mimetic kinase inhibitors (Figure 5), that represents the characteristic moiety of the three approved inhibitors [69].

The thiazole C2 amino moiety, introduced in previously synthesized CDK9 inhibitors, established a H-bond with the highly conserved Asp (Asp163 in the CDK6) residue among CDKs family of the Asp-Phe-Gly motif in the ATP-binding pocket, improving strong hydrophobic interaction of the methyl thiazole with the gatekeeper residues [70]. For this reason, the 2-amine-thiazole was introduced in C4 of the pyrimidine scaffold. The pharmacophore of the Tadesse's lead compound is the *N*-(5-(piperidin-1-yl)pyridin-2-yl)-4-(thiazol-5-yl)pyrimidine (**8–10**, Figure 5). The main modifications of the first series (**8**, Figure 5) concerned the mono or di-substitution of the amine group (R_1, R_2) with methyl, ciclopentyl, phenyl or *iso*-propyl; the introduction of a fluorine atom in C5 of pyrimidine (R_4) to optimize the pharmacokinetic properties; the N4 (R_5) of the piperazine was substituted with a variety of ionizable groups. The most active compound (**8a**, Figure 5) contains a morpholine ring and a cyclopentyl substitution of the amine (K_i CDK4 = 0.004 μM, K_i CDK6 = 0.030 μM). Its antiproliferative activity was assessed by MTT assay in human leukemia Rb positive MV4-11 (GI_{50} = 0.209 μM), and in human breast cancer Rb negative MDA-MB-453 (GI_{50} = 3.683 μM) cell lines. The SAR analysis shows that the amino group in the thiazole ring could accept only a mono-substitution and the cyclopentyl is better than alkyl chain or aromatic ring; the introduction of the electron withdrawing trifluoromethyl increases the toxicity; the substitution of the second nitrogen atom of the piperazine with carbon and the exocyclic primary amino decreases activity and selectivity, while the introduction of oxygen increases the selectivity toward CDK4/6.

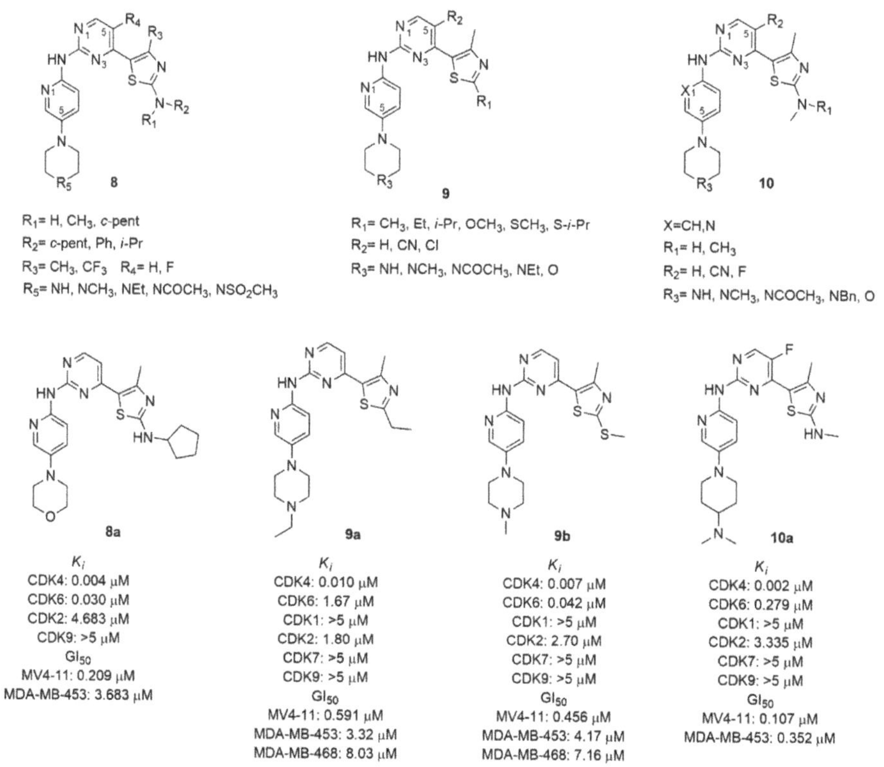

Figure 5. CDK4/6 inhibitors based on thiazolyl-pyrimidine scaffold.

In the second series of derivatives (**9**, Figure 5), the amino group on thiazole ring was replaced with alkyl, ether or thioether substituents, a cyano group or chlorine atom on C5 of pyrimidine was introduced, and the C4 of piperidine was replaced by an oxygen atom or secondary or tertiary amine substituted with alkyl or acetyl group [71]. Among the synthesized compounds, **9a** and **9b** (Figure 5) emerged with good CDK inhibition values (K_i CDK4 = 0.010 and 0.007 μM, K_i CDK6 = 1.67 and 0.042 μM, respectively) and antiproliferative activity in MV4–11 (GI_{50} = 0.591 μM and 0.456 μM, respectively). The antiproliferative activity of compounds **9a–b** was also evaluated in a panel of human cancer cell lines including breast, colon, ovary, pancreas, prostate, leukemia and melanoma. Noteworthy, the different antiproliferative activity in the MDA-MB-453 (GI_{50} = 3.32 μM and 4.17 μM, respectively) and the corrensponding Rb-deficient MDA-468 (GI_{50} = 8.03 μM and 7.16 μM, respectively) confirms the mechanism of action of these compounds which act in the presence of the intact Rb function. The potent effect on the growth of melanoma M249 (GI_{50} = 0.47 μM and 0.91 μM, respectively) and of resistant to dabrafenib M249R (GI_{50} = 0.27 μM and 0.91 μM, respectively) cell lines paves the way for a possible therapeutic use in melanoma. The SAR analysis highlighted that the presence of the nitrogen atom of the pyridine is fundamental for CDK4/6 selectivity, and the substitution of the amine group in C2 of the thiazole with alkyl, thioether or ether prevents the H-bond with the conserved Asp163, increasing the selectivity.

In another series of derivatives (**10**, Figure 5) the substitution of the pyridine with a benzene ring, the mono-substitution of the amino group of the thiazole, the introduction of fluorine atom or cyano group in C5 of pyrimidine, and the alkylation of the piperidine nitrogen or the introduction of morpholine or piperidine were studied [72]. Compound **10a** (Figure 5) was the most active in biological assays, with good CDK 4/6 inhibition

(K_i CDK4 = 0.002 μM, K_i CDK6 = 0.279 μM), selectivity over other kinases and good pharmacokinetic profile. The antiproliferative activity was tested in different cancer cell lines such as leukemia or solid cancers (breast, colorectal, melanoma, ovarian, prostate).

2.2. Benzimidazolyl-Pyrimidine Derivatives

Zha et al. focused their attention to the substitution of the abemaciclib pyridine with a benzoimidazolyl in C4 and the introduction of tetrahydro-naphthyridine as substituent of the amino linker, with the aim to discover conformationally restricted analogs sharing improved activity and selectivity [73]. Compound **11** (Figure 6), discovered through the combination of structure-based drug design and traditional medicinal chemistry approaches, retains all key contacts between abemaciclib and CDK6, such as the edge-to-face interaction of the benzimidazole ring and Phe98 of the gatekeeper and the H-bonds of the amino pyrimidine with residues in the hinge loop. The tetrahydro-naphthyridine forms an additional water-mediated H-bond between the aromatic nitrogen with His100 and a salt-bridge interaction of the physiologically protonated nitrogen and Asp104 (Figure 4D) [19,74].

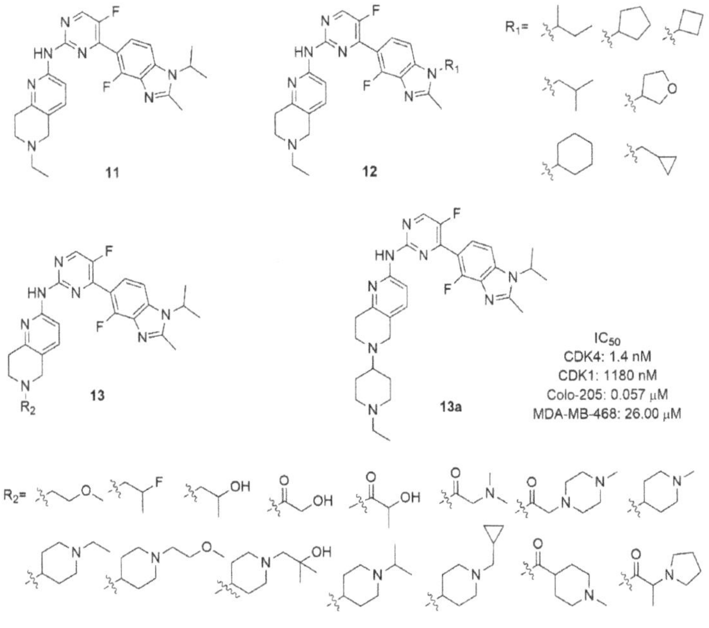

Figure 6. CDK4/6 inhibitors based on benzimidazolyl-pyrimidine scaffold.

The authors explored the removal of the nitrogen in pyridine, in 2,4-pyrimidine or the substitution with a 4,6-pyrimidine, confirming that the nitrogen atoms are fundamental for CDK6 selectivity over CDK1. Although compound **11** exhibited good activity (IC_{50} CDK4 = 1.5 nM) and a selectivity index of 311, the very poor pharmacokinetic properties required further optimization. In compounds of the series **12** (Figure 6) a cyclic or acyclic alkyl substitution of the *iso*-propyl of the imidazole of compound **11** was introduced without a substantial improvement of activity, suggesting that the hydrophobic cleft of the protein could not host rigid or bulky groups. Compounds of the series **13** (Figure 6) contain a variety of substituents on the protonable nitrogen of tetrahydro-naphthyridine. The hydrophilic substitutions maintain the inhibition potency, with amide analogues suffering from poor exposure; the introduction of a *N*-alkyl piperidine improves the inhibitory activity and selectivity. In fact, compound **13a** (Figure 6) emerged as the best compound, with enzymatic CDK4 IC_{50} of 1.4 nM and selectivity CDK1/CDK4 around 850 (IC_{50} CDK1 = 1180 nM), good antiproliferative activity in Colo-205 cell line (IC_{50} = 0.057 μM), favourable *in vitro* metabolic properties (microsomal stability and CYP isoforms inhibition) and robust pharmacokinetic properties in mice and rats.

Wang et al. synthesized and tested a library of abemaciclib analogs [75]. The tetracycle scaffold (piperazine, pyridine, pyrimidine and benzimidazole) was kept constant, while small substituents were introduced on piperazine nitrogen (ethyl, 2-fluorethyl, cyclopropyl, *iso*-propyl), in C6 of pyridine (methyl), in C5 of pyrimidine (fluorine), and in C4 of benzimidazole (fluorine). The benzimidazole ring was transformed in a tricycle by connecting N1 and C2, inserting a cyclopentyl, cyclohexyl or cycloheptene [75].

A large library of 23 compounds (**14**, Figure 7) was tested for CDK1 and CDK4/6 activity. Compounds demonstrated null activity versus CDK1, but a remarkable inhibition of CDK4/6, with IC_{50} ranging from 0.6 to 340 nM. Compound **14a** (IC_{50} CDK4 = 7.4 nM and IC_{50} CDK6 = 0.9 nM) was further tested for hERG channel inhibition, showing low heart toxicity. The pharmacokinetic parameters of **14a** (Cmax, AUC, $T_{1/2}$, MRT, CL/f, V2/F) demonstrated drug-like properties for following development. A docking study revealed that the di-methyl cyclopentyl group contributed to favourable H-bond between the nitrogen atom of the imidazole-condensed cycle and the amine group of Lys43.

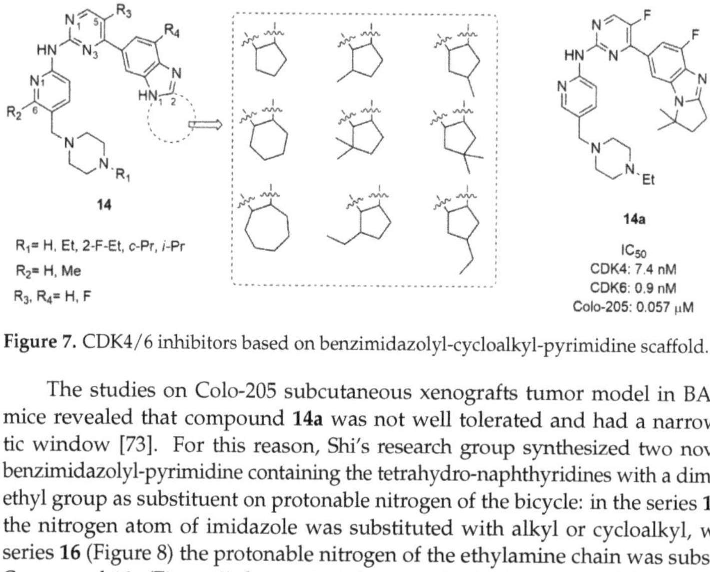

Figure 7. CDK4/6 inhibitors based on benzimidazolyl-cycloalkyl-pyrimidine scaffold.

The studies on Colo-205 subcutaneous xenografts tumor model in BALB/c nude mice revealed that compound **14a** was not well tolerated and had a narrow therapeutic window [73]. For this reason, Shi's research group synthesized two novel series of benzimidazolyl-pyrimidine containing the tetrahydro-naphthyridines with a dimethylaminoethyl group as substituent on protonable nitrogen of the bicycle: in the series **15** (Figure 8) the nitrogen atom of imidazole was substituted with alkyl or cycloalkyl, while in the series **16** (Figure 8) the protonable nitrogen of the ethylamine chain was substituted [76]. Compound **16a** (Figure 8) demonstrated nanomolar *in vitro* activity (IC_{50} CDK4 = 0.71 nM, IC_{50} CDK6 = 1.10 nM) with high kinase selectivity, excellent metabolic properties, good pharmacokinetic properties, low toxicity, and desirable antitumor efficacy in MCF-7, Colo-205, and A549 xenograft murine models. Even though compounds of series **16** possessed fair CDK4/6 activity in the range of nanomolar (IC_{50} = 0.999–6.14 nM), many of them failed in antiproliferative activity in MCF-7, T-47D, ZR-75-1, and Colo-205 cell lines.

The SAR analysis demonstrated that, with respect to *N*-*iso*-propyl (**16a**), the *N*-methyl or *N*-ethyl substitution of the imidazole decreased the activity more than others alkyl or cycloalkyl groups in terms of CDK 4/6 activity. The cycloalkyl, probably for its steric hindrance, also decreases the antiproliferative activities. Considering the substitution of *N*-methyl on the nitrogen of the ethylamine chain on tetrahydro-naphthyridine, the introduction of a bulkier group was unproductive in terms of CDK4/6 activity and selectivity over CDK2.

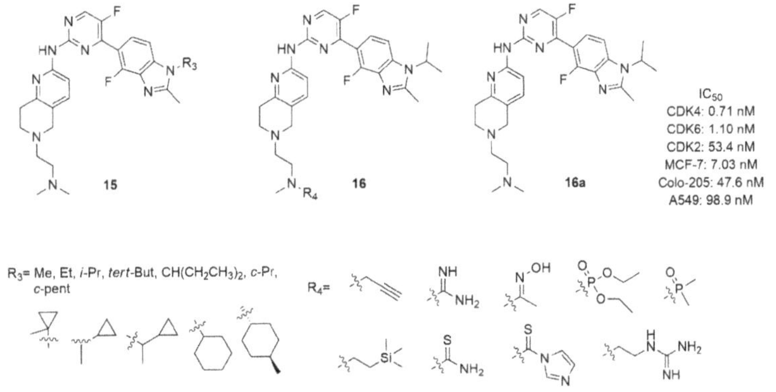

Figure 8. Structure of Shi's research group of benzimidazolyl-pyrimidine derivatives.

2.3. *Pyrido-Pyrimidine Derivatives*

Considering the pyrido [2,3-*d*]pyrimidine scaffold of palbociclib, Abbas et al. synthesized two series of 7-thienylpyrido[2,3-*d*]pyrimidines (**17** and **18**, Figure 9) and tested them for CDK6 inhibition and cytotoxicity against breast, lung, and prostate cancer cell lines [77]. In the series **17**, the 2-aryldiene hydrazinyl moiety was introduced in the scaffold and the aryl group was substituted in *para*-position. The most active compound of this series resulted **17a**, containing a *para*-methoxy group on the benzene ring. In fact, it demonstrated a CDK6 IC_{50} value of 115.38 nM and a good cytotoxicity against breast MCF-7 (IC_{50} = 1.59 μM), prostate PC-3 (IC_{50} = 0.01 μM), lung A-549 (IC_{50} = 2.48 μM) cancer cells.

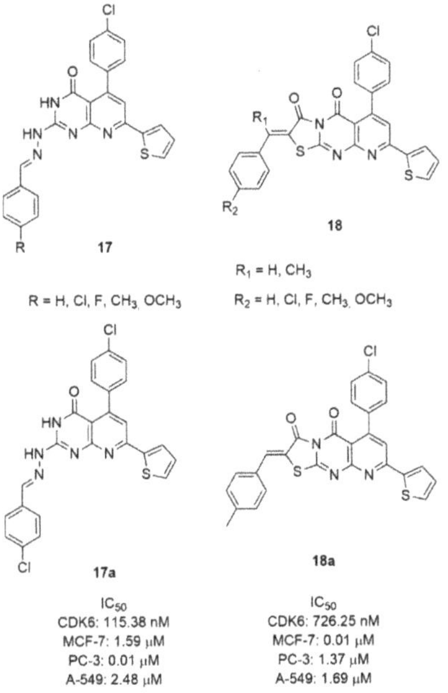

Figure 9. CDK6 inhibitors based on the pyrido-pyrimidine scaffold.

The series **18** is constituted by a fused ring to pyrimidine forming a tricyclic pyridothyazolopyrimidine, substituted in C2 with a *para*-substituted benzylidene. Compound **18a** emerged as the most potent CDK6 inhibitor (IC_{50} = 726.25 nM) and cytotoxic against

MCF-7 (IC_{50} = 0.01 μM), prostate PC-3 (IC_{50} = 1.37 μM), lung A-549 (IC_{50} = 1.69 μM) cancer cell lines.

2.4. Imidazo-Pyrido-Pyrimidine Derivatives

The pyrido-pyrimidine scaffold of palbociclib was fused with imidazole in two novel series of CDK4/6 inhibitors containing the fused tricyclic ring of imidazo[10,2′:1,6]pyrido[2,3-d]pyrimidine (**19** and **20**, Figure 10) [78].

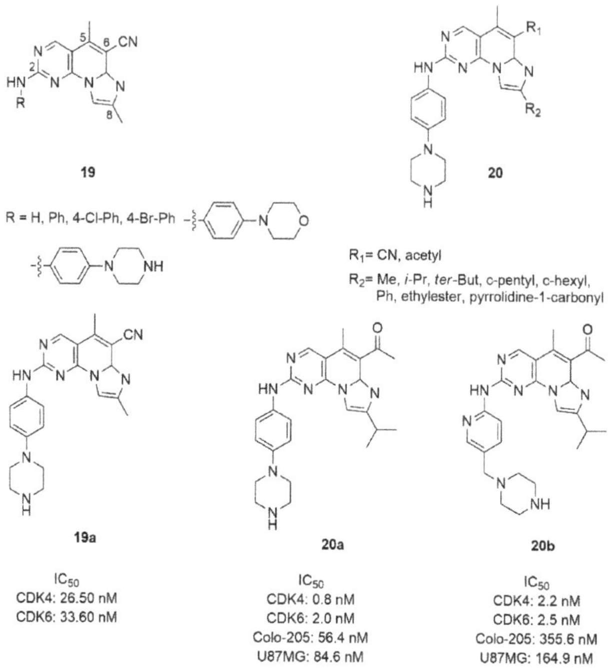

Figure 10. Structure of imidazo[10,2′:1,6]pyrido[2,3-d]pyrimidine derivatives.

In the series **19**, the fused tri-heteroaryl structure was substituted with a methyl in C5 and C8, cyano in C6, while the amino group in C2 was substituted by phenyl or para-substituted phenyl groups. This type of modification did not sufficiently improve the activity, and compound **19a** with the piperazine in *para* position showed modest inhibition values (IC_{50} CDK4 = 26.50 nM, IC_{50} CDK6 = 33.60 nM). Keeping constant the piperazine moiety, in the series **20** the C6 and C8 positions were changed by the introduction of methyl, *iso*-propyl, *terz*-butyl, cyclopentyl, cyclohexyl, phenyl, ethylester, or pyrrolidine-1-carbonyl in C8, while the cyano group in C6 was replaced with the acetyl one. Compound **20a** was the best one of the series in terms of inhibition (CDK4 IC_{50} = 0.8 nM, CDK6 IC_{50} = 2.0 nM).

The piperazine ring of compound **20a** was also replaced by saturated heterocycle, distanced by a methyl and a carbonyl linker; alternatively the piperazinyl-pyridine portion was replaced with a fused bicycle. None of these changes improved the inhibition of kinases [79]. Compound **20a** demonstrated good activities on Colo-205 (IC_{50} = 56.4 nM), and glioma U87MG (IC_{50} = 84.6 nM) cell lines, favourable *in vitro* metabolic properties (microsomal stability, CYP isoforms inhibition), acceptable pharmacokinetic profiles in mice and rats, antitumor efficacy with controllable observed side effects in xenograft in vivo studies.

2.5. Pyrazolo-Quinazoline Derivatives

Considering the inhibition activity of different kinases (Aurora-A, CDK2, Polo-like Kinase 1) of the 4,4-dimethyl-4,5-dihydro-1*H*-pyrazolo[4,3-h]quinazoline [80], Zhao et al. synthesized a series of 4,5-dihydro-1*H*-pyrazolo[4,3-h]quinazolines (**21**, Figure 11) and tested their inhibition of CDK4/6 [79]. The amine group in C2 position of the quinazoline was substituted with pyridine or benzene ring. Compounds containing the pyridine confirmed that the nitrogen atom in this position affects not only the inhibitory activity, but also the cellular activity against MCF-7 cell line. In fact, the pyridine derivatives were more active as CDK4/6 inhibitors and displayed improved cellular activity.

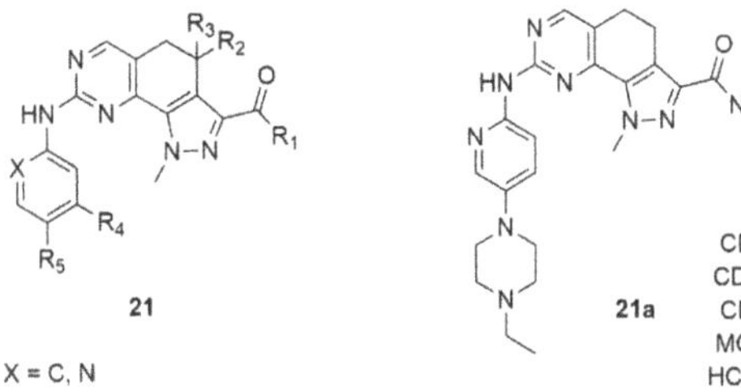

Figure 11. Structure of 4,5-dihydro-1H-pyrazolo[4,3-h]quinazoline derivatives.

Compound **21a** was the best one of this series, showing good activity on CDK4/6 (IC_{50} CDK4 = 0.01 μM, IC_{50} CDK6 = 0.026 μM) and high selectivity against CDK2 (IC_{50} CDK2 = 0.70 μM), anti-proliferative activity in MCF-7 cell line (IC_{50} = 0.19 μM) and other solid tumors (colorectal, liver, pancreatic), favorable pharmacokinetic parameters ($T_{1/2}$, CL, AUC, V, Cmax).

3. PROTACS

The therapeutic use of small-molecule inhibitors to target proteins such as transcription factors, non-enzymatic, and scaffolding proteins, has several limitations because these targets lack appropriate active site to be occupied that directly modulate protein functions [81]. Moreover, high systemic drug exposures in the use of small molecules that bind to the active site of a protein are required to achieve site occupation, which may lead to an increase in adverse effects caused by binding to off-target sites [82]. Other complications in the prolonged use of small molecule inhibitors are the possible mutation of the target protein and the establishment of resistance to the therapy, the overexpression of such protein to balance the inhibition drug-mediated, and the accumulation. These mechanisms are associated with the partial or overall suppression of the downstream signaling pathways [83].

A strategy to circumvent the problem of binding site occupancy to regulate the inhibition of a protein and the possibility of significantly expand the number of proteins that can be inhibited, is the use of small-molecule-induced protein degradation. In this way, the pharmaceutical advantages deriving from the use of small molecules are preserved and the proteins generally considered "undraggable" are removed [84]. These hybrid molecules, generally called PROteolysis-TArgeting Chimeras (PROTACs), are constituted by two small binding molecules connected by a linker (Figure 12): one domain is directed to the targeted protein, while the other domain binds E3 ubiquitin ligase. The complex allows the binding of the proteolytic ubiquitin on the target protein, and its consequent degradation of the targeted protein in proteasome. PROTACs act catalytically and are not destroyed as small molecule suicide inhibitors that permanently bind target macromolecules [85,86].

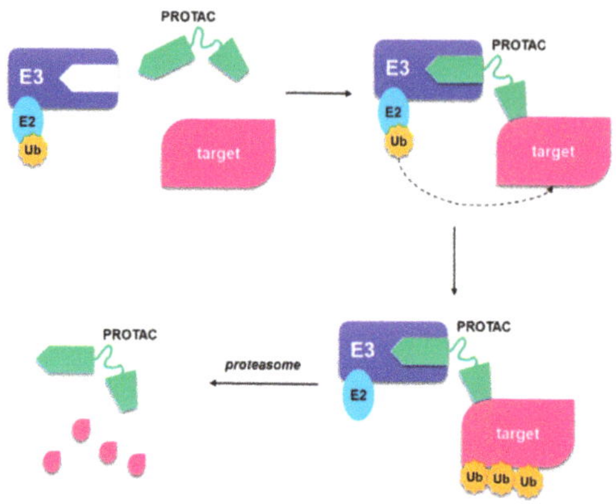

Figure 12. A schematic representation of proteolysis targeting chimera. The PROteolysis-TArgeting Chimera (PROTAC) is composed by a portion that binds to the ubiquitin ligase and a small molecule that binds to target protein, joined by a linker. When the targeted protein binds the small molecule, and the other part binds to E3 ligase, a ternary complex is formed. The following poliubiquitination of the target allows the proteasome to degrade the target protein and regenerate the PROTAC.

PROTAC strategy is widely applied to degrade proteins related to immune disorders, neurodegenerative diseases, viral infections, and cancer diseases [87–89]. In this paragraph the application of PROTAC strategy to CDK4/6 inhibitors is summarized.

The use of this approach could be exploited to selectively inhibit CDK6 with respect to CDK4, which have specific functions, could derive from the use of PROTACs. In fact, the binding site of ATP in kinases 4 and 6 possesses a high structural similarity, that could hardly be circumvented with the use of small molecules. All the reviewed studies have in common the binding of the E3-binding portion (E3 ligase ligand) to the nitrogen atom of the piperazine of the three approved CDK4/6 inhibitors. In fact, the crystallographic studies of palbociclib, ribociclib and abemaciclib show that the piperazine ring is projected towards the solvent (Figure 4B), in an optimal position to act as an anchor point.

Among the first studies reporting a PROTAC active towards CDK4/6, emerges the work of Zhao and Burgess [90], who combined palbocilib and ribocilib with pomalidomide (cereblon (CRBN), E3 ligase ligand) by means of a linker containing a triazole ring (**22a–b**, Figure 13). Studies on MDA-MB-231, a triple negative breast cancer cell line, showed that CDK4 is degraded more efficiently and PROTAC containing palbociclib (**22a**) is more potent (DC_{50} CDK4 = 12.9 nM, DC_{50} CDK6 = 34.1 nM) than **22b** (DC_{50} CDK4 = 97 nM, DC_{50} CDK6 = 300 nM). The same CDK degradation and cytotoxicity studies conducted on MCF-7 showed that **22a–b** are less efficient towards this cell line with respect to the triple negative cell line.

In the same period, Rana et al. synthesized a chimera series of palbociclib and pomalidomide by changing the length and the composition of the flexible linker (**23**, Figure 14) [91].

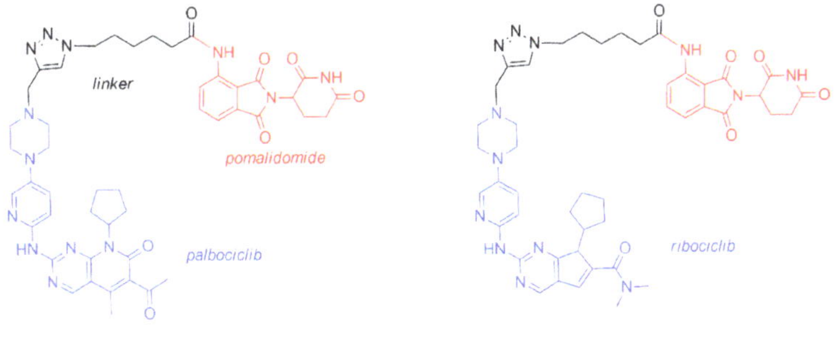

22a
DC_{50}
CDK4: 12.9 nM
CDK6: 34.1 nM

22b
DC_{50}
CDK4: 97 nM
CDK6: 300 nM

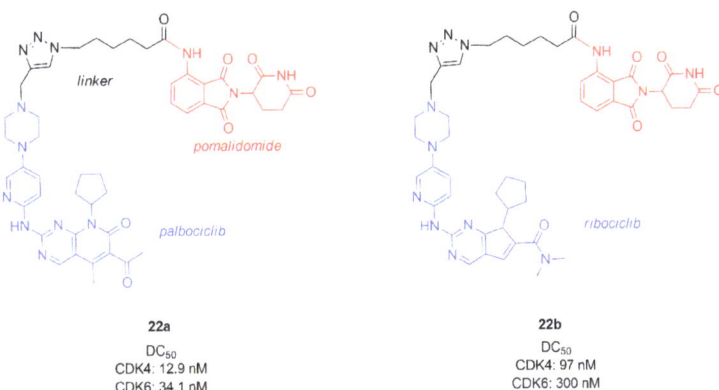

Figure 13. Chemical structures of palbociclib or ribociclib/pomalidomide PROTACs.

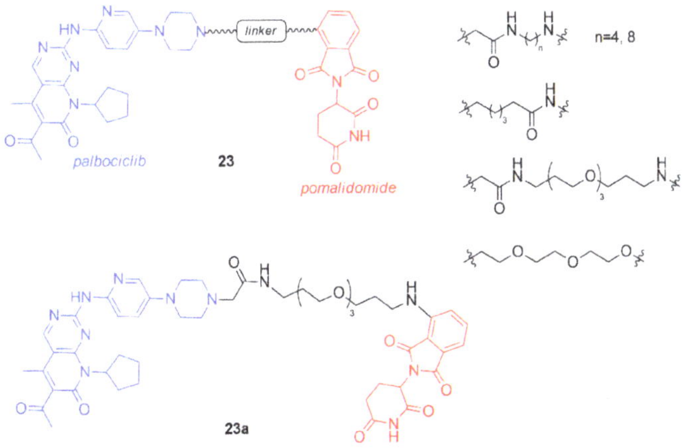

Figure 14. Chemical structures of palbociclib/pomalidomide PROTACs.

All compounds with shorter linker degrade CDK6 partly, while the PROTAC containing the longest linker (**23a**, Figure 14) selectively degraded CDK6 at the single dose of 500 nM in pancreatic cancer MiaPaCa2 cells with respect to other cyclin-dependent kinases including CDK4. Two hypotheses on the selective behavior of this PROTAC could be found in the less stable ternary complex palbociclib-E3 ligase-CDK4, that avoids the degradation, or in the fast deubiquitination of CDK4. The quantitative degradation of only CDK6 (CDK4 was not affected) was observed for compound **23a** in a dose-response study at 4 and 24 h in Human Pancreatic Nestin-Expressing ductal (HPNE) and MiaPaCa2 cells at 100 nM.

Another library of PROTACs containing CDK4/6 inhibitor and pomalidomide was synthesized by Su et al. (**24**, Figure 15), in which the influence of the length and rigidity of the linker, the spatial orientation of the target protein and the E3 ligase, and the binding affinity of PROTAC to CDK4 and 6 were studied [92].

PROTACs containing ribociclib did not degrade CDK6, while for the others best results in selectively degradation CDK6 was obtained with shorter linkers. In particular, the linker anchoring group to CDK inhibitors (amide, triazole, or methylene) did not influence the activity while to the other side, the best anchoring group to E3 ligase was the amino group, demonstrating that the flexibility of this portion is fundamental to correctly interact. The most potent PROTAC **24a** possesses a DC_{50} value of 2.1 nM in glioblastoma U251 cells and demonstrated good potency also in hematopoietic cancer cells, including multiple myeloma MM.1S (IC_{50} 10 nM).

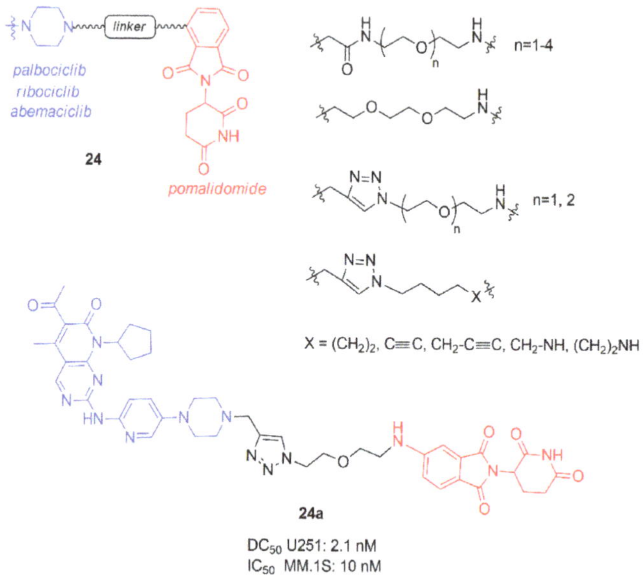

Figure 15. PROTACs containing CDK4/6 inhibitors and pomalidomide synthesized by Su et al.

Jiang and co-workers prepared a library of palbociclib, ribociclib, and abemaciclib PROTACs (**25**–**27**, Figure 16) connected to pomalidomide through an alkyl or polyethylene glycol (PEG) linker [93].

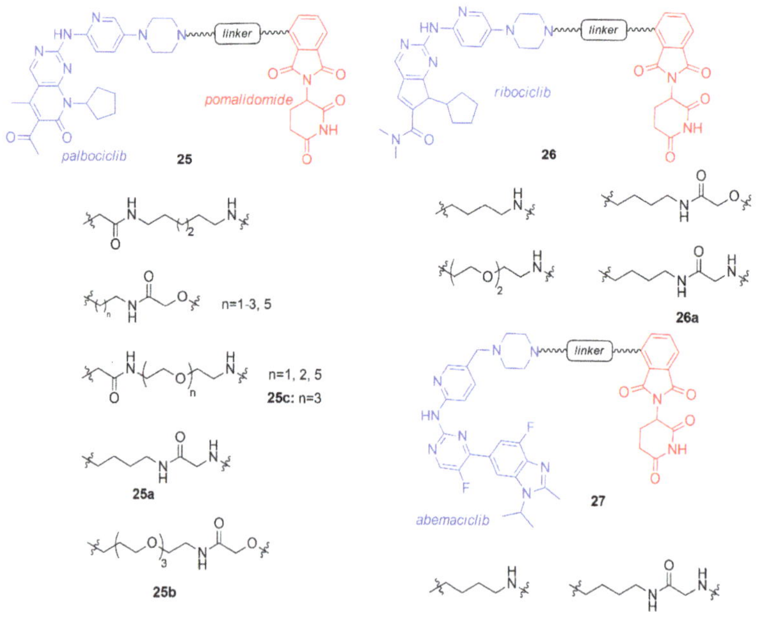

Figure 16. PROTACs containing CDK4/6 inhibitors and pomalidomide synthesized by Jiang et al.

PROTACs of each CDK4/6 inhibitor demonstrated degrading activity of both CDK4 and 6, but abemaciclib-PROTACs also induced the degradation of the off-target CDK9, that should be avoided [60]. The type of the linker (length and structure) and the CDK4/6 inhibitor of the PROTAC influenced the selectivity of degradation at 100 nM: compound **25a** (alkyl linker conjugated to palbociclib) indifferently degraded both CDK4 and CDK6, **25b** (extended PEG-3 linker conjugated to palbociclib) selectively hit CDK6, while **26a** (4-carbon alkyl linker conjugated to ribociclib) was selectively toward CDK4.

Compounds containing the imide group were tested for their capability to inhibit Ikaros (IKZF1) and Aiolos (IKZF3), well-established targets of imide-based degraders [94–96]. Compounds **25a–b** and **26a** degraded also IKZF1/3, resulting in an enhnanced anti-proliferative effect on mantle cell lymphoma lines.

Compound **25c** was previously synthesized by Brand and co-workers and studied for its ability to selectively degrade CDK6 over CDK4, in particular the correlation between the use of the CDK6 degrader in acute myeloid leukemia cells was investigated [97].

In a recent study, Anderson et al. evaluated the effect of other E3 ligase, such as von Hippel-Lindau (VHL) and Inhibitor of Apoptosis (IAP) instead of CRBN, on the selective degradation of CDK4/6, maintaining the anchoring on the nitrogen of piperazine of palbociclib and using different types of linkers (**28**, Figure 17) [98].

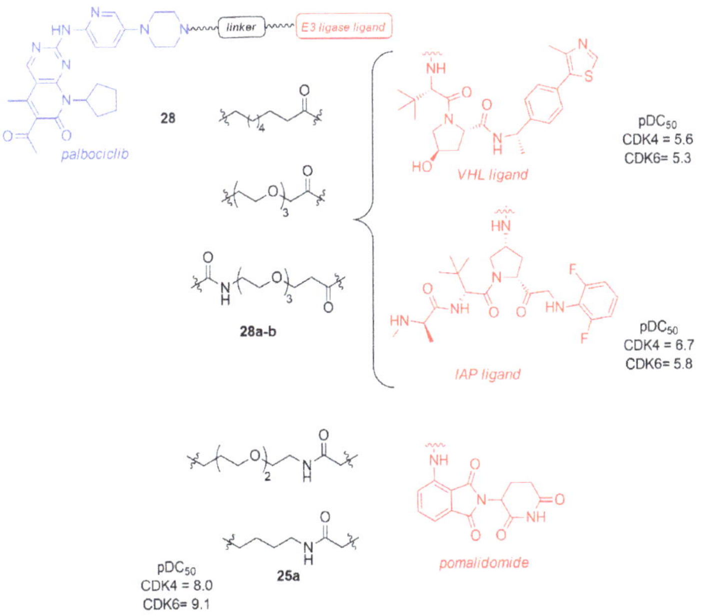

Figure 17. PROTACs palbociclib and E3 ligase ligands, such as von Hippel-Lindau (VHL) and Inhibitor of Apoptosis (IAP) ligands and pomalidomide.

The dose-response study in Jurkat cells after 24 h revealed that the degradation of CDK4 and CDK6 occurred independently of the type of E3 ligases (VHL, CRBN, and IAP binder), with a CDK4 pDC_{50} in the range of 6.2–8.0 and CDK6 pDC_{50} in the range of 7.7–9.1. It is important to note that all of them show a greater degradation power towards CDK6, probably due to a better stability of the formed ternary complex.

Compounds **28a–b**, containing VHL and IAP, are the less potent degraders (**28a**: pDC_{50} CDK4 = 5.6; pDC_{50} CDK6 = 5.3; **28b**: pDC_{50} CDK4 = 6.7; pDC_{50} CDK6 = 5.8), probably due to the linker nature. The most potent CDK4/6 degrader is **25a**, previously reported by Jiang (pDC_{50} CDK4 = 8.0, pDC_{50} CDK6 = 9.1) [93].

Compounds **25a** was taken into account by Steinbach et al. to synthesize novel palbociclib based PROTACs by changing the E3 ligase portion and inserting various linkers (**29–31**, Figure 18) [99]. In the series **29**, pomalidomide was linked by an amide linker to the palbociclib piperidine, avoiding the protonation of the previously synthesized tertiary amine that could affect activity and selectivity. The linkers were polyethylene or alkyl chain of different size. These compounds were tested in multiple myeloma (MM.1S) cell lines at 0.1 μM and the activity of PROTACs was shown as the percentage of remaining CDK levels (D). The degradation percentage (D) of CDK6 for compounds **29a–c** was in the range of 7.7–8.4 and the selectivity over CDK4 in the range of 1.9–3.3. In the series **30** and **31**, palbociclib was linked to VHL ligand functionalized in two different positions to create an amide or a phenoxy group in the E3 ligase ligand side, while in the other side of the linker there was an amine group. Compound **30a** showed a degradation percentage 1.7 and a selectivity CDK4 ratio of 19, while compound **31a** showed a comparable degradation activity (D CDK6 = 1.4) but an improved selectivity (D_{CDK4}/D_{CDK6} = 31). PROTACs **30a** and **31a** were also tested in different cancer cell lines (multiple mieloma, acute myeloid leukemia, acute lymphoid blastic leukemia) inhibiting cell proliferation.

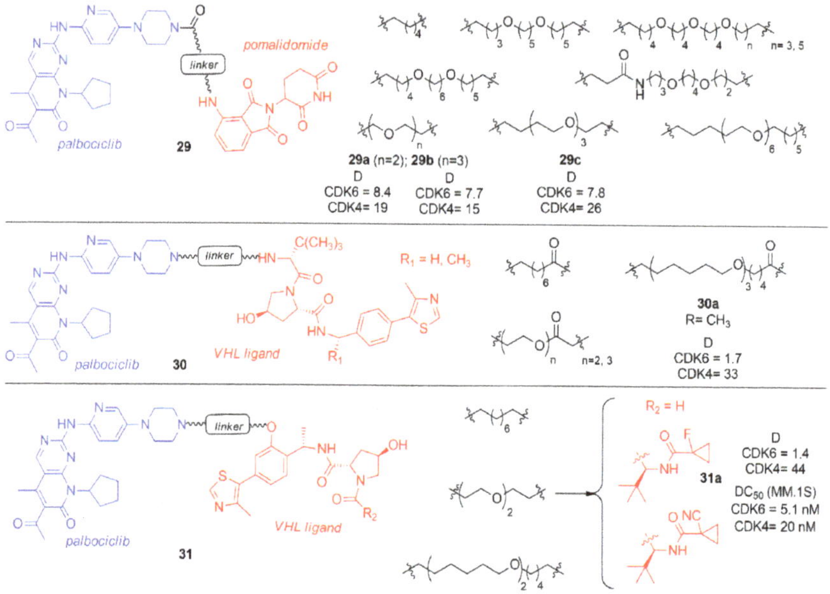

Figure 18. PROTACs containing palbociclib and E3 ligase ligand, such as pomalidomide and VHL ligand.

4. Conclusions

Since 2015, the arsenal of drug against breast cancer is enriched with third-generation CDK4/6 inhibitors. Three compounds (palbociclib, ribociclib, abemaciclib) have been approved by the FDA for the treatment of breast cancer in association with endocrine therapy. These ATP-competitive compounds share a common portion interacting with the ATP-binding site; in fact, they contain the pyridine-amine-pyrimidine scaffold, that determines the formation of more than one H-bond with the hinge residue of the target kinases.

In the last five years, a number of small molecule inhibitors have been synthesized and tested in order to identify compounds more potent, selective, and with improved pharmacokinetic parameters. The main heteroaromatic scaffold, that represents the central part of the molecule, was kept constant, while different groups or additional cycles were introduced on the terminal portions.

The use of PROTACs (proteolysis targeting chimeras), composed combining the CDK4/6 inhibitor small molecule and an E3 ligase ligand, is a novel approach to selectively degrade the targeted kinases. The anchoring point in CDK inhibitor is the nitrogen of the piperazine, which is extended towards the outside of the binding site, without interfering with the ATP-binding site. The majority of studies have been done on palbociclib and pomalidomide, by varying the type (nature and length) of the linker, although studies on the other two approved CDK inhibitors and different E3 ligases are reported. These studies have shown that it is possible to selectively degrade CDK4 or CDK6, depending on the type of inhibitor and linker, although the single inhibitor acts to a comparable extent on the two kinases.

Moreover, in addition to the study on breast cancer, the actions on other cancer cell lines have been explored. The development of new CDK inhibitors or degraders will certainly continue over the next years and possibly will allow to treat other forms of cancer with improved potency and less side effects.

Author Contributions: Conceptualization and supervision: M.F.; literature review: M.F., A.A., M.A., B.D.F. figures: M.F., A.A., M.A., B.D.F. writing and review: M.F., A.A., M.A., B.D.F. All authors have read and agreed to the published version of the manuscript.

Funding: This research received no external funding. The APC was funded by MDPI.

Data Availability Statement: The data presented in this study are available in this article.

Conflicts of Interest: The authors declare no conflict of interest.

Abbreviations

AIs	Aromatase Inhibitors
BC	Breast Cancer
CDK4/6	Cyclin-Dependent Kinase 4/6
CDKs	Cyclin-Dependent Kinases
ER	Estrogen Receptor
ER+	Estrogen-Receptor Positive
ERE	Estrogen Responsive Element
FDA	Food and Drug Administration
HER2	Human Epidermal Growth Factor Receptor 2
HPNE	Human Pancreatic Nestin-Expressing ductal
INK4	INhibitor of CDK4
KIP	CDK-Kinase Inhibitory Protein
MMP	Matrix-Metallo-Proteinase
mTOR	Mammalian Target Of Rapamycin
PI3K	PhosphatidylInositol 3-Kinase
PR	Progesterone Receptor
SERD	Selective ER Down-regulators
SERM	Selective ER Modulators
SMI	Small Molecule Inhibitor
TN	Triple Negative

References

1. Bray, F.; Ferlay, J.; Soerjomataram, I.; Siegel, R.L.; Torre, L.A.; Jemal, A. Global cancer statistics 2018: GLOBOCAN estimates of incidence and mortality worldwide for 36 cancers in 185 countries. *CA Cancer J. Clin.* **2018**, *68*, 394–424. [CrossRef]
2. Dai, X.; Li, T.; Bai, Z.; Yang, Y.; Liu, X.; Zhan, J.; Shi, B. Breast cancer intrinsic subtype classification, clinical use and future trends. *Am. J. Cancer. Res.* **2015**, *5*, 2929–2943.
3. Hu, Z.; Fan, C.; Oh, D.S.; Marron, J.S.; He, X.; Qaqish, B.F.; Livasy, C.; Carey, L.A.; Reynolds, E.; Dressler, L.; et al. The molecular portraits of breast tumors are conserved across microarray platforms. *BMC Genom.* **2006**, *7*, 96. [CrossRef]
4. Lehmann, B.D.; Bauer, J.A.; Chen, X.; Sanders, M.E.; Chakravarthy, A.B.; Shyr, Y.; Pietenpol, J.A. Identification of human triple-negative breast cancer subtypes and preclinical models for selection of targeted therapies. *J. Clin. Investig.* **2011**, *121*, 2750–2767. [CrossRef] [PubMed]
5. Tao, M.; Song, T.; Du, W.; Han, S.; Zuo, C.; Li, Y.; Wang, Y.; Yang, Z. Classifying breast cancer subtypes using multiple kernel learning based on bmics data. *Genes* **2019**, *10*, 200. [CrossRef] [PubMed]
6. Aggelis, V.; Johnston, S.R.D. Advances in endocrine-based therapies for estrogen receptor-positive metastatic breast cancer. *Drugs* **2019**, *79*, 1849–1866. [CrossRef] [PubMed]

7. Jordan, V.C.; O'Malley, B.W. Selective estrogen-receptor modulators and antihormonal resistance in breast cancer. *J. Clin. Oncol.* **2007**, *25*, 5815–5824. [CrossRef]
8. Gombos, A. Selective oestrogen receptor degraders in breast cancer: A review and perspectives. *Curr. Opin. Oncol.* **2019**, *31*, 424–429. [CrossRef]
9. Early Breast Cancer Trialists' Collaborative Group. Aromatase inhibitors versus tamoxifen in early breast cancer: Patient-level meta-analysis of the randomised trials. *Lancet* **2015**, *386*, 1341–1352. [CrossRef]
10. Portman, N.; Alexandrou, S.; Carson, E.; Wang, S.; Lim, E.; Caldon, E. Overcoming CDK4/6 inhibitor resistance in ER-positive breast cancer. *Endocr. Relat. Cancer.* **2019**, *26*, R15–R30. [CrossRef]
11. Dutta, U.; Pant, K. Aromatase inhibitors: Past, present and future in breast cancer therapy. *Med. Oncol.* **2008**, *25*, 113–124. [CrossRef]
12. Kharb, R.; Haider, K.; Neha, K.; Yar, M.S. Aromatase inhibitors: Role in postmenopausal breast cancer. *Arch. Pharm.* **2020**, *353*, e2000081. [CrossRef]
13. Ghosh, D.; Lo, J.; Morton, D.; Valette, D.; Xi, J.; Griswold, J.; Hubbell, S.; Egbuta, C.; Jiang, W.; An, J.; et al. Novel aromatase inhibitors by structure-guided design. *J. Med. Chem.* **2012**, *55*, 8464–8476. [CrossRef]
14. Fantacuzzi, M.; De Filippis, B.; Gallorini, M.; Ammazzalorso, A.; Giampietro, L.; Maccallini, C.; Aturki, Z.; Donati, E.; Ibrahim, R.S.; Shawky, E.; et al. Synthesis, biological evaluation, and docking study of indole arylsulfonamides as aromatase inhibitors. *Eur. J. Med. Chem.* **2020**, *185*, 111815. [CrossRef] [PubMed]
15. Di Matteo, M.; Ammazzalorso, A.; Andreoli, F.; Caffa, I.; De Filippis, B.; Fantacuzzi, M.; Giampietro, L.; Maccallini, C.; Nencioni, A.; Parenti, M.D.; et al. Synthesis and biological characterization of 3-(imidazole-1-ylmethyl) piperidine sulfonamides as aromatase inhibitors. *Bioorg. Med. Chem. Lett.* **2016**, *26*, 3192–3194. [CrossRef] [PubMed]
16. Ammazzalorso, A.; Gallorini, M.; Fantacuzzi, M.; Gambacorta, N.; De Filippis, B.; Giampietro, L.; Maccallini, C.; Nicolotti, O.; Cataldi, A.; Amoroso, R. Design, synthesis and biological evaluation of imidazole and triazole-based carbamates as novel aromatase inhibitors. *Eur. J. Med. Chem.* **2021**, *211*, 113115. [CrossRef] [PubMed]
17. The Cancer Genome Atlas Network. Comprehensive molecular portraits of human breast tumours. *Nature* **2012**, *490*, 61–70. [CrossRef]
18. Hanker, A.B.; Sudhan, D.R.; Arteaga, C.L. Overcoming endocrine resistance in breast cancer. *Cancer Cell* **2020**, *37*, 496–513. [CrossRef]
19. Kalra, S.; Joshi, G.; Munshi, A.; Kumar, R. Structural insights of cyclin dependent kinases: Implications in design of selective inhibitors. *Eur. J. Med. Chem.* **2017**, *142*, 424–458. [CrossRef]
20. Zhang, J.; Yang, P.L.; Gray, N.S. Targeting cancer with small molecule kinase inhibitors. *Nat. Rev. Cancer* **2009**, *9*, 28–39. [CrossRef]
21. Scheiblecker, L.; Kollmann, K.; Sexl, V. CDK4/6 and MAPK-crosstalk as opportunity for cancer treatment. *Pharmaceuticals* **2020**, *13*, 418. [CrossRef] [PubMed]
22. Malumbres, M. Cyclin-dependent kinases. *Genome Biol.* **2014**, *15*, 122. [CrossRef]
23. Malumbres, M.; Harlow, E.; Hunt, T.; Hunter, T.; Lahti, J.M.; Manning, G.; Morgan, D.O.; Tsai, L.H.; Wolgemuth, D.J. Cyclin-dependent kinases: A family portrait. *Nat. Cell Biol.* **2009**, *11*, 1275–1276. [CrossRef]
24. Kollmann, K.; Heller, G.; Schneckenleithner, C.; Warsch, W.; Scheicher, R.; Ott, R.G.; Schafer, M.; Fajmann, S.; Schlederer, M.; Schiefer, A.I.; et al. A kinase-independent function of CDK6 links the cell cycle to tumor angiogenesis. *Cancer Cell* **2013**, *24*, 167–181. [CrossRef] [PubMed]
25. Roovers, K.; Assoian, R.K. Integrating the MAP kinase signal into the G1 phase cell cycle machinery. *BioEssays* **2000**, *22*, 818–826. [CrossRef]
26. Xiong, Y.; Li, T.; Assani, G.; Ling, H.; Zhou, Q.; Zeng, Y.; Zhou, F.; Zhou, Y. Ribociclib, a selective cyclin D kinase 4/6 inhibitor, inhibits proliferation and induces apoptosis of human cervical cancer in vitro and in vivo. *Biomed. Pharmacother.* **2019**, *112*, 108602–108613. [CrossRef] [PubMed]
27. Roskoski, R., Jr. Cyclin-dependent protein kinase inhibitors including palbociclib as anticancer drugs. *Pharmacol. Res.* **2016**, *107*, 249–275. [CrossRef]
28. Lynce, F.; Shajahan-Haq, A.N.; Swain, S.M. CDK4/6 inhibitors in breast cancer therapy: Current practice and future opportunities. *Pharmacol. Ther.* **2018**, *191*, 65–73. [CrossRef] [PubMed]
29. Peyressatre, M.; Prével, C.; Pellerano, M.; Morris, M.C. Targeting cyclin-dependent kinases in human cancers: From small molecules to peptide inhibitors. *Cancers* **2015**, *7*, 179–237. [CrossRef]
30. Asghar, U.; Witkiewicz, A.K.; Turner, N.C.; Knudsen, E.S. The history and future of targeting cyclin-dependent kinases in cancer therapy. *Nat. Rev. Drug Discov.* **2015**, *14*, 130–146. [CrossRef]
31. Pernas, S.; Tolaney, S.M.; Winer, E.P.; Goel, S. CDK4/6 inhibition in breast cancer: Current practice and future directions. *Ther. Adv. Med. Oncol.* **2018**, *10*, 1758835918786451. [CrossRef]
32. Goel, S.; DeCristo, M.J.; McAllister, S.S.; Zhao, J.J. CDK4/6 inhibition in cancer: Beyond cell cycle arrest. *Trends Cell Biol.* **2018**, *28*, 911–925. [CrossRef]
33. Dos Santos Paparidis, N.F.; Canduri, F. The emerging picture of CDK11: Genetic, functional and medicinal aspects. *Curr. Med. Chem.* **2018**, *25*, 880–888. [CrossRef] [PubMed]
34. Shazzad Hossain Prince, G.M.; Yang, T.-Y.; Lin, H.; Chen, M.-C. Mechanistic insight of cyclin-dependent kinase 5 in modulating lung cancer growth. *Chin. J. Physiol.* **2019**, *62*, 231–240. [CrossRef]

35. Pozo, K.; Bibb, J.A. The emerging role of Cdk5 in cancer. *Trends Cancer* **2016**, *2*, 606–618. [CrossRef]
36. Xi, M.; Chen, T.; Wu, C.; Gao, Z.; Wu, Y.; Luo, X.; Du, K.; Yu, L.; Cai, T.; Shen, R.; et al. CDK8 as a therapeutic target for cancers and recent developments in discovery of CDK8 inhibitors. *Eur. J. Med. Chem.* **2019**, *164*, 77–91. [CrossRef] [PubMed]
37. Eyvazis, S.; Hejazi, M.S.; Kahora, H.; Abasi, M.; Zamiri, R.E.; Tarhriz, V. CDK9 as an appealing target for therapeutic interventions. *Curr. Drug Targets* **2019**, *20*, 453–464. [CrossRef]
38. Bose, P.; Simmons, G.L.; Grant, S. Cyclin-dependent kinase inhibitor therapy for hematologic malignancies. *Expert Opin. Investig. Drugs* **2013**, *22*, 723–738. [CrossRef]
39. Blum, K.A.; Ruppert, A.S.; Woyach, J.A.; Jones, J.A.; Andritsos, L.; Flynn, J.M.; Rovin, B.; Villalona-Calero, M.; Ji, J.; Phelps, M.; et al. Risk factors for tumor lysis syndrome in patients with chronic lymphocytic leukemia treated with the cyclin-dependent kinase inhibitor, flavopiridol. *Leukemia* **2011**, *25*, 1444–1451. [CrossRef]
40. Le Tourneau, C.; Faivre, S.; Laurence, V.; Delbaldo, C.; Vera, K.; Girre, V.; Chiao, J.; Armour, S.; Frame, S.; Green, S.R.; et al. Phase I evaluation of seliciclib (R-roscovitine), a novel oral cyclin-dependent kinase inhibitor, in patients with advanced malignancies. *Eur. J. Cancer* **2010**, *46*, 3243–3250. [CrossRef]
41. Payton, M.; Chung, G.; Yakowec, P.; Wong, A.; Powers, D.; Xiong, L.; Zhang, N.; Leal, J.; Bush, T.L.; Santora, V.; et al. Discovery and evaluation of dual CDK1 and CDK2 inhibitors. *Cancer Res.* **2006**, *66*, 4299–4308. [CrossRef] [PubMed]
42. Parry, D.; Guzi, T.; Shanahan, F.; Davis, N.; Prabhavalkar, D.; Wiswell, D.; Seghezzi, W.; Paruch, K.; Dwyer, M.P.; Doll, R.; et al. Dinaciclib (SCH 727965), a novel and potent cyclin-dependent kinase inhibitor. *Mol. Cancer Ther.* **2010**, *9*, 2344–2353. [CrossRef] [PubMed]
43. Teng, Y.; Lu, K.; Zhang, Q.; Zhao, L.; Huang, Y.; Ingarra, A.M.; Galons, H.; Li, T.; Cui, S.; Yu, P.; et al. Recent advances in the development of cyclin-dependent kinase 7 inhibitors. *Eur. J. Med. Chem.* **2019**, *183*, 1116412. [CrossRef] [PubMed]
44. Czudor, Z.; Balogh, M.; Bánhegyi, P.; Boros, S.; Breza, N.; Dobos, J.; Fábián, M.; Horváth, Z.; Illyés, E.; Markó, P.; et al. Novel compounds with potent CDK9 inhibitory activity for the treatment of myeloma. *Bioorg. Med. Chem. Lett.* **2018**, *28*, 769–773. [CrossRef]
45. Dukelow, T.; Kishan, D.; Khasraw, M.; Murphy, C.G. CDK4/6 inhibitors in breast cancer. *Anticancer Drugs* **2015**, *26*, 797–806. [CrossRef] [PubMed]
46. Poratti, M.; Marzaro, G. Third-generation CDK inhibitors: A review on the synthesis and binding modes of palbociclib, ribociclib and abemaciclib. *Eur. J. Med. Chem.* **2019**, *172*, 143–153. [CrossRef]
47. Beaver, J.A.; Amiri-Kordestani, L.; Charlab, R.; Chen, W.; Palmby, T.; Tilley, A.; Zirkelbach, J.F.; Yu, J.; Liu, Q.; Zhao, L.; et al. FDA approval: Palbociclib for the treatment of postmenopausal patients with estrogen receptor-positive, HER2-negative metastatic breast cancer. *Clin. Cancer Res.* **2015**, *21*, 4760–4766. [CrossRef]
48. Syed, Y.Y. Ribociclib: First global approval. *Drugs* **2017**, *77*, 799–807. [CrossRef] [PubMed]
49. Patnaik, A.; Rosen, L.S.; Tolaney, S.M.; Tolcher, A.W.; Goldman, J.W.; Gandhi, L.; Papadopoulos, K.P.; Beeram, M.; Rasco, D.W.; Hilton, J.F.; et al. Efficacy and safety of abemaciclib, an inhibitor of CDK4 and CDK6, for patients with breast cancer, non-small cell lung cancer, and other solid tumors. *Cancer Discov.* **2016**, *6*, 740–753. [CrossRef]
50. Tan, A.R.; Wright, G.S.; Thummala, A.R.; Danso, M.A.; Popovic, L.; Pluard, T.J.; Han, H.S.; Vojnović, Ž.; Vasev, N.; Ma, L.; et al. Trilaciclib plus chemotherapy versus chemotherapy alone in patients with metastatic triple-negative breast cancer: A multicentre, randomised, open-label, phase 2 trial. *Lancet Oncol.* **2019**, *20*, 1587–1601. [CrossRef]
51. Hart, L.L.; Ferrarotto, R.; Andric, Z.G.; Beck, J.T.; Subramanian, J.T.; Radosavljevic, D.Z.; Zaric, B.; Hanna, W.T.; Aljumaily, R.; Owonikoko, T.K.; et al. Myelopreservation with trilaciclib in patients receiving topotecan for small cell lung cancer: Results from a randomized, double-blind, placebo-controlled phase II study. *Adv. Ther.* **2021**, *38*, 350–365. [CrossRef]
52. Bisi, J.E.; Sorrentino, J.A.; Roberts, P.J.; Tavares, F.X.; Strum, J.C. Preclinical characterization of G1T28: A novel CDK4/6 inhibitor for reduction of chemotherapy-induced myelosuppression. *Mol. Cancer Ther.* **2016**, *15*, 783–793. [CrossRef] [PubMed]
53. He, S.; Roberts, P.J.; Sorrentino, J.A.; Bisi, J.E.; Storrie-White, H.; Tiessen, R.G.; Makhuli, K.M.; Wargin, W.A.; Tadema, H.; van Hoogdalem, E.J.; et al. Transient CDK4/6 inhibition protects hematopoietic stem cells from chemotherapy-induced exhaustion. *Sci. Transl. Med.* **2017**, *9*, eaal3986. [CrossRef]
54. Bisi, J.E.; Sorrentino, J.A.; Jordan, J.L.; Darr, D.D.; Roberts, P.J.; Tavares, F.X.; Strum, J.C. Preclinical development of G1T38: A novel, potent and selective inhibitor of cyclin dependent kinases 4/6 for use as an oral antineoplastic in patients with CDK4/6 sensitive tumors. *Oncotarget* **2017**, *8*, 42343–42358. [CrossRef] [PubMed]
55. Stice, J.P.; Wardell, S.E.; Norris, J.D.; Yllanes, A.P.; Alley, H.M.; Haney, V.O.; White, H.S.; Safi, R.; Winter, P.S.; Cocce, K.J.; et al. CDK4/6 therapeutic intervention and viable alternative to taxanes in CRPC. *Mol. Cancer Res.* **2017**, *15*, 660–669. [CrossRef] [PubMed]
56. Long, F.; He, Y.; Fu, H.; Li, Y.; Bao, X.; Wang, Q.; Wang, Y.; Xie, C.; Lou, L. Preclinical characterization of SHR6390, a novel CDK 4/6 inhibitor, in vitro and in human tumor xenograft models. *Cancer Sci.* **2019**, *110*, 1420–1430. [CrossRef]
57. Wang, J.; Li, Q.; Yuan, J.; Wang, J.; Chen, Z.; Liu, Z.; Li, Z.; Lai, Y.; Gao, J.; Shen, L. CDK4/6 inhibitor-SHR6390 exerts potent antitumor activity in esophageal squamous cell carcinoma by inhibiting phosphorylated Rb and inducing G1 cell cycle arrest. *J. Transl. Med.* **2017**, *15*, 127. [CrossRef]
58. Wang, Y.; Wang, J.; Ding, L. Benzimidazole Derivatives, Preparation Methods and Uses Thereof. PCT. International Patent WO2016145622A1, 22 September 2016.

59. Gelbert, L.M.; Cai, S.; Lin, X.; Sanchez-Martinez, C.; del Prado, M.; Lallena, M.J.; Torres, R.; Ajamie, R.T.; Wishart, G.N.; Flack, R.S.; et al. Preclinical characterization of the CDK4/6 inhibitor LY2835219: In-vivo cell cycle-dependent/independent anti-tumor activities alone/in combination with gemcitabine. *Investig. New Drugs* **2014**, *32*, 825–837. [CrossRef] [PubMed]
60. Tate, S.C.; Cai, S.; Ajamie, R.T.; Burke, T.; Beckmann, R.P.; Chan, E.M.; De Dios, A.; Wishart, G.N.; Gelbert, L.M.; Cronier, D.M. Semi-mechanistic pharmacokinetic/pharmacodynamic modeling of the antitumor activity of LY2835219, a new cyclin-dependent kinase 4/6 inhibitor, in mice bearing human tumor xenografts. *Clin. Cancer Res.* **2014**, *20*, 3763. [CrossRef]
61. Rader, J.; Russell, M.R.; Hart, L.S.; Nakazawa, M.S.; Belcastro, L.T.; Martinez, D.; Li, Y.; Carpenter, E.L.; Attiyeh, E.F.; Diskin, S.J.; et al. Dual CDK4/CDK6 inhibition induces cell-cycle arrest and senescence in neuroblastoma. *Clin. Cancer Res.* **2013**, *19*, 6173. [CrossRef]
62. Chen, P.; Lee, N.V.; Hu, W.; Xu, M.; Ferre, R.A.; Lam, H.; Bergqvist, S.; Solowiej, J.; Diehl, W.; He, Y.A.; et al. Spectrum and degree of CDK drug interactions predicts clinical performance. *Mol. Cancer Ther.* **2016**, *15*, 2273. [CrossRef] [PubMed]
63. Tsai, C.J.; Nussinov, R. The molecular basis of targeting protein kinases in cancer therapeutics. *Semin. Cancer Biol.* **2013**, *23*, 235–242. [CrossRef]
64. Hojjat-Farsangi, M. Small-molecule inhibitors of the receptor tyrosine kinases: Promising tools for targeted cancer therapies. *Int. J. Mol. Sci.* **2014**, *15*, 13768–13801. [CrossRef]
65. Zhou, M.; Wang, R. Small-molecule regulators of autophagy and their potential therapeutic applications. *ChemMedChem* **2013**, *8*, 694–707. [CrossRef] [PubMed]
66. Roskoski, R., Jr. A historical overview of protein kinases and their targeted small molecule inhibitors. *Pharmacol. Res.* **2015**, *100*, 1–23. [CrossRef] [PubMed]
67. Roskoski, R., Jr. Properties of FDA-approved small molecule protein kinase inhibitors. *Pharmacol. Res.* **2019**, *144*, 19–50. [CrossRef]
68. Meisel, J.E.; Chang, M. Selective small-molecule inhibitors as chemical tools to define the roles of matrix metalloproteinases in disease. *BBA Mol. Cell Res.* **2017**, *1864*, 2001–2014. [CrossRef]
69. Tadesse, S.; Yu, M.; Mekonnen, L.B.; Lam, F.; Islam, S.; Tomusange, K.; Rahaman, M.H.; Noll, B.; Basnet, S.K.C.; Teo, T.; et al. Highly potent, selective, and orally bioavailable 4-thiazol *N*-(pyridin-2-yl)pyrimidin-2-amine cyclin-dependent kinases 4 and 6 inhibitors as anticancer drug candidates: Design, synthesis, and evaluation. *J. Med. Chem.* **2017**, *60*, 1892–1915. [CrossRef]
70. Shao, H.; Shi, S.; Huang, S.; Hole, A.J.; Abbas, A.Y.; Baumli, S.; Liu, X.; Lam, F.; Foley, D.W.; Fischer, P.M.; et al. Substituted 4-(thiazol-5-yl)-2-(phenylamino)pyrimidines are highly active CDK9 inhibitors: Synthesis, X-ray crystal structures, structure-activity relationship, and anticancer activities. *J. Med. Chem.* **2013**, *56*, 640–659. [CrossRef]
71. Tadesse, S.; Zhu, G.; Mekonnen, L.B.; Lenjisa, J.L.; Yu, M.; Brown, M.P.; Wang, S. A novel series of *N*-(pyridin-2-yl)-4-(thiazol5-yl)pyrimidin-2-amines as highly potent CDK4/6 inhibitors. *Future Med. Chem.* **2017**, *9*, 1495–1506. [CrossRef]
72. Tadesse, S.; Bantie, L.; Tomusange, K.; Yu, M.; Islam, S.; Bykovska, N.; Noll, B.; Zhu, G.; Li, P.; Lam, F.; et al. Discovery and pharmacological characterization of a novel series of highly selective inhibitors of cyclin-dependent kinases 4 and 6 as anticancer agents. *Br. J. Pharmacol.* **2018**, *175*, 2399–2413. [CrossRef]
73. Zha, C.; Deng, W.; Fu, Y.; Tang, S.; Lan, X.; Ye, Y.; Su, Y.; Jiang, L.; Chen, Y.; Huang, Y.; et al. Design, synthesis and biological evaluation of tetrahydronaphthyridine derivatives as bioavailable CDK4/6 inhibitors for cancer therapy. *Eur. J. Med. Chem.* **2018**, *148*, 140–153. [CrossRef]
74. Fu, Y.; Tang, S.; Su, Y.; Lan, X.; Ye, Y.; Zha, C.; Li, L.; Cao, J.; Chen, Y.; Jiang, L.; et al. Discovery of a class of diheteroaromatic amines as orally bioavailable CDK1/4/6 inhibitors. *Bioorg. Med. Chem. Lett.* **2017**, *27*, 5332–5336. [CrossRef]
75. Wang, Y.; Liu, W.-J.; Yin, L.; Li, H.; Chen, Z.-H.; Zhu, D.-X.; Song, X.-Q.; Cheng, Z.-Z.; Song, P.; Wang, Z.; et al. Design and synthesis of 4-(2,3-dihydro-1H-benzo[d]pyrrolo[1,2-a] imidazol-7-yl)-*N*-(5-(piperazin-1-ylmethyl) pyridine-2-yl)pyrimidin-2-amine as a highly potent and selective cyclin-dependent kinases 4 and 6 inhibitors and the discovery of structure-activity relationships. *Bioorg. Med. Chem. Lett.* **2018**, *28*, 974–978. [CrossRef]
76. Shi, C.; Wang, Q.; Liao, X.; Ge, H.; Huo, G.; Zhang, L.; Chen, N.; Zhai, X.; Hong, Y.; Wang, L.; et al. Discovery of 6-(2-(dimethylamino)ethyl)-*N*-(5-fluoro-4-(4-fluoro-1-isopropyl-2-methyl-1H-benzo[d]imidazole-6-yl)pyrimidin-2-yl)-5,6,7,8-tetrahydro-1,6-naphthyridin-2-amine as a highly potent cyclin-dependent kinase 4/6 inhibitor for treatment of cancer. *Eur. J. Med. Chem.* **2019**, *178*, 352–364. [CrossRef]
77. Abbas, S.E.-S.; George, R.F.; Samir, E.M.; Aref, M.M.A.; Abdel-Aziz, H.A. Synthesis and anticancer activity of some pyrido[2,3-*d*]pyrimidine derivatives as apoptosis inducers and cyclin-dependent kinase inhibitors. *Future Med. Chem.* **2019**, *11*, 2395–2414. [CrossRef]
78. Shi, C.; Wang, Q.; Liao, X.; Ge, H.; Huo, G.; Zhang, L.; Chen, N.; Zhai, X.; Hong, Y.; Wang, L.; et al. Discovery of a novel series of imidazo[10,2′:1,6]pyrido[2,3-*d*]pyrimidin derivatives as potent cyclin-dependent kinase 4/6 inhibitors. *Eur. J. Med. Chem.* **2020**, *193*, 112239. [CrossRef]
79. Zhao, H.; Hu, X.; Cao, K.; Zhang, Y.; Zhao, K.; Tang, C.; Feng, B. Synthesis and SAR of 4,5-dihydro-1H-pyrazolo[4,3-h]quinazoline derivatives as potent and selective CDK4/6 inhibitors. *Eur. J. Med. Chem.* **2018**, *157*, 935–945. [CrossRef] [PubMed]
80. Garg, M.; Chauhan, M.; Singh, P.K.; Alex, J.M.; Kumar, R. Pyrazoloquinazolines: Synthetic strategies and bioactivities. *Eur. J. Med. Chem.* **2015**, *97*, 444–461. [CrossRef] [PubMed]
81. Toure, M.; Crews, C.M. Small-molecule PROTACS: New approaches to protein degradation. *Angew. Chem. Int. Ed. Engl.* **2016**, *55*, 1966–1973. [CrossRef] [PubMed]

82. Lai, A.C.; Crews, C.M. Induced protein degradation: An emerging drug discovery paradigm. *Nat. Rev. Drug Discov.* **2017**, *16*, 101–114. [CrossRef]
83. Marak, B.N.; Dowarah, J.; Khiangte, L.; Singh, V.P. A comprehensive insight on the recent development of cyclic dependent kinase inhibitors as anticancer agents. *Eur. J. Med. Chem.* **2020**, *203*, 112571. [CrossRef] [PubMed]
84. Crews, C.M. Targeting the undruggable proteome: The small molecules of my dreams. *Chem. Biol.* **2010**, *17*, 551–555. [CrossRef]
85. Li, X.; Song, Y. Proteolysis-targeting chimera (PROTAC) for targeted protein degradation and cancer therapy. *J. Hematol. Oncol.* **2020**, *13*, 50. [CrossRef] [PubMed]
86. Gadd, M.S.; Testa, A.; Lucas, X.; Chan, K.-H.; Chen, W.; Lamont, D.J.; Zengerle, M.; Ciulli, A. Structural basis of PROTAC cooperative recognition for selective protein degradation. *Nat. Chem. Biol.* **2017**, *13*, 514–521. [CrossRef] [PubMed]
87. Gao, H.; Sun, X.; Rao, Y. PROTAC technology: Opportunities and challenges. *ACS Med. Chem. Lett.* **2020**, *11*, 237–240. [CrossRef] [PubMed]
88. Robb, C.M.; Contreras, J.I.; Kour, S.; Taylor, M.A.; Abid, M.; Sonawane, Y.A.; Zahid, M.; Murry, D.J.; Natarajan, A.; Rana, S. Chemically induced degradation of CDK9 by a proteolysis targeting chimera (PROTAC). *Chem. Commun.* **2017**, *53*, 7577–7580. [CrossRef]
89. Hatcher, J.M.; Wang, E.S.; Johannessen, L.; Kwiatkowski, N.; Sim, T.; Gray, N.S. Development of highly potent and selective steroidal inhibitors and degraders of CDK8. *ACS Med. Chem. Lett.* **2018**, *9*, 540–545. [CrossRef]
90. Zhao, B.; Burgess, K. PROTACs suppression of CDK4/6, crucial kinases for cell cycle regulation in cancer. *Chem. Commun.* **2019**, *55*, 2704–2707. [CrossRef]
91. Rana, S.; Bendjennat, M.; Kour, S.; King, H.M.; Kizhake, S.; Zahid, M.; Natarajan, A. Selective degradation of CDK6 by a palbociclib based PROTAC. *Bioorg. Med. Chem. Lett.* **2019**, *29*, 1375–1379. [CrossRef]
92. Su, S.; Yang, Z.; Gao, H.; Yang, H.; Zhu, S.; An, Z.; Wang, J.; Li, Q.; Chandarlapaty, S.; Deng, H.; et al. Potent and preferential degradation of CDK6 via proteolysis targeting chimera degraders. *J. Med. Chem.* **2019**, *62*, 7575–7582. [CrossRef]
93. Jiang, B.; Wang, E.S.; Donovan, K.A.; Liang, Y.; Fischer, E.S.; Zhang, T.; Gray, N.S. Development of dual and selective degraders of cyclin-dependent kinases 4 and 6. *Angew. Chem. Int. Ed.* **2019**, *58*, 6321–6326. [CrossRef]
94. Lu, G.; Middleton, R.E.; Sun, H.; Naniong, M.; Ott, C.J.; Mitsiades, C.S.; Wong, K.K.; Bradner, J.E.; Kaelin, W.G., Jr. The myeloma drug lenalidomide promotes the cereblon-dependent destruction of Ikaros proteins. *Science* **2014**, *343*, 305–309. [CrossRef] [PubMed]
95. Kronke, J.; Udeshi, N.D.; Narla, A.; Grauman, P.; Hurst, S.N.; McConkey, M.; Svinkina, T.; Heckl, D.; Comer, E.; Li, X.; et al. Lenalidomide causes selective degradation of IKZF1 and IKZF3 in multiple myeloma cells. *Science* **2014**, *343*, 301–305. [CrossRef] [PubMed]
96. Huang, T.; Dobrovolsky, D.; Paulk, J.; Yang, G.; Weisberg, E.L.; Doctor, Z.M.; Buckley, D.L.; Cho, J.H.; Ko, E.; Jang, J.; et al. A chemoproteomic approach to query the degradable kinome using a multi-kinase degrader. *Cell Chem. Biol.* **2018**, *25*, 88–99.e6. [CrossRef]
97. Brand, M.; Jiang, B.; Bauer, S.; Donovan, K.A.; Liang, Y.; Wang, E.S.; Nowak, R.P.; Yuan, J.C.; Zhang, T.; Kwiatkowski, N.; et al. Homolog-selective degradation as a strategy to probe the function of CDK6 in AML. *Cell Chem. Biol.* **2019**, *26*, 300–306. [CrossRef]
98. Anderson, N.A.; Cryan, J.; Ahmed, A.; Dai, H.; McGonagle, G.A.; Rozier, C.; Benowitz, A.B. Selective CDK6 degradation mediated by cereblon, VHL, and novel IAP-recruiting PROTACs. *Bioorg. Med. Chem. Lett.* **2020**, *30*, 127106. [CrossRef]
99. Steinebach, C.; Ng, Y.L.D.; Sosič, I.; Lee, C.-S.; Chen, S.; Lindner, S.; Vu, L.P.; Bricelj, A.; Haschemi, R.; Monschke, M.; et al. Systematic exploration of different E3 ubiquitin ligases: An approach towards potent and selective CDK6 degraders. *Chem. Sci.* **2020**, *11*, 3474–3486. [CrossRef] [PubMed]

molecules

MDPI

Article

A Series of Isatin-Hydrazones with Cytotoxic Activity and CDK2 Kinase Inhibitory Activity: A Potential Type II ATP Competitive Inhibitor

Huda S. Al-Salem [1,*], Md Arifuzzaman [2], Hamad M. Alkahtani [1], Ashraf N. Abdalla [3], Iman S. Issa [1], Aljawharah Alqathama [4], Fatemah S. Albalawi [1] and A. F. M. Motiur Rahman [1,*]

1 Department of Pharmaceutical Chemistry, College of Pharmacy, King Saud University, Riyadh 11451, Saudi Arabia; ahamad@ksu.edu.sa (H.M.A.); iman_issa69@yahoo.com (I.S.I.); fsalbalawi@ksu.edu.sa (F.S.A.)

2 College of Pharmacy, Yeungnam University, Gyeongsan 38541, Korea; arifmilon2016@gmail.com

3 Department of Pharmacology and Toxicology, Faculty of Pharmacy, Umm Al-Qura University, Makkah 21955, Saudi Arabia; ashraf_abdalla@hotmail.com

4 Department of Pharmacognosy, Faculty of Pharmacy, Umm Al-Qura University, Makkah 21955, Saudi Arabia; aaqathama@uqu.edu.sa

* Correspondence: hhalsalem@ksu.edu.sa (H.S.A.-S.); afmrahman@ksu.edu.sa (A.F.M.M.R.); Tel.: +966-11-29-52740 (H.S.A.); +966-11-46-70237 (A.F.M.M.R.)

Academic Editor: Marialuigia Fantacuzzi

Received: 2 September 2020; Accepted: 18 September 2020; Published: 25 September 2020

Abstract: Isatin derivatives potentially act on various biological targets. In this article, a series of novel isatin-hydrazones were synthesized in excellent yields. Their cytotoxicity was tested against human breast adenocarcinoma (MCF7) and human ovary adenocarcinoma (A2780) cell lines using MTT assay. Compounds **4j** (IC_{50} = 1.51 ± 0.09 μM) and **4k** (IC_{50} = 3.56 ± 0.31) showed excellent activity against MCF7, whereas compound **4e** showed considerable cytotoxicity against both tested cell lines, MCF7 (IC_{50} = 5.46 ± 0.71 μM) and A2780 (IC_{50} = 18.96± 2.52 μM), respectively. Structure-activity relationships (SARs) revealed that, halogen substituents at 2,6-position of the C-ring of isatin-hydrazones are the most potent derivatives. In-silico absorption, distribution, metabolism and excretion (ADME) results demonstrated recommended drug likeness properties. Compounds **4j** (IC_{50} = 0.245 μM) and **4k** (IC_{50} = 0.300 μM) exhibited good inhibitory activity against the cell cycle regulator CDK2 protein kinase compared to imatinib (IC_{50} = 0.131 μM). A molecular docking study of **4j** and **4k** confirmed both compounds as type II ATP competitive inhibitors that made interactions with ATP binding pocket residues, as well as lacking interactions with active state DFG motif residues.

Keywords: isatin-hydrazones; cytotoxicity; CDK2 inhibitor; ATP competitive inhibitor; ADME analysis

1. Introduction

Development of anticancer drugs is essential due to the increasing number of morbidity and mortality by cancer day-by-day all over the world. According to the International Agency for Research on Cancer, in 2018, around 18 million people were infected; 9.6 million people among them had died due to life threatening cancer [1,2]. It is rather alarming that cancer morbidity cases may increase to 29.5 million by 2040 [3]. Having said that, it is very much challenging to develop an anticancer drug due to the long and expensive synthesis/isolation process and the huge lack of opportunities to conduct clinical trials. Moreover, most of the anticancer drugs currently available are lacking specificity and have adverse effects. In this context, developing novel anticancer agents with great efficacy and high specificity becomes imperative. To overcome these challenges, researchers should develop a drug molecule with potent biological activity and low/no toxicity, study its mode of action, in silico properties and in vitro/vivo metabolism, conduct a toxicity evaluation [4,5], study its topoisomerase inhibitory activity [6–8] and enzyme inhibitory activity [9], etc., all of which are some of the key evaluation practices for the development of potential anticancer therapeutics. Regarding enzyme inhibitory activities, cyclin-dependent kinases (CDKs) are considered as a vital feature, inciting various key transitions in the cell cycle for cancer cells, in addition to instructing apoptosis, transcription and exocytosis. CDKs are active only when bound to their regulator proteins, cyclins. CDK activity is tightly controlled for successful cell division. Since abnormal cell division represents cancer pathology, controlling CDK activity has been shown as a promising therapeutic strategy. In particular, CDK2 plays an important role in DNA replication. Therefore, therapeutic strategies based on the inhibition of CDKs work as an encouraging viewpoint for anticancer drug discovery. With that being said, to consider a compound, such as a drug molecule, as a treatment, it is still necessary to first test their drug likeness properties as well as analyze their physiological descriptors, such as absorption, distribution, metabolism and excretion (ADME). ADME is an important physiological descriptor of chemical compounds used for selecting potential drug targets. However, testing a wide range of compounds directly in the clinical or pre-clinical phase is extensively time consuming and costly. Moreover, ADME is considered as the last step of drug development, where many drugs (approximately 60%) fail after all the procedures. To tackle these problems, recent experiments have utilized in silico ADME tools as the first step to shortlist the amount of target compounds by calculating predicted ADME properties and discarding the compounds with unsatisfactory ADME values from the drug designing pipeline [10].

Isatin (**1**) is an organic compound first discovered in 1840 by Erdmann and Laurent from the oxidation of indigo dye [11,12]. It was considered as a synthetic product until isolated from natural sources, such as *Couroupita guianensis* [13], *Isatis tinctoria* [14] and *Calanthe discolor* [15], and from many other sources [16–18]. It has been reported that tryptophan obtained from food sources is usually converted to indole by gastrointestinal bacteria, which is further oxidized in the liver by CYP450 to isatin, therefore, isatin is present as an endogenous molecule in humans [19,20]. Various substituents on the isatin nucleus displayed numerous biological activities [21–36], including antimicrobial activity[31,37], topoisomerase inhibitory activity [7,38], epidermal growth factor receptor (EGFR) inhibitory activity [39], inhibitory activities on histone deacetylase (HDAC) [40,41], carbonic anhydrase [42–44], tyrosine kinase [45–47], cyclin-dependent kinases (CDKs) [9,48,49], adenylate cyclase inhibition [50] and protein tyrosine phosphatase (Shp2) [51]. A number of isatin-based marketed drugs and potential anticancer agents [41] are illustrated in Figure 1. Considering the importance of the development of anticancer therapeutics and the various biological properties of isatin and isatin nucleus-containing derivatives, a series of isatin-hydrazones were designed and synthesized, their cytotoxicities against two different cancer cell lines, namely MCF7 (human breast adenocarcinoma) and A2780 (human ovary adenocarcinoma), were evaluated, their structure–activity relationships (SARs) were studied, their ADME properties were studied using in silico ADME tools and cyclin-dependent kinases 2 inhibitory activities were performed using an enzyme inhibition assay. Additionally, docking simulations were conducted in order to explore the behavior of the synthesized compounds within the active site of CDK2 to justify its binding mechanism.

2. Results and Discussion

2.1. Synthesis of Isatin-Hydrazones (4)

Synthesis of 3-((substituted)benzylidene)hydrazono)indolin-2-one (**4**) was straightforward, as illustrated in Scheme 1 [36,52]. In the first step, a mixture of isatin (**1**) and hydrazine hydrate was refluxed in ethanol and isatin monohydrazone (**2**) was obtained in quantitative yields (~99%). Subsequently, the isatin monohydrazone (**2**) was refluxed with substituted aryl aldehydes (**3**) in the presence of a catalytic amount of glacial acetic acid in absolute ethanol to obtain 3-((substituted)benzylidene)hydrazono)indolin-2-one (**4**) in good to excellent yields (75–98%). The structures of the synthesized compounds were confirmed using IR, NMR (^{1}H and ^{13}C) and mass spectral data, as well as reported values that are known.

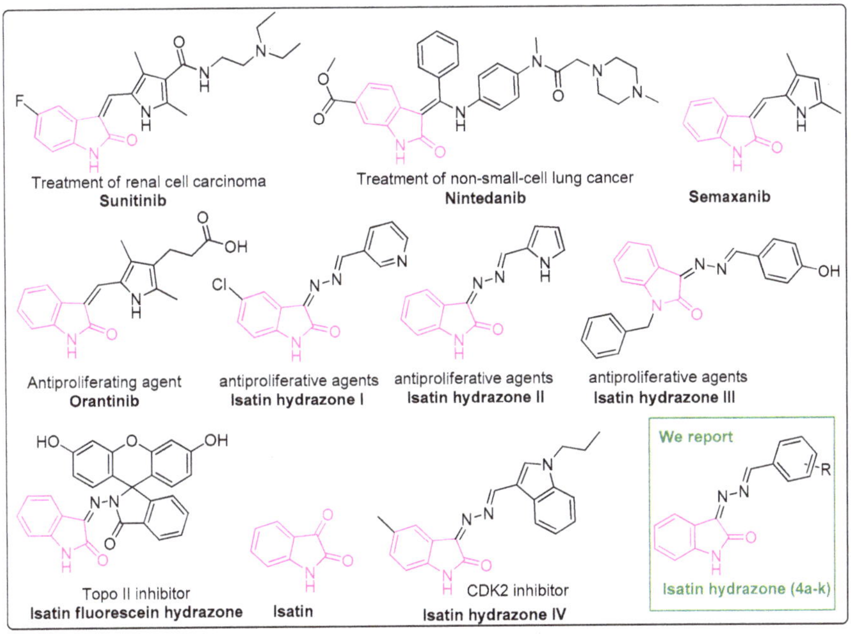

Figure 1. Isatin moiety containing active and potential drugs.

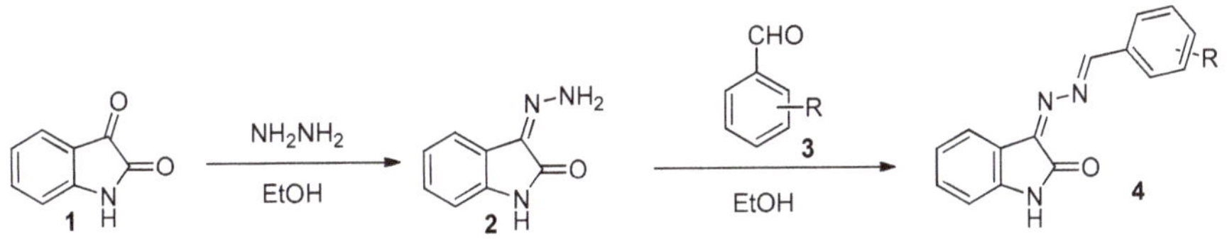

a	b	c	d	e	f	g	h	i	j	k
2-CH_3	3-CH_3	4-CH_3	4-SCH_3	2-Br	3-Br	4-Br	2,6-di-CH_3,4-OCH_3	2-OH,4-OCH_3	2,6-di-Cl	2-Cl, 6-F

Scheme 1. Synthesis of 3-((substituted)benzylidene)hydrazono)indolin-2-one (4).

2.2. *Biological Evaluation*

2.2.1. Cytotoxicity

The cytotoxicity of the synthesized compounds **4a–k** was evaluated against two different cancer cell lines, namely MCF7 and A2780, and the results are summarized in Table 1. Among the tested compounds, the isatin-hydrazone **4j** exhibited the highest inhibitory activity against MCF7 cell lines (1.51 ± 0.09 μM). It should be noted that **4k** (3.56 ± 0.31), **4e** (5.46 ± 0.71), **4i** (7.77 ± 0.008) and **4f** (9.07 ± 0.59) showed moderate inhibitory activity against MCF7 cell lines. In the case of A2780 cell lines, however, only the halogen-substituted compounds **4e, 4j, 4k** and **4f** showed a little inhibitory activity. Nevertheless, all of the tested compounds were more sensitive towards MCF7 compared to A2780 cell lines.

Table 1. Cytotoxicity of **4a–k** against MCF7 and A2780 cell lines.

Compound	IC_{50} (μM)	
	MCF7	**A2780**
4a	10.82 ± 0.05	>50
4b	14 ± 1.33	>50
4c	32.48 ± 0.52	>50
4d	24 ± 2.61	>50
4e	5.46 ± 0.71	19 ± 2.52
4f	9.07 ± 0.59	25 ± 2.82
4g	15.70 ± 0.78	>50
4h	25.78 ± 0.13	>50
4i	7.77 ± 0.008	>50
4j	1.51 ± 0.09	26 ± 2.24
4k	3.56 ± 0.31	27 ± 3.20
Doxorubicin	3.10 ± 0.29	0.20 ± 0.03

Figure 2 shows the dose–response curves for compounds **4j** and **4k,** which were the most cytotoxic compounds against the breast cancer cells lines (MCF7) at a concentration of 1.51 and 3.56 μM, respectively. The IC_{50} values interpolated from dose–response data with five different concentrations were 0.1, 1, 10, 25 and 50 μM.

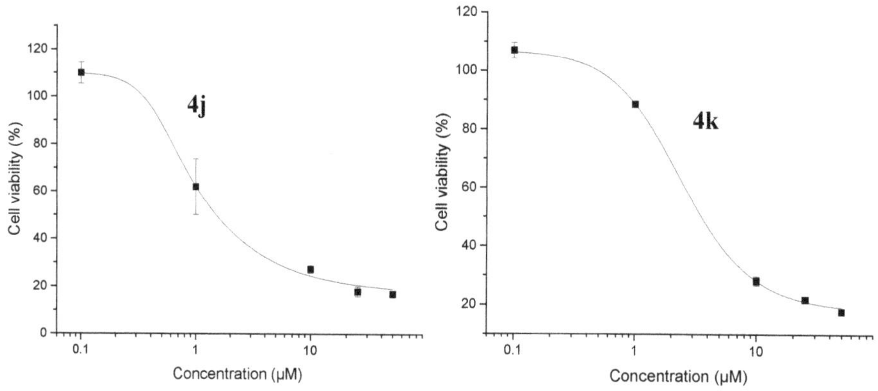

Figure 2. Dose–response curve of the most cytotoxic compounds against MCF7 cell lines.

2.2.2. Structure–Activity Relationships (SARs) Study of **4a–k**

The SARs study revealed that the cytotoxicity of **4a–k** increased or decreased in the same fashion as increases or decreases in halogen substitution in the aromatic C-ring. It is also related to the position of the substituents. As depicted in Figure 3, the bromo substituent at 4-position of the C-ring gave IC_{50} = 15.7 μM against MCF7 cell lines (Table 1, entry **4g**), while at 3-position, it increased to IC_{50} = 9.07 μM (Table 1, entry **4f**). Interestingly, the bromo substituent's cytotoxicity at 2-position, increased dramatically to IC_{50} = 5.46 μM (Table 1, entry **4e**). Surprisingly, while 2- and 6-positions of the C-ring having respective chloro- and fluoro- substituents, the IC_{50} of compound **4k** was 3.56 μM (Table 1, entry **4k**). More surprisingly, with both 2- and 6-positions of the C-ring with chloro- substituents, compound **4j** exhibited the highest cytotoxicity of IC_{50} = 1.51 μM (Table 1, entry **4j**) which is two-fold more than the control anticancer drug doxorubicin (IC_{50} = 3.1 μM) (Table 1, entry doxorubicin). On the other hand, the methyl substituent at the C-ring also affects cytotoxicity against MCF7 cell lines. The methyl substituent at 4-position gave IC_{50} = 32.48 μM (Table 1, entry **4c**) and it increased at 3-position to IC_{50} = 14.65 μM (Table 1, entry **4b**), whereas at 2-position, the IC_{50} value was 10.82 μM

(Table 1, entry **4a**). On the other hand, A2780 cell lines were inhibited by the halogenated derivatives **4e**, **4j**, **4k** and **4f**. In this case, 2-bromo substituted derivatives showed higher activity than the other three.

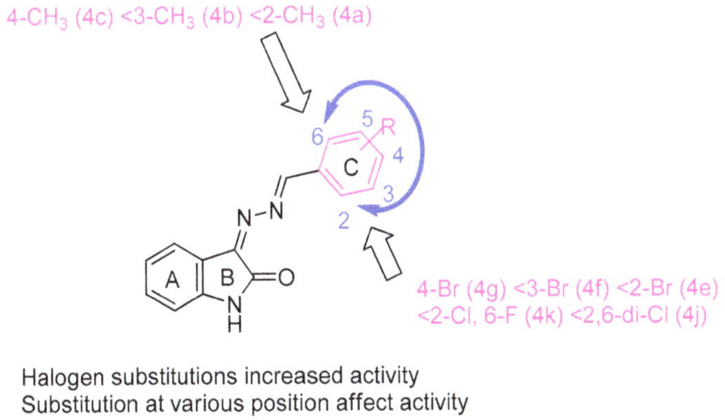

Figure 3. Structure–activity relationship (SAR) analysis of compounds **4a–k**.

2.2.3. CDK2 Protein Kinase Inhibitory Activity of **4a–k**

The promising cytotoxicity of **4**, especially **4j** and **4k**, motivated us to study further inhibitory activities against CDK2 protein kinase. As summarized in Table 2, **4j** and **4k** exhibited good inhibitory activity against cyclin-dependent kinase 2 (CDK2), which is half of that of the known kinase inhibitor imatinib.

Table 2. Inhibitory activities of compounds **4j** and **4k** against CDK2 protein kinase.

Compounds	CDK2 Protein Kinase (IC_{50} in μM) *
4j	0.2456
4k	0.3006
Imatinib	0.1312

* IC_{50} values are the mean ± SD of triplicate measurements.

2.3. In Silico Drug Likeness Property Analysis

Rational drug designing is the most significant part in modern drug discovery approaches. In this regard, computational ADME (absorption, distribution, metabolism and excretion) analysis can help us select the best drug in terms of cost, time and efficiency. Applying computational chemistry tools, in vitro and in vivo ADME prediction is now much more convenient and it can aid pharmaceutical industries to screen thousands of compounds within a short time [53]. Here, synthesized compounds (**4a–k**) were screened for predicted ADME values and the results are summarized in Table 3. Since high molecular weight compounds are always less effective in terms of intestinal absorption [54,55], our designed and synthesized isatin-hydrazones' (**4a–k**) molecular weights were kept low, in between 263–328 Da. Compounds **4a–k** showed hydrogen bond donor (HBD) values of 1, except **4i** which had a HBD value of 2 (recommended value = <5), and hydrogen bond acceptor (HBA) values of 5, except **4i** which had HBA value = 6.5, **4h** with a HBA value = 5.75 and **4d** with **a** HBA value = 5.5 (recommended value = <10). On the other hand, doxorubicin (Doxo) showed a HBD value of 5 and HBA value of 15, which indicates that synthesized isatin-hydrazones are superior to Doxo in respect to HBD and HBA values. A parameter was established in 2002 to check the bioavailability of a drug using octanol/water partition coefficient and solubility scoring (recommended values for octanol/water partition coefficient are −2 – 6.5 and solubility scoring are −6.5 – 0.5 mol/dm−3) [56]. The octanol/water partition coefficient for hydrazones **4a–k** is in between 1.79–3.12 and solubility score is −3.39 – −4.35, respectively. Doxo showed a score within the reference values of −0.49 and −2.37, respectively. The hERG K^+ channel blockers are potentially toxic for the heart, thus the recommended range for predicted $logIC_{50}$ values for blockage of hERG K^+ channels (loghERG) is > −5 [57]. Intriguingly, **4a–c** and **4e–k** showed higher values for loghERG score (> −5.58—−5.91) than Doxo (−6.02), except **4d,** which was similar to Doxo, which proved their **(4a–k)** toxicity to be lower than Doxo. The Caco-2 cell, considered as the reliable in vitro model to estimate oral drug absorption and transdermal delivery [58], was high (>1310) for all compounds except **4i** (487). Interestingly, Doxo had a much lower value (2.29) than **4a–k**, which signifies the improved oral drug absorption and transdermal delivery efficiency of the studied compounds compared to Doxo.

Table 3. Analysis of drug likeness and pharmacokinetic properties by QikProp for compounds **4a–k**.

No.	MW [a]	HBD [b]	HBA [c]	logPo/w [d]	logS [e]	logP	HERG [f]	Caco-2 [g]	BBB [h]	MDCK [i]	HOA(%) [j]
4a	263	1	5	2.59	−3.82	9.8	−5.84	1324	−0.49	670	100
4b	263	1	5	2.62	−3.95	9.7	−5.89	1317	−0.51	666	100
4c	263	1	5	2.62	−3.95	9.7	−5.89	1317	−0.51	666	100
4d	295	1	5.5	2.93	−4.31	10.0	-6.03	1310	−0.49	1126	100
4e	328	1	5	2.83	−4.06	9.9	−5.90	1323	−0.33	1584	100
4f	328	1	5	2.88	−4.19	9.8	−5.91	1317	−0.32	1766	100
4g	328	1	5	2.88	−4.19	9.8	−5.91	1317	−0.32	1766	100
4h	307	1	5.75	2.89	−4.14	9.8	−5.58	1760	−0.44	911	100
4i	295	2	6.5	1.79	−3.39	12.4	−5.74	487	−1.07	227	86
4j	318	1	5	3.12	−4.35	9.6	−5.67	1616	−0.13	3162	100
4k	302	1	5	2.90	−4.17	9.7	−5.75	1432	−0.24	2158	100
Doxo [k]	544	5	15	-0.49	−2.37	24.2	−6.02	2.29	−2.95	0.766	0

[a] Molecular weight in Daltons (acceptable range: <500); [b] hydrogen bond donor (acceptable range: ≤5); [c] hydrogen bond acceptor (acceptable range: ≤10); [d] predicted octanol/water partition coefficient (acceptable range: −2–6.5); [e] predicted aqueous solubility, S in mol/dm−3 (acceptable range: −6.5–0.5); [f] predicted IC_{50} value for blockage of hERG K+ channels (concern: below −5); [g] Caco−2 value, permeability to Caco−2 (human colorectal carcinoma) cells in vitro; [h] blood−brain barrier permeability (acceptable range: ~−0.4); [i] predicted apparent Madin–Darby canine kidney (MDCK) cell permeability in nm/sec, QPPMDCK= >500 is great, <25 is poor; [j] predicted human oral absorption on 0% to 100% scale (<25% is poor and >80% is high); [k] Doxo = Doxorubicin.

The blood–brain barrier separates the CNS from blood, and a successful compound must pass into the blood stream, which depends on several factors, such as molecular weight, which must be below 480 [59]. Since our synthesized compounds have low molecular weights and fall within the recommended values, this, therefore, showed significant results. Madin–Darby canine kidney (MDCK) cell permeability is considered as the measurement of blood–brain barrier permeability, where greater than 500 is of great value and less than 25 indicates a very poor result according to Jorgensen's rule of 3 [60]. Except compound **4i** (227), all the other compounds gave much higher MDCK values (> 666 to 3162) than Doxo (0.766 only). The synthesized compounds also gave a predicted human oral absorption rate of 100%, except compound **4i** which gave 86%. On the other hand, Doxo showed a predicted human oral absorption rate of 0%. Taken together, all the designed compounds, **4a–k**, of this study showed higher predicted ADME values than Doxo.

2.4. Architecture of the CDK2 Active Site

Developing new inhibitors against CDK2 mainly involves designing compounds that can act as ATP competitive inhibitors by binding to the ATP binding cleft of CDK2. According to the active and inactive state of the protein kinase, two different types of inhibitors can be designed: type I and type II inhibitors. Type I inhibitors mainly bind to the ATP binding pocket of an active kinase, whereas type II inhibitors bind to the inactive kinase [61]. From the recently published crystal structure of CDK2 in a complex with the inhibitor CVT-313, it was found that active kinase inhibition depends solely on the interaction with the DFG motif, which comprises Asp145-Phe146- Gly147. Leu83, Asp86 and Asp145 form the ATP binding site of CDK2 through hydrogen bonds, where Asp145 belongs to the DFG motif. Outside of the active site, the residues Glu81–Leu83 hinge linker sequence is responsible for flexibility of the kinase. The phosphorylation of the C-terminal domain contains the catalytic residue (Glu51) required for the phosphorylation of Thr160 in the T-loop for its activation.

The activation segment is composed of the conserved DFG motif (Asp145-Phe146- Gly147) and the APE motif (Ala170-Pro171-Glu172). The unique PSTAIRE motif (Pro45–Glu51) in CDK2 that has a key role in its interaction with the cyclin subunit is found in the N-terminal domain [61]. To investigate whether the synthesized compounds (**4j** and **4k**, based on best cytotoxicity assay and enzyme inhibition assay against CDK2 protein kinase) are type I or type II inhibitors, and also to check their binding mechanism with CDK2, we performed a molecular docking analysis.

2.5. *In Silico Binding Mechanism Analysis*

From the docking analysis of compounds **4j** and **4k** with CDK2, it was clearly observed that both compounds interacted with the ATP binding pocket residues Leu83 and Asp86 but not with Asp145 of the DFG motif (Figure 4A,D). **4j** and **4k** thus can act as ATP competitive type II inhibitor by binding to inactive kinase [61]. Moreover, both the compounds showed a similar fashion of interactions, which involved several hydrogen bonds and ionic interactions with the binding site cavity surrounding residues, such as Ile10, Val18, Ala31, Val64, Glu81, Phe82, Leu134 and Ala144, which is consistent with the molecular docking analysis of 3,6-disubstituted pyridazines; 6-N,6-N-dimethyl-9-(2-phenylethyl)purine-2,6-diamine as CDK2 inhibitors (2, 3) [62,63]. However, compound **4j** formed one additional interaction with Lys89, which was absent in case of compound **4k**. It may bind to inactive kinase, which can be analyzed by finding no interaction between the compounds with catalytic residue Glu51 that is responsible for the phosphorylation of Thr160 for activation of kinase function. The interacting residues, although they do not belongs to the ATP binding pocket, formed a pathway for the compounds to bind properly to the ATP binding pocket. Glu81 to Leu83, on the other hand, forms the hinge region responsible for the flexibility of the protein kinase. From Figure 4C,F, it is visible how these residues form the binding cleft and pathway for the compounds to occupy the ATP binding site of CDK2 protein kinase. Figure 4B,E show the 3D interaction pattern and formation of binding cleft. From the docking analysis, it can be concluded that both **4j** and **4k** served as ATP competitive type II inhibitors by interacting with ATP binding pocket residues and with the residues that paved the way for the compounds to bind to the CDK2 ATP binding pocket. Table 4 summarizes the compounds and names the interacting residues, along with the types of interactions and the docking score of each compound.

Table 4. Docking score, interacting residues and types of interaction mediated by **4j** and **4k** with the ATP binding pocket of CDK2 protein kinase.

Compounds	Docking Score	Interacting Residues	Types of Interaction
4j	−6.5	Ile10, Val18, Ala31, Val64, Glu81, Phe82, Leu83, Asp86, Lys89, Leu134 and Ala144	Hydrogen π-Alkyl Halogen π-σ
4k	−5.9	Ile10, Val18, Ala31, Val64, Glu81, Phe82, Leu83, Asp86, Leu134 and Ala144	Hydrogen σ-Alkyl Halogen

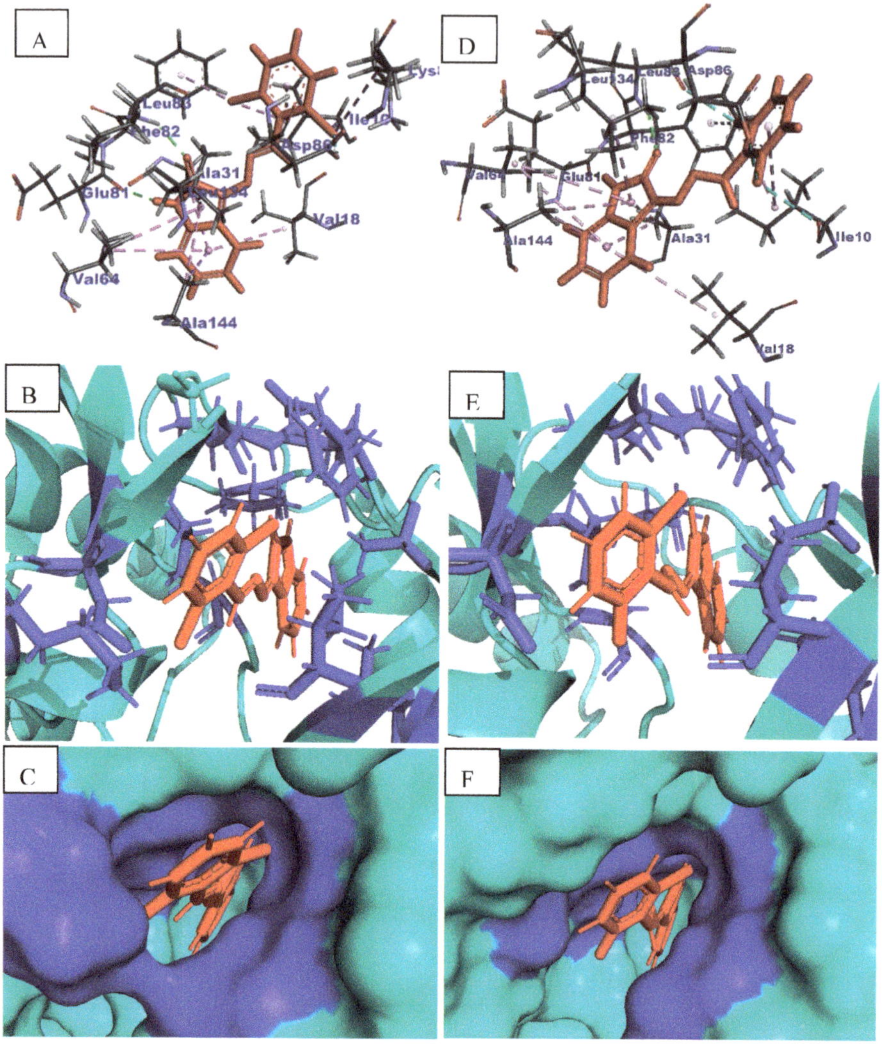

Figure 4. (**A**) 2D docking pose of **4j** within the active site of CDK2; (**B**) 3D docking pose of **4j** within the active site of CDK2; (**C**) binding pocket formed by interacting residues of active site of CDK2 surrounding **4j**; (**D**) 2D docking pose of **4k** within the active site of CDK2; (**E**) 3D docking pose of **4k** within the active site of CDK2; (**F**) binding pocket formed by interacting residues of active site of CDK2 surrounding **4k**. Compounds are shown in red color, protein in cyan and interacting residues in blue color.

3. Materials and Methods

3.1. General

Chemicals and solvents were of commercial reagent grade (Sigma-Aldrich, St. Louis, MO, USA) and were used without further purification. The progress of reactions and purity of reactants and products were checked using pre-coated silica gel 60 aluminum TLC sheets with fluorescent indicator

UV254 of Macherey-Nagel, and detection was carried out with an ultraviolet light (254 nm) (Merck, Darmstadt, Germany). Melting points were measured using an Electrothermal IA9100 melting point apparatus (Stone, Stafforshire, ST15 OSA, UK). Infrared (IR) spectra (as KBr pellet) were recorded on a FT-IR Spectrum BX device from Perkin Elmer (Ayer Rajah Crescent, Singapore). ^{1}H NMR spectra were recorded using a Bruker 600 MHz spectrometer (Reinstetten, Germany) and DMSO-d_6 was used as a solvent. Chemical shifts were expressed in parts per million (ppm) relative to TMS as an internal standard. Mass spectra were taken with an Agilent 6410 Triple Quad mass spectrometer fitted with an electrospray ionization (ESI) ion source (Agilent Technologies, Palo Alto, CA, USA).

3.2. *(Z)-3-Hydrazonoindolin-2-one* (**2**)

A mixture of isatin (0.1 mole) and hydrazine hydrate (1.2 equiv.) in methanol was refluxed for 1h and cooled to room temperature. The precipitate was filtered, washed with cold methanol and dried at room temperature in open air to give isatin monohydrazone in quantitative yield (~99%). A yellow powder was obtained (~99%). Mp. = 230–231 °C (Lit. [64] Mp. = 231–232 °C).

3.3. *General Procedure for the Synthesis of 3-[benzylidene(substituted)hydrazono]indolin-2-ones* ***4a–k***

A mixture of isatin monohydrazone (**2**, 5 mmol) and 4-methylbenzaldehyde (**3a**, 5 mmol) in absolute ethanol (15 mL) was added to a few drops of glacial acetic acid. The reaction mixture was refluxed for 4 h. The completion of the reaction was monitored by TLC. The precipitate solid was filtered, washed with cold ethanol and air dried, and was then further purified by recrystallization using ethanol, obtained **4a** as yellow powder. Please see in Supplementary Materials for NMR (^{1}H & ^{13}C) and MS spectra of compound **4** (in Supplementary Materials).

3.3.1. 3-((2-Methylbenzylidene)hydrazono)indolin-2-one (**4a**)

Yellow powder (80%). Mp. = 198–199 °C. IR (KBr) ν_{max}(cm^{-1}): 3238 (N-H), 2910 (C-H), 1728 (C=O), 1612 (C=N). ^{1}H NMR (DMSO-d_6, 600 MHz) (ppm), δ 2.52 (s, 3H, -CH_3), 6.89 (t, 1H, ArH), 7.01 (t, 1H, ArH), 7.32–7.44 (m, 4H, ArH), 7.89 (t, 1H, ArH), 8.06 (t, 1H, ArH), 8.80 (s, 1H), 10.88 (s, 1H, -NH). ^{13}C NMR (DMSO-d_6, 150 MHz) (ppm), δ 165.02, 159.58, 150.71, 145.45, 139.72, 134.20, 132.31, 131.78, 129.00, 127.96, 127.06, 122.83, 116.81, 111.35 and 19.58. ESI mass *m/z* = 264 [M + H]$^+$; 286 [M + Na]$^+$.

3.3.2. 3-((3-Methylbenzylidene)hydrazono)indolin-2-one (**4b**)

Yellow powder (82%). Mp. = 183–184 °C. ^{1}H NMR (DMSO-d_6, 600 MHz) (ppm), δ 2.39 (s, 3H, -CH_3), 6.89 (t, 1H, ArH), 7.02 (t, 1H, ArH), 7.39 (m, 2H, ArH). 7.44 (t, 1H, ArH), 7.56 (m, 2H, ArH), 7.88 (t, 1H, ArH), 8.53 (s, 1H), 10.86 (s, 1H, -NH). ^{13}C NMR (DMSO-d_6, 150 MHz) (ppm), δ 164.93, 160.61, 150.64, 145.46, 139.02, 134.19, 133.83, 133.28, 129.87, 129.58, 129.20, 126.34, 122.86, 116.82, 111.32 and 21.36. ESI mass *m/z* = 264 [M + H]$^+$; 286 [M + Na]$^+$.

3.3.3. 3-((4-Methylbenzylidene)hydrazono)indolin-2-one (**4c**)

Orange powder (75%). Mp. = 230–231 °C. (Lit. [65] mp. = 231 °C) IR (KBr) ν_{max}(cm^{-1}): 3182 (N-H), 2839 (C-H), 1716 (C=O), 1612 (C=N). ^{1}H NMR (DMSO-d_6, 600 MHz) (ppm), δ 2.38 (s, 3H, -CH_3), 6.88 (t, 1H, ArH), 7.02 (t, 1H, ArH), 7.37 (m, 3H, ArH), 7.86 (m, 2H, ArH), 7.93 (t, 1H, ArH), 8.58 (s, 1H), 10.86 (s, 1H, -NH). ^{13}C NMR (DMSO-d_6, 150 MHz) (ppm), δ 165.02, 161.34, 150.91, 145.4, 142.96, 134.11, 131.29, 130.3, 129.39, 129.26, 122.83, 116.91, 111.28 and 21.73. ESI mass *m/z* = 264 [M + H]$^+$; 286 [M + Na]$^+$.

3.3.4. 3-((4-(Methylthio)benzylidene)hydrazono)indolin-2-one (**4d**)

Red crystals (79%). Mp. = 204–205 °C. IR (KBr) ν_{max}(cm^{-1}): 3278 (N-H), 2920 (C-H), 1732 (C=O), 1612 (C=N). ^{1}H NMR (DMSO-d_6, 600 MHz) (ppm), δ 2.53 (s, 3H, S-CH_3), 6.88 (t, 1H, ArH), 7.02 (t, 1H, ArH), 7.33–7.50 (m, 3H, ArH). 7.77–7.95 (m, 3H, ArH). 8.59 (s, 1H), 10.84 (s, 1H, -NH). ^{13}C NMR

(DMSO-d_6, 150 MHz) (ppm), δ 165.07, 161.47, 151.01, 145.40, 144.69, 134.09, 130.09, 129.75, 129.28, 129.13, 126.05, 125.93, 122.79, 116.97, 111.27 and 14.50. ESI mass *m/z* = 296 $[M + H]^+$; 318 $[M + Na]^+$.

3.3.5. 3-((2-Bromobenzylidene)hydrazono)indolin-2-one (**4e**)

Yellow powder (93%). Mp. = 233–234 °C. IR (KBr) $\nu_{max}(cm^{-1})$: 3194 (N-H), 2818 (C-H), 1730 (C=O), 1535 (C=N). ^{1}H NMR (DMSO-d_6, 600 MHz) (ppm), δ 6.89 (d, *J*=1.2 Hz, 1H, ArH), 7.02 (t, 1H, ArH), 7.40 (t, 1H, ArH), 7.51 (t, 1H, ArH), 7.59 (t, 1H, ArH), 7.80–7.58 (m, 2H, ArH), 7.22 (t, 1H, ArH), 8.72 (s, 1H), 10.90 (s, 1H, -NH). ^{13}C NMR (DMSO-d_6, 150 MHz) (ppm), δ 164.75, 158.16, 150.99, 145.73, 134.56, 134.18, 134.13, 132.23, 129.25, 129.09, 125.60, 122.93, 116.62 and 111.45. ESI mass *m/z* = 328 $[M(^{79}Br) + H]^+$, 330 $[M(^{81}Br) + H]^+$; 350 $[M(^{79}Br) + Na]^+$, 352 $[M(^{81}Br) + Na]^+$.

3.3.6. 3-((3-Bromobenzylidene)hydrazono)indolin-2-one (**4f**)

Yellowish brown powder (92%). Mp. = 182–183 °C. IR (KBr) $\nu_{max}(cm^{-1})$: 3412 (N-H), 2920 (C-H), 1714 (C=O), 1676 (C=N). ^{1}H NMR (DMSO-d_6, 600 MHz) (ppm), δ 6.89 (t, 1H, ArH), 7.01 (t, 1H, ArH), 7.39–7.53 (m, 2H, ArH), 7.71–7.87 (m, 2H, ArH), 7.99–8.10 (m, 1H, ArH), 8.54 (s, 1H), 10.91 (s, 1H, -NH). ^{13}C NMR (DMSO-d_6, 150 MHz) (ppm), δ 164.77, 161.07, 158.28, 150.52, 145.60, 136.16, 134.98, 134.42, 131.97, 131.84, 131.60, 131324, 129.16, 127.72, 127.56, 122.92, 116.64 and 111.41. ESI mass *m/z* = 328 $[M(^{79}Br) + H]^+$, 330 $[M(^{81}Br) + H]^+$; 350 $[M(^{79}Br) + Na]^+$, 352 $[M(^{81}Br) + Na]^+$.

3.3.7. 3-((4-Bromobenzylidene)hydrazono)indolin-2-one (**4g**)

Orange powder (90%). Mp. = 267–268 °C. IR (KBr) $\nu_{max}(cm^{-1})$: 3169 (N-H), 2879 (C-H), 1735 (C=O), 1616 (C=N). ^{1}H NMR (DMSO-d_6, 600 MHz) (ppm), δ 6.89 (t, 1H, ArH), 7.01 (t, 1H, ArH), 7.39 (t, 1H, ArH), 7.77 (t, 2H, ArH), 7.83 (t, 1H, ArH), 7.90 (t, 2H, ArH), 8.58 (s, 1H), 10.89 (s, 1H, -NH). ^{13}C NMR (DMSO-d_6, 150 MHz) (ppm), δ 164.87, 159.42, 150.73, 145.52, 134.35, 133.01, 132.75, 131.05, 129.25, 126.18, 122.90, 116.72 and 111.38. ESI mass *m/z* = 328 $[M(^{79}Br) + H]^+$, 330 $[M(^{81}Br) + H]^+$; 350 $[M(^{79}Br) + Na]^+$, 352 $[M(^{81}Br) + Na]^+$.

3.3.8. 3-((4-Methoxy-2,6-dimethylbenzylidene)hydrazono)indolin-2-one (**4h**)

Orange powder (90%). Mp. = 251–252 °C. IR (KBr) $\nu_{max}(cm^{-1})$: 3182 (N-H), 2839 (C-H), 1716 (C=O), 1612 (C=N). ^{1}H NMR (DMSO-d_6, 600 MHz) (ppm), δ 2.18 (s, 3H, $-CH_3$) 2.52 (s, 3H, $-CH_3$) 3.85 (t, 3H, OCH_3), 6.88 (d, *J* = 9, 2H, ArH), 7.03 (t, 1H, ArH), 7.36 (t, 1H, ArH), 7.85 (t, 1H, ArH), 8.02 (t, 1H, ArH), 8.78 (s, 1H), 10.82 (s, 1H, -NH). ^{13}C NMR (DMSO-d_6, 150 MHz) (ppm), δ 165.32, 161.75, 160.97, 150.83, 145.19, 140.40, 133.81, 130.36, 129.01, 124.59, 123.77, 122.79, 117.04, 113.28, 111.17, 56.06, 19.70 and 16.19. ESI mass *m/z* = 308 $[M + H]^+$; 330 $[M + Na]^+$.

3.3.9. 3-((2-Hydroxy-4-methoxybenzylidene)hydrazono)indolin-2-one (**4i**)

Reddish brown (98%). Mp. = 242–243 °C. IR (KBr) $\nu_{max}(cm^{-1})$: 3188 (O-H), 2910 (C-H), 1724 (C=O), 1620 (C=N). ^{1}H NMR (DMSO-d_6, 600 MHz) (ppm), δ 3.81 (s, 3H, OCH_3), 6.52 (t, 1H, ArH), 6.59 (t, 1H, ArH), 6.87 (t, 1H, ArH), 7.04 (t, 1H, ArH), 7.40 (t, 1H, ArH), 7.55 (t, 1H, ArH), 7.60 (t, 1H, ArH), 8.97 (s, 1H), 10.9 (s, 1H, -NH), 12.31 (s, 1H, -OH). ^{13}C NMR (DMSO-d_6, 150 MHz) (ppm), δ 167.89, 165.07, 163.03, 159.79, 150.21, 144.64, 135.36, 133.90, 122.69, 120.40, 111.69, 111.20, 108.06, 101.54 and 56.08. ESI mass *m/z* = 296 $[M + H]^+$; 318 $[M + Na]^+$.

3.3.10. 3-((2,6-Dichlorobenzylidene)hydrazono)indolin-2-one (**4j**)

Orange powder (98%). Mp. = 286–287 °C. IR (KBr) $\nu_{max}(cm^{-1})$: 3165 (N-H), 2812 (C-H), 1730 (C=O), 1618 (C=N). ^{1}H NMR (DMSO-d_6, 600 MHz) (ppm), δ 6.89 (t, 1H, ArH), 6.97 (t, 1H, ArH), 7.39–7.55 (m, 2H, ArH), 7.65 (t, 2H, ArH), 7.83 (t, 1H, ArH), 8.71 (s, 1H), 10.91 (s, 1H, -NH). ^{13}C NMR (DMSO-d_6, 150 MHz) (ppm), δ 164.67, 155.50, 150.49, 145.80, 134.76, 134.72, 133.03, 129.98, 128.85,

122.77, 116.48 and 111.46. ESI mass *m/z* = 318 [M(^{35}Cl) + H]$^+$, 320 [M(^{37}Cl) + H]$^+$; 340 [M(^{35}Cl) + Na]$^+$, 342 [M(^{37}Cl) + Na]$^+$.

3.3.11. 3-((2-Chloro-6-fluorobenzylidene)hydrazono)indolin-2-one (**4k**)

Reddish brown (75%). Mp. = 277–778 °C. IR (KBr) ν_{max}(cm^{-1}): 3165 (N-H), 2852 (C-H), 1732 (C=O), 1620 (C=N). ^{1}H NMR (DMSO-d_6, 600 MHz) (ppm), δ 6.89 (t, 1H, ArH), 6.99 (t, 1H, ArH), 7.39–7.45 (m, 2H, ArH), 7.52 (t, 1H, ArH), 7.62 (t, 1H, ArH), 7.94 (t, 1H, ArH), 8.73 (s, 1H), 10.90 (s, 1H, -NH). ^{13}C NMR (DMSO-d_6, 150 MHz) (ppm), δ 164.80, 162.18, 160.46, 154.25, 150.99, 145.77, 135.57, 134.74, 134.35, 134.29, 128.86, 127.07, 122.78, 119.84, 119.76, 116.67, 116.58, 116.44 and 111.43. ESI mass *m/z* = 302 [M(^{35}Cl) + H]$^+$, 304 [M(^{37}Cl) + H]$^+$ 324 [M(^{35}Cl) + H]$^+$, 326 [M(^{37}Cl) + H]$^+$.

3.4. *Cytotoxicity*

The cytotoxicity of the synthesized compounds was evaluated by MTT assay, as previously described [66]. Two cancer cell lines, MCF7 (human breast adenocarcinoma) and A2780 (human ovary adenocarcinoma), were used in this study, which were obtained from the ATCC (Rockville, MD, USA). They were sub-cultured in RPMI-1640 media (supplemented with 10% FBS and 1% antibiotics) at 37 °C and 5% CO_2. Additionally, compounds were prepared at the same medium to obtain serial dilutions (50, 25, 19,1 and 0.1 μM). The two cell lines were separately cultured in 96-well plates (3 × 10^3/well) and incubated at 37 °C overnight. The following day, before treating the cells with the compounds, each well of the T0 plate was treated with 50 μL MTT solution (2 mg/mL in phosphate buffered saline) and then incubated for 2–4 h. The media were aspirated, and the formazan crystals were solubilized by adding 150 μL DMSO. Absorbance was read on a multi-plate reader (BioRad) at 550 mm. Optical density of the purple formazan A550 was proportional to the number of viable cells. Compound concentration causing 50% inhibition (IC_{50}) compared to control cell growth (100%) was determined. The data were obtained from triplicates and analyzed using statistical software.

3.5. *In Vitro Cyclin Dependent Kinase2 (CDK2) Inhibitory Activity*

The CDK2 Assay Kit is designed to measure CDK2/CyclinA2 activity for screening and profiling applications, using Kinase-Glo® MAX as a detection reagent. The CDK2 Assay Kit comes in a convenient 96-well format, with enough purified recombinant CDK2/CyclinA2 enzyme, CDK substrate peptide, ATP and kinase assay buffer for 100 enzyme reactions [67]. The assay was performed according to the protocol supplied from the CDK2 Assay kit #79599. The CDK2/CyclinA2 activity at a single dose concentration of 10μM was performed, where the Kinase-Glo MAX luminescence kinase assay kit (Promega#V6071) was used. The compounds were diluted in 10% DMSO and 5 μL of the dilution was added to a 50 μL reaction so that the final concentration of DMSO was 1% in all of the reactions. All of the enzymatic reactions were conducted at 30 °C for 40 min. The 50 μL reaction mixture contained 40 mM Tris, pH 7.4, 10 mM $MgCl_2$, 0.1 mg/mL BSA, 1 mM DTT, 10 mM ATP, Kinase substrate and the enzyme (CDK2/CyclinA2). After the enzymatic reaction, 50 μL of Kinase-Glo® MAX Luminescence kinase assay solution was added to each reaction and the plates were incubated for 5 min at room temperature. Luminescence signal was measured using a Bio Tek Synergy 2 microplate reader.

3.6. *Molecular Docking and In-Silico ADME Analysis*

For molecular docking purposes, the Protein Data Bank (PDB) structure corresponding to the CDK2 protein kinase was downloaded from the Research Collaboratory for Structural Bioinformatics (RCSB) PDB database (https://www.rcsb.org/) in PDB format. The PDB ID used for CDK2 protein kinase was 2BHY. Proteins and compounds were prepared for docking by using an established procedure [68]. Discovery Studio was used for making 2D interaction figures. Pymol was used to generate the 3D and surface representation figures. For the in silico ADME analysis, all the compounds' structures were prepared with the LigPrep module of Schrodinger Maestro and ADME was calculated by the Qikprop module of the same software package [69].

4. Conclusions

A series of novel isatin-hydrazones (**4a–b and 4d–k**), with a known compound **4c,** were designed and synthesized with good to moderate yields for cytotoxicity evaluation for the development of potent anticancer therapeutics. Among the compounds, **4j** showed a two-fold increase in cytotoxicity compared to the known cancer drug doxorubicin, and **4k** showed a similar cytotoxicity. The IC_{50} value of compound **4j** was 1.51 and for **4k** it was 3.56 μM, whereas doxorubicin had a 3.1 μM concentration against human breast adenocarcinoma (MCF7) cell lines. The most active compounds, **4j** and **4k,** were further evaluated for their inhibitory activities against CDK2 protein kinase. As expected, **4j** and **4k** exhibited good inhibitory activity against cyclin-dependent kinase 2 (CDK2) 0.2456 and 0.3006 μM, respectively, which is comparable to kinase imatinib 0.1512 μM. Highly recommended predicted ADME values were obtained than the known doxorubicin. The molecular docking study of **4j** and **4k** with CDK2 protein kinase revealed that they interacted with ATP binding pocket residues and lacked interactions with the active state DFG motif residues; therefore, **4j** and **4k** can be considered as ATP competitive type II inhibitors against CDK2 protein kinase. In conclusion, these simple molecules, isatin-hydrazones **4j** and **4k,** can be used as potential agents for anticancer therapeutics in further mechanism and toxicity studies.

Supplementary Materials: The following are available online, Figure S1.: Proton (^{1}H) Spectra of **4a**, Figure S2.: Carbon (^{13}C) Spectra of **4a,** Figure S3.: Proton (^{1}H) Spectra of **4g**, Figure S4.: Carbon (^{13}C) Spectra of **4g,** Figure S5.: Proton (^{1}H) Spectra of **4h**, Figure S6.: Carbon (^{13}C) Spectra of **4h,** Figure S7.: Proton (^{1}H) Spectra of **4i**, Figure S8.: Carbon (^{13}C) Spectra of **4i,** Figure S9.: Proton (^{1}H) Spectra of **4j**, Figure S10.: Carbon (^{13}C) Spectra of **4j,** Figure S11.: Proton (^{1}H) Spectra of **4k**, Figure S12.: Carbon (^{13}C) Spectra of **4k,** Figure S13.: Mass Spectra of **4a**, Figure S14.: Mass Spectra of **4b**, Figure S15.: Mass Spectra of **4c**, Figure S16.: Mass Spectra of **4d**, Figure S17.: Mass Spectra of **4e**, Figure S18.: Mass Spectra of **4f**, Figure S19.: Mass Spectra of **4g**, Figure S20.: Mass Spectra of **4g**, Figure S21.: Mass Spectra of **4i**, Figure S22.: Mass Spectra of **4j**, Fifure S23.: Mass Spectra of **4k**.

Author Contributions: Conceptualization, H.S.A.-S. and A.F.M.M.R.; methodology, I.S.I., F.S.A., H.M.A., M.A., A.N.A. and A.A.; software, M.A.; validation, A.F.M.M.R. and H.S.A.-S.; formal analysis, I.S.I., F.S.A., H.M.A., A.N.A. and A.A.; investigation, H.S.A.-S. and A.F.M.M.R.; resources, H.S.A.-S.; data curation, M.A., I.S.I., F.S.A., H.M.A., M.A. and A.N.A.; writing—original draft preparation, A.F.M.M.R.; writing—review and editing, A.F.M.M.R. and H.S.A.-S.; visualization, I.S.I., F.S.A., H.M.A., M.A., A.N.A. and M.A.; supervision, A.F.M.M.R.; project administration, H.S.A.-S.; funding acquisition, H.S.A.-S. All authors have read and agreed to the published version of the manuscript.

Funding: This research was funded by the King Saud University, Research Center of the Female Campus for Scientific and Medical Studies.

Acknowledgments: This research project was supported by a grant from the research center of the Female Campus for Scientific and Medical Studies, King Saud University, Riyadh, Saudi Arabia. The authors are thankful to Mrs. Yin Wencui for English editing.

Conflicts of Interest: The authors declare no conflict of interest.

References

1. Cancer Control: Knowledge into ACTION. Available online: http://www.who.int/cancer/modules/en/ (accessed on 20 August 2020).
2. Latest Global Cancer Data. Available online: https://www.iarc.fr/featured-news/latestglobal-cancer-data-cancer-burden-rises-to-18-1-million-new-casesand-9-6-million-cancer-deaths-in-2018/ (accessed on 20 August 2020).
3. Cancer Tomorrow. Available online: https://gco.iarc.fr/tomorrow/graphic-isotype?type=0&population=900&mode=population&sex=0&cancer=39&age_group=value&apc_male=0&apc_female=0 (accessed on 20 August 2020).
4. Alsubi, T.A.; Attwa, M.W.; Bakheit, A.H.; Darwish, H.W.; Abuelizz, H.A.; Kadi, A.A. In silico and in vitro metabolism of ribociclib: A mass spectrometric approach to bioactivation pathway elucidation and metabolite profiling. *RSC Adv.* **2020**, *10*, 22668–22683. [CrossRef]

5. Attwa, M.W.; Kadi, A.A.; Abdelhameed, A.S. Phase I metabolic profiling and unexpected reactive metabolites in human liver microsome incubations of X-376 using LC-MS/MS: Bioactivation pathway elucidation and in silico toxicity studies of its metabolites. *RSC Adv.* **2020**, *10*, 5412–5427. [CrossRef]
6. Islam, M.S.; Park, S.; Song, C.; Kadi, A.A.; Kwon, Y.; Rahman, A.F.M.M. Fluorescein hydrazones: A series of novel non-intercalative topoisomerase IIα catalytic inhibitors induce G1 arrest and apoptosis in breast and colon cancer cells. *Eur. J. Med. Chem.* **2017**, *125*, 49–67. [CrossRef]
7. Rahman, A.F.M.M.; Park, S.-E.; Kadi, A.A.; Kwon, Y. Fluorescein Hydrazones as Novel Nonintercalative Topoisomerase Catalytic Inhibitors with Low DNA Toxicity. *J. Med. Chem.* **2014**, *57*, 9139–9151. [CrossRef]
8. Ahmad, P.; Woo, H.; Jun, K.-Y.; Kadi, A.A.; Abdel-Aziz, H.A.; Kwon, Y.; Rahman, A.F.M.M. Design, synthesis, topoisomerase I & II inhibitory activity, antiproliferative activity, and structure–activity relationship study of pyrazoline derivatives: An ATP-competitive human topoisomerase IIα catalytic inhibitor. *Bioorganic Med. Chem.* **2016**, *24*, 1898–1908. [CrossRef]
9. Al-Warhi, T.; Abo-Ashour, M.F.; Almahli, H.; Alotaibi, O.J.; Al-Sanea, M.M.; Al-Ansary, G.H.; Ahmed, H.Y.; Elaasser, M.M.; Eldehna, W.M.; Abdel-Aziz, H.A. Novel [(N-alkyl-3-indolylmethylene)hydrazono]oxindoles arrest cell cycle and induce cell apoptosis by inhibiting CDK2 and Bcl-2: Synthesis, biological evaluation and in silico studies. *J. Enzym. Inhib. Med. Chem.* **2020**, *35*, 1300–1309. [CrossRef]
10. Islam, M.S.; Al-Majid, A.M.; El-Senduny, F.F.; Badria, F.A.; Rahman, A.F.M.M.; Barakat, A.; Elshaier, Y.A.M.M. Synthesis, Anticancer Activity, and Molecular Modeling of New Halogenated Spiro[pyrrolidine-thiazolo-oxindoles] Derivatives. *Appl. Sci.* **2020**, *10*, 2170. [CrossRef]
11. Erdmann, O.L. Untersuchungen über den Indigo. *J. Prakt. Chem.* **1840**, *19*, 321–362. [CrossRef]
12. Laurent, A. Recherches sur l'indigo. *Ann. Chim. Phys.* **1840**, *3*, 40.
13. Bergman, J.; Lindström, J.-O.; Tilstam, U. The structure and properties of some indolic constituents in Couroupita guianensis aubl. *Tetrahedron* **1985**, *41*, 2879–2881. [CrossRef]
14. Guo, Y.; Chen, F. TLC-UV spectrophotometric and TLC-scanning determination of isatin in leaf of Isatis. *Zhong Cao Yao* **1986**, *17*, 8–11.
15. Yoshikawa, M.; Murakami, T.; Kishi, A.; Sakurama, T.; Matsuda, H.; Nomura, M.; Matsuda, H.; Kubo, M. Novel indoles, o-bisdesmoside, calanthoside, the precursor glycoside of tryptanthrin, indirubin, and isatin, with increasing skin blood flow promoting effects, from two calanthe species (orchidaceae). *Chem. Pharm. Bull.* **1998**, *46*, 886–888. [CrossRef]
16. Popp, P.D. The Chemistry of Isatin. In *Advances in Heterocyclic Chemistry*; Katritzky, A.R., Boulton, A.J., Eds.; Academic Press: London, UK, 1975; Volume 18, pp. 1–58.
17. Silva, J.F.M.d.; Garden, S.J.; Pinto, A.C. The chemistry of isatins: A review from 1975 to 1999. *J. Braz. Chem. Soc.* **2001**, *12*, 273–324. [CrossRef]
18. Sumpter, W.C. The Chemistry of Isatin. *Chem. Rev.* **1944**, *34*, 393–434. [CrossRef]
19. Minami, M.; Hamaue, N.; Endo, T.; Hirafuji, M.; Terado, M.; Ide, H.; Yamazaki, N.; Yoshioka, M.; Ogata, A.; Tashiro, K. Effects of isatin, an endogenous MAO inhibitor, on dopamine (DA) and acetylcholine (ACh) concentrations in rats. *Folia Pharmacol. Jpn.* **1999**, *114*, 186–191. [CrossRef]
20. Gillam, E.M.J.; Notley, L.M.; Cai, H.; De Voss, J.J.; Guengerich, F.P. Oxidation of Indole by Cytochrome P450 Enzymes. *Biochemistry* **2000**, *39*, 13817–13824. [CrossRef]
21. Pervez, H.; Ahmad, M.; Zaib, S.; Yaqub, M.; Naseer, M.M.; Iqbal, J. Synthesis, cytotoxic and urease inhibitory activities of some novel isatin-derived bis-Schiff bases and their copper(II) complexes. *MedChemComm* **2016**, *7*, 914–923. [CrossRef]
22. Ibrahim, H.S.; Abou-seri, S.M.; Ismail, N.S.M.; Elaasser, M.M.; Aly, M.H.; Abdel-Aziz, H.A. Bis-isatin hydrazones with novel linkers: Synthesis and biological evaluation as cytotoxic agents. *Eur. J. Med. Chem.* **2016**, *108*, 415–422. [CrossRef]
23. Han, K.; Zhou, Y.; Liu, F.; Guo, Q.; Wang, P.; Yang, Y.; Song, B.; Liu, W.; Yao, Q.; Teng, Y.; et al. Design, synthesis and in vitro cytotoxicity evaluation of 5-(2-carboxyethenyl)isatin derivatives as anticancer agents. *Bioorg. Med. Chem. Lett.* **2014**, *24*, 591–594. [CrossRef]
24. Vine, K.L.; Matesic, L.; Locke, J.M.; Ranson, M.; Skropeta, D. Cytotoxic and anticancer activities of isatin and its derivatives: A comprehensive review from 2000–2008. *Anti-Cancer Agents Med. Chem.* **2009**, *9*, 397–414. [CrossRef]

25. Matesic, L.; Locke, J.M.; Bremner, J.B.; Pyne, S.G.; Skropeta, D.; Ranson, M.; Vine, K.L. N-Phenethyl and N-naphthylmethyl isatins and analogues as in vitro cytotoxic agents. *Bioorg. Med. Chem.* **2008**, *16*, 3118–3124. [CrossRef]
26. Medvedev, A.; Igosheva, N.; Crumeyrolle-Arias, M.; Glover, V. Isatin: Role in stress and anxiety. *Stress* **2005**, *8*, 175–183. [CrossRef]
27. Eldehna, W.M.; Altoukhy, A.; Mahrous, H.; Abdel-Aziz, H.A. Design, synthesis and QSAR study of certain isatin-pyridine hybrids as potential anti-proliferative agents. *Eur. J. Med. Chem.* **2015**, *90*, 684–694. [CrossRef]
28. Dweedar, H.E.; Mahrous, H.; Ibrahim, H.S.; Abdel-Aziz, H.A. Analogue-based design, synthesis and biological evaluation of 3-substituted-(methylenehydrazono)indolin-2-ones as anticancer agents. *Eur. J. Med. Chem.* **2014**, *78*, 275–280. [CrossRef]
29. Pakravan, P.; Kashanian, S.; Khodaei, M.M.; Harding, F.J. Biochemical and pharmacological characterization of isatin and its derivatives: From structure to activity. *Pharmacol. Rep. PR* **2013**, *65*, 313–335. [CrossRef]
30. Medvedev, A.; Buneeva, O.; Gnedenko, O.; Ershov, P.; Ivanov, A. Isatin, an endogenous nonpeptide biofactor: A review of its molecular targets, mechanisms of actions, and their biomedical implications. *BioFactors* **2018**, *44*, 95–108. [CrossRef]
31. Guo, H. Isatin derivatives and their anti-bacterial activities. *Eur. J. Med. Chem.* **2019**, *164*, 678–688. [CrossRef]
32. Vine, K.L.; Locke, J.M.; Ranson, M.; Pyne, S.G.; Bremner, J.B. In vitro cytotoxicity evaluation of some substituted isatin derivatives. *Bioorganic Med. Chem.* **2007**, *15*, 931–938. [CrossRef]
33. Vine, K.L.; Locke, J.M.; Ranson, M.; Pyne, S.G.; Bremner, J.B. An Investigation into the Cytotoxicity and Mode of Action of Some Novel N-Alkyl-Substituted Isatins. *J. Med. Chem.* **2007**, *50*, 5109–5117. [CrossRef]
34. Vine, K.L.; Matesic, L.; Locke, J.M.; Skropeta, D. Recent highlights in the development of isatin-based anticancer agents. *Adv. Anticancer Agents Med. Chem.* **2013**, *2*, 254–312.
35. Nikalje, A.P.; Ansari, A.; Bari, S.; Ugale, V. Synthesis, Biological Activity, and Docking Study of Novel Isatin Coupled Thiazolidin-4-one Derivatives as Anticonvulsants. *Archiv. Pharm.* **2015**, *348*, 433–445. [CrossRef]
36. Shingade, S.G.; Bari, S.B.; Waghmare, U.B. Synthesis and antimicrobial activity of 5-chloroindoline-2,3-dione derivatives. *Med. Chem. Res.* **2012**, *21*, 1302–1312. [CrossRef]
37. Pandeya, S.; Smitha, S.; Jyoti, M.; Sridhar, S. Biological activities of isatin and its derivatives. *Acta Pharm.* **2005**, *55*, 27–46.
38. Saha, S.; Acharya, C.; Pal, U.; Chowdhury, S.R.; Sarkar, K.; Maiti, N.C.; Jaisankar, P.; Majumder, H.K. A Novel Spirooxindole Derivative Inhibits the Growth of *Leishmania donovani* Parasites both In Vitro and In Vivo by Targeting Type IB Topoisomerase. *Antimicrob. Agents Ch.* **2016**, *60*, 6281–6293. [CrossRef]
39. Ganguly, S.; Debnath, B. Molecular docking studies and ADME prediction of novel isatin analogs with potent anti-EGFR activity. *Med. Chem.* **2014**, *4*, 558–568. [CrossRef]
40. Singh, A.; Raghuwanshi, K.; Patel, V.K.; Jain, D.K.; Veerasamy, R.; Dixit, A.; Rajak, H. Assessment of 5-substituted Isatin as Surface Recognition Group: Design, Synthesis, and Antiproliferative Evaluation of Hydroxamates as Novel Histone Deacetylase Inhibitors. *Pharm. Chem. J.* **2017**, *51*, 366–374. [CrossRef]
41. Varun; Sonam; Kakkar, R. Isatin and its derivatives: A survey of recent syntheses, reactions, and applications. *MedChemComm* **2019**, *10*, 351–368. [CrossRef]
42. Abo-Ashour, M.F.; Eldehna, W.M.; Nocentini, A.; Ibrahim, H.S.; Bua, S.; Abou-Seri, S.M.; Supuran, C.T. Novel hydrazido benzenesulfonamides-isatin conjugates: Synthesis, carbonic anhydrase inhibitory activity and molecular modeling studies. *Eur. J. Med. Chem.* **2018**, *157*, 28–36. [CrossRef]
43. Eldehna, W.M.; Abo-Ashour, M.F.; Nocentini, A.; Gratteri, P.; Eissa, I.H.; Fares, M.; Ismael, O.E.; Ghabbour, H.A.; Elaasser, M.M.; Abdel-Aziz, H.A.; et al. Novel 4/3-((4-oxo-5-(2-oxoindolin-3-ylidene) thiazolidin-2-ylidene)amino) benzenesulfonamides: Synthesis, carbonic anhydrase inhibitory activity, anticancer activity and molecular modelling studies. *Eur. J. Med. Chem.* **2017**, *139*, 250–262. [CrossRef]
44. Eldehna, W.M.; Fares, M.; Ceruso, M.; Ghabbour, H.A.; Abou-Seri, S.M.; Abdel-Aziz, H.A.; Abou El Ella, D.A.; Supuran, C.T. Amido/ureidosubstituted benzenesulfonamides-isatin conjugates as low nanomolar/subnanomolar inhibitors of the tumor-associated carbonic anhydrase isoform XII. *Eur. J. Med. Chem.* **2016**, *110*, 259–266. [CrossRef] [PubMed]
45. O'Donnell, A.; Padhani, A.; Hayes, C.; Kakkar, A.J.; Leach, M.; Trigo, J.M.; Scurr, M.; Raynaud, F.; Phillips, S.; Aherne, W.; et al. A Phase I study of the angiogenesis inhibitor SU5416 (semaxanib) in solid tumours, incorporating dynamic contrast MR pharmacodynamic end points. *Br. J. Cancer* **2005**, *93*, 876–883. [CrossRef] [PubMed]

46. Molina, A.M.; Feldman, D.R.; Ginsberg, M.S.; Kroog, G.; Tickoo, S.K.; Jia, X.; Georges, M.; Patil, S.; Baum, M.S.; Reuter, V.E.; et al. Phase II trial of sunitinib in patients with metastatic non-clear cell renal cell carcinoma. *Investig. New Drugs* **2012**, *30*, 335–340. [CrossRef] [PubMed]
47. Hoff, P.M.; Wolff, R.A.; Bogaard, K.; Waldrum, S.; Abbruzzese, J.L. A Phase I study of escalating doses of the tyrosine kinase inhibitor semaxanib (SU5416) in combination with irinotecan in patients with advanced colorectal carcinoma. *Jpn. J. Clin. Oncol.* **2006**, *36*, 100–103. [CrossRef]
48. Marko, D.; Schätzle, S.; Friedel, A.; Genzlinger, A.; Zankl, H.; Meijer, L.; Eisenbrand, G. Inhibition of cyclin-dependent kinase 1 (CDK1) by indirubin derivatives in human tumour cells. *Br. J. Cancer* **2001**, *84*, 283–289. [CrossRef] [PubMed]
49. Bramson, H.N.; Corona, J.; Davis, S.T.; Dickerson, S.H.; Edelstein, M.; Frye, S.V.; Gampe, R.T.; Harris, P.A.; Hassell, A.; Holmes, W.D.; et al. Oxindole-Based Inhibitors of Cyclin-Dependent Kinase 2 (CDK2): Design, Synthesis, Enzymatic Activities, and X-ray Crystallographic Analysis. *J. Med. Chem.* **2001**, *44*, 4339–4358. [CrossRef] [PubMed]
50. Medvedev, A.; Crumeyrolle-Arias, M.; Cardona, A.; Sandler, M.; Glover, V. Natriuretic peptide interaction with [3H]isatin binding sites in rat brain. *Brain Res.* **2005**, *1042*, 119–124. [CrossRef]
51. Lawrence, H.R.; Pireddu, R.; Chen, L.; Luo, Y.; Sung, S.-S.; Szymanski, A.M.; Yip, M.L.R.; Guida, W.C.; Sebti, S.M.; Wu, J.; et al. Inhibitors of Src Homology-2 Domain Containing Protein Tyrosine Phosphatase-2 (Shp2) Based on Oxindole Scaffolds. *J. Med. Chem.* **2008**, *51*, 4948–4956. [CrossRef]
52. Al-Salem, H.S.; Abuelizz, H.A.; Issa, I.S.; Mahmoud, A.Z.; AlHoshani, A.; Arifuzzaman, M.; Rahman, A.F.M.M. Synthesis of Novel Potent Biologically Active N-Benzylisatin-Aryl Hydrazones in Comparison with Lung Cancer Drug 'Gefitinib'. *Appl. Sci.* **2020**, *10*, 3669. [CrossRef]
53. Ekins, S.; Waller, C.L.; Swaan, P.W.; Cruciani, G.; Wrighton, S.A.; Wikel, J.H. Progress in predicting human ADME parameters in silico. *J. Pharmacol. Toxicol. Methods* **2000**, *44*, 251–272. [CrossRef]
54. Lipinski, C.A.; Lombardo, F.; Dominy, B.W.; Feeney, P.J. Experimental and computational approaches to estimate solubility and permeability in drug discovery and development settings. *Adv. Drug Deliv. Rev.* **1997**, *23*, 3–25. [CrossRef]
55. Ghose, A.K.; Viswanadhan, V.N.; Wendoloski, J.J. A Knowledge-Based Approach in Designing Combinatorial or Medicinal Chemistry Libraries for Drug Discovery. 1. A Qualitative and Quantitative Characterization of Known Drug Databases. *J. Comb. Chem.* **1999**, *1*, 55–68. [CrossRef]
56. Jorgensen, W.L.; Duffy, E.M. Prediction of drug solubility from structure. *Adv. Drug Deliv. Rev.* **2002**, *54*, 355–366. [CrossRef]
57. Chemi, G.; Gemma, S.; Campiani, G.; Brogi, S.; Butini, S.; Brindisi, M. Computational Tool for Fast in silico Evaluation of hERG K+ Channel Affinity. *Front. Chem.* **2017**, *5*, 7. [CrossRef]
58. Kulkarni, A.; Han, Y.; Hopfinger, A.J. Predicting Caco-2 Cell Permeation Coefficients of Organic Molecules Using Membrane-Interaction QSAR Analysis. *J. Chem. Inf. Comput. Sci.* **2002**, *42*, 331–342. [CrossRef] [PubMed]
59. Clark, D.E. In silico prediction of blood-brain barrier permeation. *Drug Discov. Today* **2003**, *8*, 927–933. [CrossRef]
60. Lionta, E.; Spyrou, G.; Vassilatis, D.K.; Cournia, Z. Structure-based virtual screening for drug discovery: Principles, applications and recent advances. *Curr. Top Med. Chem.* **2014**, *14*, 1923–1938. [CrossRef] [PubMed]
61. Talapati, S.R.; Nataraj, V.; Pothuganti, M.; Gore, S.; Ramachandra, M.; Antony, T.; More, S.S.; Krishnamurthy, N.R. Structure of cyclin-dependent kinase 2 (CDK2) in complex with the specific and potent inhibitor CVT-313. *Acta Crystallogr. Sect. F Struct. Biol. Commun.* **2020**, *76*, 350–356. [CrossRef]
62. Sabt, A.; Eldehna, W.M.; Al-Warhi, T.; Alotaibi, O.J.; Elaasser, M.M.; Suliman, H.; Abdel-Aziz, H.A. Discovery of 3,6-disubstituted pyridazines as a novel class of anticancer agents targeting cyclin-dependent kinase 2: Synthesis, biological evaluation and in silico insights. *J. Enzym. Inhib. Med. Chem.* **2020**, *35*, 1616–1630. [CrossRef]
63. Mohammad, T.; Batra, S.; Dahiya, R.; Baig, M.H.; Rather, I.A.; Dong, J.-J.; Hassan, I. Identification of high-affinity inhibitors of cyclin-dependent kinase 2 towards anticancer therapy. *Molecules* **2019**, *24*, 4589. [CrossRef]
64. Coffey, K.E.; Moreira, R.; Abbas, F.Z.; Murphy, G.K. Synthesis of 3,3-dichloroindolin-2-ones from isatin-3-hydrazones and (dichloroiodo)benzene. *Org. Biomol. Chem.* **2015**, *13*, 682–685. [CrossRef]

65. Afsah, E.M.; Elmorsy, S.S.; Abdelmageed, S.M.; Zaki, Z.E. Synthesis of some new mixed azines, Schiff and Mannich bases of pharmaceutical interest related to isatin. *Z. Nat. B J. Chem. Sci.* **2015**, *70*, 393–402. [CrossRef]
66. Bkhaitan, M.M.; Mirza, A.Z.; Abdalla, A.N.; Shamshad, H.; Ul-Haq, Z.; Alarjah, M.; Piperno, A. Reprofiling of full-length phosphonated carbocyclic 2′-oxa-3′-aza-nucleosides toward antiproliferative agents: Synthesis, antiproliferative activity, and molecular docking study. *Chem. Biol. Drug Des.* **2017**, *90*, 679–689. [CrossRef] [PubMed]
67. Asghar, U.; Witkiewicz, A.K.; Turner, N.C.; Knudsen, E.S. The history and future of targeting cyclin-dependent kinases in cancer therapy. *Nat. Rev. Drug Discov.* **2015**, *14*, 130–146. [CrossRef] [PubMed]
68. Arifuzzaman, M.; Hamza, A.; Zannat, S.S.; Fahad, R.; Rahman, A.; Hosen, S.M.Z.; Dash, R.; Hossain, M.K. Targeting galectin-3 by natural glycosides: A computational approach. *Netw. Modeling Anal. Health Inform. Bioinform.* **2020**, *9*, 14. [CrossRef]
69. Zhu, K.; Day, T.; Warshaviak, D.; Murrett, C.; Friesner, R.; Pearlman, D. Antibody structure determination using a combination of homology modeling, energy-based refinement, and loop prediction. *Proteins Struct. Funct. Bioinform.* **2014**, *82*, 1646–1655. [CrossRef]

Sample Availability: Samples of the compounds **4a–k** are available from the authors.

molecules

MDPI

Article

Tamoxifen and the PI3K Inhibitor: LY294002 Synergistically Induce Apoptosis and Cell Cycle Arrest in Breast Cancer MCF-7 Cells

Mohamed E. Abdallah [1], Mahmoud Zaki El-Readi [1,2,*], Mohammad Ahmad Althubiti [1], Riyad Adnan Almaimani [1], Amar Mohamed Ismail [3], Shakir Idris [4], Bassem Refaat [4], Waleed Hassan Almalki [5], Abdullatif Taha Babakr [1], Mohammed H. Mukhtar [1], Ashraf N. Abdalla [5,6,*] and Omer Fadul Idris [3]

1 Department of Biochemistry, Faculty of Medicine, Umm Al-Qura University, Makkah 21955, Saudi Arabia; mezubier@uqu.edu.sa (M.E.A.); mathubiti@uqu.edu.sa (M.A.A.); ramaimani@uqu.edu.sa (R.A.A.); atbabakr@uqu.edu.sa (A.T.B.); mhmukhtar@uqu.edu.sa (M.H.M.)
2 Department of Biochemistry, Faculty of Pharmacy, Al-Azhar University, Assiut 71524, Egypt
3 Department of Biochemistry and Molecular Biology, Faculty of Science and Technology, Al-Neelain University, Khartoum 11121, Sudan; amarqqqu@yahoo.com (A.M.I.); ibnomer57@yahoo.com (O.F.I.)
4 Department of Laboratory Medicine, Faculty of Applied Medical Sciences, Umm Al-Qura University, Makkah 7607, Saudi Arabia; siidris@uqu.edu.sa (S.I.); barefaat@uqu.edu.sa (B.R.)
5 Department of Pharmacology and Toxicology, Faculty of Pharmacy, Umm Al-Qura University, Makkah 21955, Saudi Arabia; whmalki@uqu.edu.sa
6 Department of Pharmacology and Toxicology, Medicinal and Aromatic Plants Research Institute, National Center for Research, Khartoum 2404, Sudan
* Correspondence: mzreadi@uqu.edu.sa or zakielreadi@azhar.edu.eg (M.Z.E.-R.); anabdrabo@uqu.edu.sa (A.N.A.); Tel.: +96-625-270-000/4347 (M.Z.E.-R.); +96-653-890-3316 (A.N.A.)

Academic Editors: Marialuigia Fantacuzzi and Alessandra Ammazzalorso
Received: 27 June 2020; Accepted: 21 July 2020; Published: 24 July 2020

Abstract: Breast cancer is considered as one of the most aggressive types of cancer. Acquired therapeutic resistance is the major cause of chemotherapy failure in breast cancer patients. To overcome this resistance and to improve the efficacy of treatment, drug combination is employed as a promising approach for this purpose. The synergistic cytotoxic, apoptosis inducing, and cell cycle effects of the combination of LY294002 (LY), a phosphatidylinositide-3-kinase (PI3K) inhibitor, with the traditional cytotoxic anti-estrogen drug tamoxifen (TAM) in breast cancer cells (MCF-7) were investigated. LY and TAM exhibited potent cytotoxic effect on MCF-7 cells with IC_{50} values 0.87 μM and 1.02 μM. The combination of non-toxic concentration of LY and TAM showed highly significant synergistic interaction as observed from isobologram (IC_{50}: 0.17 μM, combination index: 0.18, colony formation: 9.01%) compared to untreated control. The percentage of early/late apoptosis significantly increased after treatment of MCF-7 cells with LY and TAM combination: 40.3%/28.3% ($p < 0.001$), compared to LY single treatment (19.8%/11.4%) and TAM single treatment (32.4%/5.9%). In addition, LY and TAM combination induced the apoptotic genes Caspase-3, Caspase-7, and p53, as well as p21 as cell cycle promotor, and significantly downregulated the anti-apoptotic genes Bcl-2 and survivin. The cell cycle assay revealed that the combination induced apoptosis by increasing the pre-G_1: 28.3% compared to 1.6% of control. pAKT and Cyclin D1 protein expressions were significantly more downregulated by the combination treatment compared to the single drug treatment. The results suggested that the synergistic cytotoxic effect of LY and TAM is achieved by the induction of apoptosis and cell cycle arrest through cyclin D1, pAKT, caspases, and Bcl-2 signaling pathways.

Keywords: breast cancer; tamoxifen; LY294002; synergism; apoptosis; cell cycle

1. Introduction

Worldwide, breast cancer (BC) has the highest incidence rate (24.2%) of all cancers in women with more than two million newly diagnosed cases and almost 627,000 deaths (15%) occurred in 2018 [1]. In Saudi Arabia, BC has the largest number of incidences between females (3629 cases: 29.7% of total malignancies) [2]. Nevertheless, frequent tumor recurrence results in poor prognosis of BC patient of which less than 5% survive for more than ten years [3]. Discovering new therapies with improved pharmacokinetics is therefore required for improving the outcome of BC treatment [4].

BC is classified according to the gene expression of estrogen receptor (ER) and human epidermal growth factor receptor 2 (HER2) into five major molecular subtypes, which are different in growth and prognosis. Theses subtypes include luminal A ($ER^+/HER2^-$/low levels of Ki-67 protein), luminal B ($ER^+/HER2^{-/+}$/high levels of Ki-67 protein), triple-negative/basal-like ($ER^-/HER2^-$), HER2 enriched ($HR^-/HER2^+$), and normal-like BC, which is similar to luminal A, but with poor prognosis [5]. Luminal A and luminal B breast cancer are the most dominant subtype, affecting more than 73% of total BC patients [6].

Tamoxifen (TAM) is the oldest and most-prescribed selective estrogen receptor modulator, that has been approved to treat women and men diagnosed with hormonal receptor (HR^+), early-stage BC after surgery to reduce the risk of the cancer recurrence as well as treatment of advanced-stage or metastatic HR^+ BC patients [7–9]. The combination of high efficacy in both pre- and postmenopausal women and a good tolerability profile of TAM lead to maintain its position as drug of choice for most patients with HR^+ breast cancer [7]. In addition, TAM has been used as chemopreventive agent to reduce breast cancer risk in women, who haven't been diagnosed, but are at higher-than-average risk for incidence of BC [10]. These high therapeutic benefits of TAM by binding with the ER causing apoptotic effect on the mammary cells [7,11].

The development of both de novo and acquired resistance to TAM is a significant problem. Recent advances in our understanding of the molecular mechanisms that contribute to resistance have provided means to predict patient responses to TAM and develop rational approaches for combining therapeutic agents with TAM to avoid or desensitize the resistant phenotype [12]. Overcoming the anti ER drug resistance can be achieved by the introduction of new drug classes and combinations that can synergistically improve the efficacy and decrease the effective dose, hence decrease the side effects. Long term estrogen deprivation (LTED) treatment among ER+ BC cells results in adaptive increase in ER expression, which is followed by activation of multiple tyrosine kinases. Combination therapy with the ER down-regulator fulvestrant and the broad kinase inhibitor dasatinib exhibited synergistic activity against LTED cells, by a reduction of cell proliferation, survival, and invasion [13].

In addition, the phosphatidylinositide-3-kinase (PI3K)/Akt signaling pathway is considered as the ideal pathway to explain the transmission of anti-apoptotic signals for cancer cell survival and regulate cell growth, proliferation, transcription, and metabolic processes [14]. The activation of PI3K/Akt signaling pathway is associated with poor prognosis in BC [14]. Inhibitors of PI3K/Akt have undergone pre-clinical evaluation with encouraging results and considered to be one of the most promising targeted therapies for cancer treatment [15]. LY294002 (LY) is a morpholine containing compound with potent inhibitory action for numerous proteins, and a strong inhibition of PI3Ks, which causes induction of apoptosis in tumor cells, but the precise mechanism of its antitumor activity is not completely well understood, as it was also shown to inhibit the invasiveness of cancer cells by downregulating the expression of MMP-2, MMP-9, and VEGF, and reducing MVD [16]. LY, among other PI3K inhibitors, did not reach the clinical trials phase because of its weak drug ability and toxicity [17].

This study was conducted to show the effects of LY or TAM alone or in combination against MCF-7 (ER^+) cells. The underlying mechanisms of the possible synergistic effects of this combination are further explored in order to develop a novel and effective therapeutic combination against BC and to reduce the toxicity and resistance of LY and TAM.

2. Results

2.1. LY294002 and Tamoxifen Synergistically Inhibited Breast Cancer Cells Proliferation

The ability of LY to improve the cytotoxicity of tamoxifen on MCF-7 breast cancer was evaluated using an MTT assay. Figure 1A shows dose-response curve of MTT assay. The down deviation of curve was observed in MCF-7 cell treated with LY + TAM combination comparing to each of LY or TAM alone. The combination showed significant synergistic interaction with decrease in IC_{50} in MCF-7 cells (0.17 μM) comparing to LY (0.87 μM) and TAM (1.02 μM) treated cells (Figure 1B). Non-toxic concentration 100 nM (85% live cells) from LY and TAM was selected to use in all experimental sets. The synergistic effect of the combination was elucidated from isobologram and combination index value (0.18) Figure 1C. To confirm the synergistic interaction of LY and TAM, the plate colony formation assay was performed. As shown in Figure 2, the combination of LY and TAM exhibited a significant lower percentage of colony formation (9.1%) compared to the control, where LY treated cells showed (27.3%) and TAM showed (36.4%) compared to the control MCF-7 cells. A non-significant difference between LY and TAM treated cells was observed.

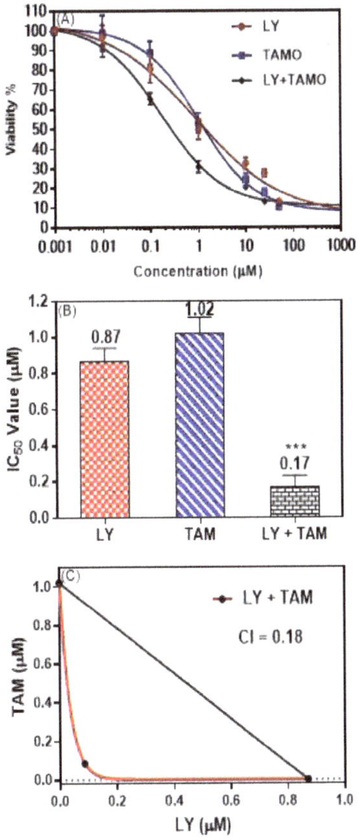

Figure 1. (**A**): Dose response curve, (**B**): IC_{50} values, (**C**): isobolgram and combination index of MCF-7 cells treated with different concentrations of LY, TAM, and LY + TAM combination for 72 h. The IC_{50} was calculated using GraphPad Prism V6 by fitting of sigmodal four parameter curve. The data expressed as mean ± SD ($n = 3$, of three experiments). Statistical differences, compared with the control cells, were assessed by a one-way ANOVA with the Tukey's post-hoc multiple comparison test (GraphPad Prism). $p < 0.001$ (***) was taken as significant.

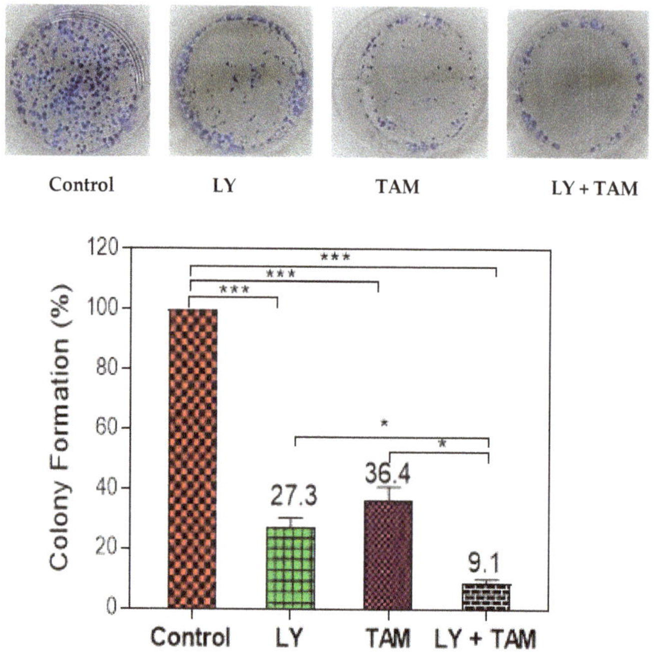

Figure 2. Colony formation assay of MCF-7 cells treated with LY, TAM, and LY + TAM combination. MCF-7 cells were treated for 24 h with the experimental set and cells were seeded in 6-well plates (200 cells/well) and incubated for 14 days. The colonies were counted after staining with methylene blue. The colony formation of the treatment set was quantified as a percentage related to untreated control. Statistical differences, compared with the control cells, were assessed by a one-way ANOVA with the Tukey's post-hoc multiple comparison test (GraphPad Prism).). $p < 0.05$ (*), $p < 0.001$ (***) was taken as significant.

2.2. *LY294002 and Tamoxifen Induced Apoptosis in Breast Cancer Cells*

In order to elucidate the underlying mechanism of the synergistic inhibition of BC cell growth by LY and TAM combination, apoptosis analysis was performed through annexin V FITC/PI double staining. The data revealed that each of LY and TAM were able to induce early/late apoptosis 19.8%/11.4% and 32.4/5.9%, respectively (Figure 3). However, the combination of LY with TAM significantly increased the early/late apoptosis to 40.3/28.3% ($p < 0.001$). To explore the molecular mechanism of increasing in the apoptotic MCF-7 cells, anti-apoptotic and apoptotic genes were measured by immunofluorescence in MCF-7 cells. As shown in Figure 4, the treatment of MCF-7 cells by LY + TAM increased the expression of Caspase-3 and decreased the expression of Bcl-2 compared to the cells treated with either LY or TAM alone. In addition, Figure 5A shows that LY +TAM significantly increased the expression of Caspase-3 3.2 and 9.2-times more compared to TAM and LY alone, respectively. Moreover, caspase-7 was overexpressed in MCF-7 cells 3.4 and 12.6 times higher in treated cells with LY +TAM compared to cells treated with TAM and LY single treatment, respectively. The combination also significantly induced the expression of both p53 and p21: 4 and 2 times more compared to LY, and 6.3 and 3.6 times more compared to TAM, respectively. Additionally, the combination decreased the Bcl-2, BAX, and survivin 2.8 times, 2.5 times, and 3 times more than single treatment with TAM, and 3.1 times, 2.8 times, and 4.46 times more than single treatment LY, respectively. Finally, LY and TAM did not exhibit any change in HER-2 gene, while the combination decreased the expression of HER-2 to 0.45 folds compared to untreated control (Figure 5B)

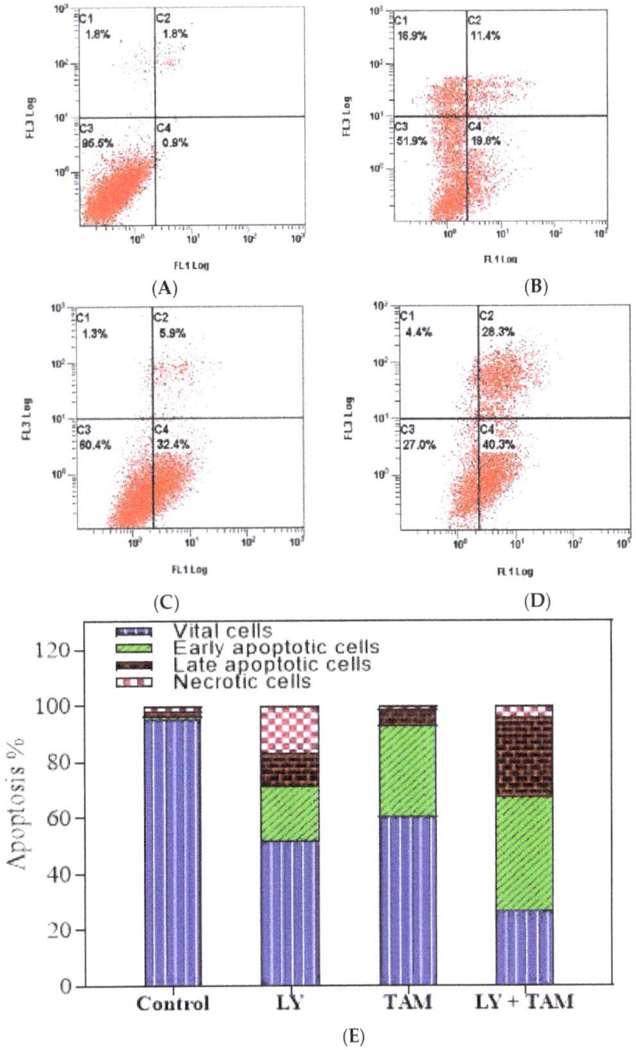

Figure 3. The induction of apoptosis in MCF-7 cells treated with (**A**): control, (**B**): LY, (**C**): TAM, and (**D**): LY + TAM combination for 24 h. Followed by Annexin V FITC/PI staining. The scattered plot *X* axis: FL1 for Annexin V, *Y* axis: FL3 for PI. (**E**): Columns represent the flow cytometry data analysis as means of the percentages of vital, early apoptotic, late apoptotic, and narcotic cells ($n = 3$ of three independent experiments).

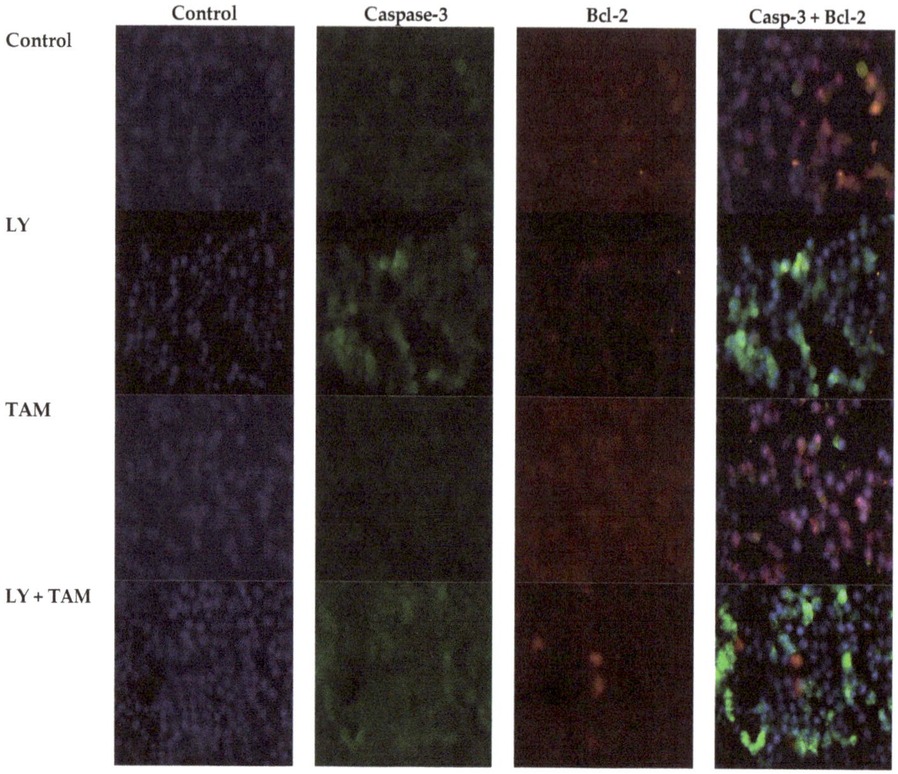

Figure 4. The induction of apoptosis in MCF-7 cells treated with LY, TAM, and LY + TAM combination 24 h. Images taken with confocal microscope (EVOS FL, scale bar 20 nM) to evaluate the expression of apoptotic (Caspase-3) and antiapoptotic (Bcl-2) markers. The images show green and red color staining for Caspase-3 and Bcl-2, respectively. Overlay images represent the fluorescence intensity of both apoptotic markers.

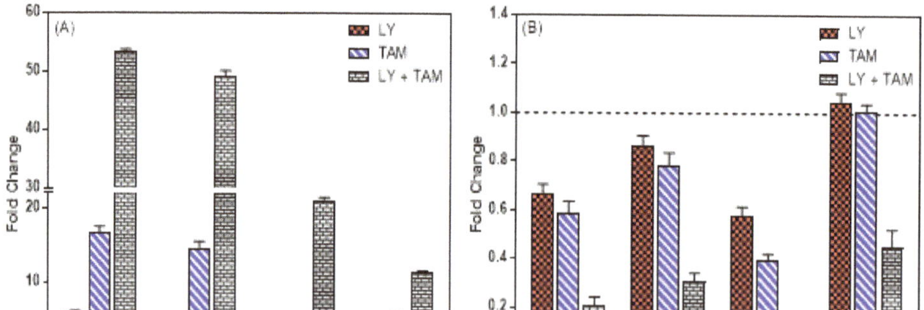

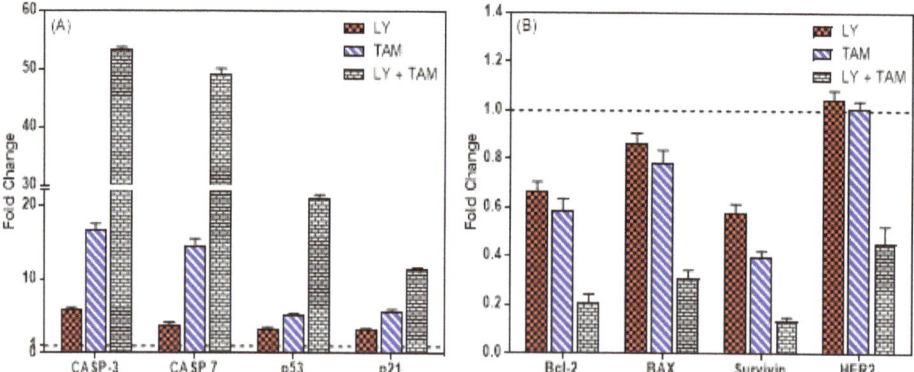

Figure 5. The expression of apoptosis genes in MCF-7 cell after treatment with LY, TAM, and LY+ TAM combination for 24 h. The total RNA was extracted and the mRNA levels of upregulated genes (**A**) and downregulated genes (**B**) was quantified using RT-PCR. The data represented the mean of the fold change related to untreated control (fold change = 1 dashed line).

2.3. *LY294002 and Tamoxifen Induced Cell Cycle Arrest in Breast Cancer Cells*

The effect of LY, TAM, and LY + TAM combination on the DNA content of MCF-7 cells was assessed using PI staining. The treatments lead to a significant increase in the apoptotic pre-G1cell population phase from 1.6% (untreated control) to 8.1%, 9.8%, and 28.3% in the treated cells with LY, TAM, and LY + TAM, respectively as shown in Figure 6. The cell population of G_0/G_1 phase decreased from 69.6% to 53.2%, 55.4%, and 50.6% after treatment with LY, TAM, and their combination, respectively. A non-significant decrease in S phase cell population was observed in all experimental set compared to untreated cells (6.8%). The G_2/M cell population was reduced in cells treated with LY (23.7%), TAM (13.7%, $p < 0.05$), and combination (12%, $p < 0.05$) compared to untreated cells (19.1%) (Figure 6).

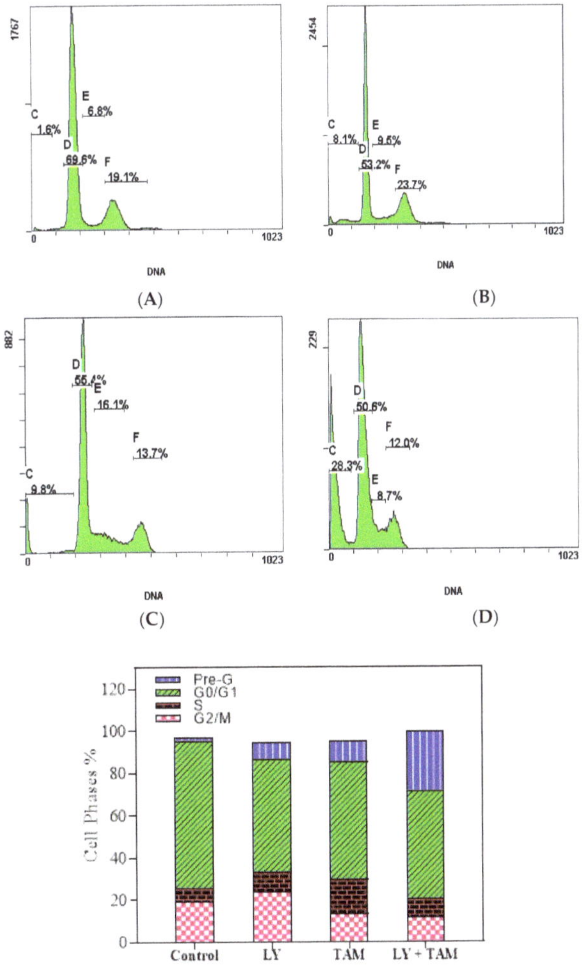

(E)

Figure 6. Histograms represent DNA cell cycle distribution in MCF-7 cells treated with (**A**): control, (**B**): LY, (**C**): TAM, and (**D**): LY + TAM combination for 24 h. (**E**): columns represent the flow cytometry data analysis as means of the percentages of pre-G_1, G_0/G_1, S, and G_2/M ($n = 3$, three independent experiments).

2.4. pAKT and Cyclin D1 Decreased in MCF-7 Cells Treated with LY294002 and Tamoxifen

To explore the molecular targeting of PI3K signaling, AKT, pAKT, and cyclin D1 were assessed after 24 h of the treatment with combination. A Significant decrease of pAKT and cyclin D1 was seen after treatment with LY, ATM, and LY + TAM combination compared to untreated control (Figure 7).

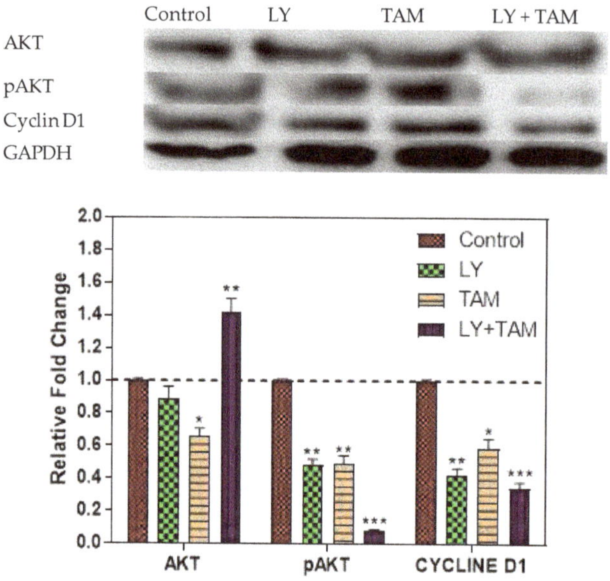

Figure 7. MCF-7 cells were incubated with control, LY, TAM, and LY + TAM for 24 h. Proteins from total cell lysate were separated by SDS-PAGE gel electrophoresis, and immunoblotted with antibodies against AKT, phosphorylated AKT, and cyclin D1. The color density was quantified using densitometry). Statistical differences, compared with the control cells, were assessed by a one-way ANOVA with the Tukey's post-hoc multiple comparison test (GraphPad Prism). $p < 0.05$ (*), $p < 0.01$ (**) and $p < 0.001$ (***) were taken as significant.

3. Discussion

The phosphatidylinositide-3-kinase (PI3K)/Akt signaling pathway regulates many biological processes including cancer cell growth and metastasis [18,19]. Consequently, aberrant activation of the PI3K/Akt signaling pathway is frequently associated with progressive BC, which could be resistant to anticancer therapies [20]. It has been estimated that upregulation of PI3K signalling is involved in around 70% of BC cases [21]. Several PI3K/Akt signaling inhibitors have been effective in inhibiting progression of tumors during pre-clinical and clinical trials and approved by United States Food and Drug Administration (FDA) [22,23]. However, most of these inhibitors have demonstrated only modest clinical efficacy as monotherapies in BC because of drawbacks in their pharmacokinetics and tolerability [23]. Therefore, the combination of PI3K/Akt signaling inhibitors with radiation or chemotherapy is considered as a dynamic research area, approached to overcome therapeutic resistance and enhance treatment efficacy [24]. In a previous study, the tumor associated macrophages were shown to accelerate the endocrine resistance of MCF-7 cells treated with TAM, due to activation of the PI3K/Akt/mTOR signaling pathway [25]. Thus, the co-targeting of ER and PI3K/Akt pathway may stand as a new therapeutic target.

This study was conducted to evaluate the possible synergistic cytotoxic combination effect of LY: as a specific phosphatidylinositide-3-kinase (PI3K) inhibitor, and TAM: as an established BC/ER$^+$ drug. MCF-7 cells were used as a model of ER$^+$ BC. Our results uncovered that the non-toxic dose of LY and TAM synergistically enhanced their cytotoxicity and clonogenecity against MCF-7 with a significant decrease in IC_{50} and combination index (Figures 1 and 2). The cytotoxicity of LY and TAM as single treatments and in combination were previously evaluated on A2780 (ovarian cancer) and MRC-5 (normal fibroblast). The IC_{50} of LY were 21.2 μM and 35.7 μM, and for TAM were 10.4 μM and 11.4 μM, and for the combination of LY and TAM were 4.7 and 24.2 μM, respectively [26–28]. When that result was compared with the result of this study, LY and TAM were found to be more effective in MCF-7 cells compared to A2780 cells. In other previous studies, the co-treatment of LY and TAM significantly enhanced the cytotoxicity against lung and brain cancer cells compared to treatment with TAM alone [27,29].

In the second part of this study, the underlying mechanism of the synergistic apoptosis-inducing effect resulting from the treatment of MCF-7 cells with LY and TAM combination, could be explained by the increase of released apoptotic molecules or the decrease of released anti-apoptotic ones. Some of these key apoptotic molecules, which are used as indicators of apoptosis in BC are caspase-3, -7, and p53 [30–33] and p21 as cell cycle promotors [34]. In addition to the Bcl-2 family, which are also considered as important anti-apoptotic genes, their overexpression is frequently related to cancer development [35]. The LY and TAM combination decreased the expression of Bcl-2 and increased the expression of caspase-3 in MCF-7 cells as observed from immunofluorescence experiment (Figure 4). These data were confirmed by determination of mRNA levels of apoptosis genes Bcl-2, BAX, surviving, HER2, p53, p21, caspase-3, and caspse-7 after treatment of MCF-7 cells with LY, TAM, and their combination (Figure 5).

The downregulation of Bcl-2 and survivin was more significant by treatment with the combination more compared to single treatments, which may partly explain the weaker effect of LY or TAM on the induction of apoptosis. While, the non-significant downregulation of BAX might be explained by indirect interaction of LY, TAM or combination with BID/BIM, which required to initiate membrane permeabilization and apoptosis [36]. Survivin is a pro-survival gene and its overexpression is observed in most cancers. It is associated with resistance to chemotherapy and radiation, thus possibly leading to the failure of therapy and poor prognosis [37,38]. Therefore, through the downregulation of anti-apoptotic genes (Bcl-2 and surviving) and overexpression of apoptotic genes (p53 and caspases) the resistance against TAM in breast cancer cells can be reversed.

In this study, the treatment with LY, TAM, and their combination increased the expression of caspase-3 in MCF-7 cells. There are debate in the expression of caspase-3 in MCF-7. Several studies measured levels of caspase-3 indirectly via fluorometric assay systems and by western blotting analyses and reported that directly the presence of this protease in MCF-7 cells [39,40]. However, other reports stated that MCF-7 cells do not express caspase-3 [41]. Our results supposed that the expression of caspase-3 is deficient in untreated MCF-7 cells, but by treatment with LY, TAM, and their combination, the expression of genes was increased as an indication of apoptosis induction by their treatment.

In this study, the induction of apoptosis by LY, TAM, and their combination was confirmed by annexin V/PI double staining using flow cytometry (Figure 3). The pattern of cell death in LY treated cells was suggest necrosis rather than apoptosis Figure 3B. The LY dose (100 nM) that was used in this experiment might be too high to induce necrosis. Previously, it has been reported that LY induced apoptosis and necrosis in mice depending on the treated dose [42].

The combination of LY and TAM increased the percentage of cells in pre-G_1 cell cycle phase and decreased the percentage of cells in G_0/G_1, S and G_2/M phases compared to untreated cells (Figure 6), thus indicating the down regulation of the cell cycle regulation genes. It has been previously reported that one of major problems in BC is the occurrence of cross-resistance that develops due to the change in the expression of DNA damage repair or cell cycle genes [43]. The phosphorylation of AKT can mediate BC resistance to therapy [44,45]. We have shown in this study a significant decrease in the levels of pAKT and cyclin D1 after treatment with LY and TAM combination better than the decreasing effect of LY or TAM alone (Figure 7). These results indicated that the downregulation of the pAKT signaling pathway could also be responsible for the synergistic cytotoxic effect of LY and TAM combination in MCF-7.

4. Materials and Methods

4.1. Compounds and Reagents

LY294002 and tamoxifen were purchased from Selleckchem, Houston, TX, USA. All reagents and kits used in this study were purchased from Sigma-USA, unless other manufacturer is mentioned.

4.2. Cell Culture

MCF-7 cells (breast adenocarcinoma) was obtained from the ATCC. For sub-culture, RPMI-1640 media (10% FBS; 1% Antibiotic-Antimycotic, Gibco) was used. Cells were kept at 95% humidity, 37 °C, and 5% CO_2 for up to 10 passages. Mycoplasma was tested monthly using the bio-luminescence kit (Lonza, Visp, witzerland) and read by a multi-plate reader.

4.3. Cytotoxicity and Combination Studies

MTT assay was used for evaluation the cytotoxic effects of LY and TAM and their combination according to previous reports [46,47]. MCF-7 cells were cultured in 96-well (1×10^3/well). Cells were treated with several concentrations (0.001–50 μM) of LY and TAM. Cells were incubated for 72 h, followed by addition of MTT for 3 h (Life technologies). The formazan crystals were dissolved in DMSO (100 μL) and the light absorbance was measured used BIORAD PR 4100 microplate reader at λmax 570 nm. IC_{50} were calculated using GraphPad Prism. Nontoxic concentrations (~80% of viable cells) from LY (100 nM) and TAM (100 nM) were used for all combination experiments of this study.

4.4. Clonogenic Survival Assay

The cytotoxicity of LY, TAM and the synergistic cytotoxic effect of their combination was confirmed by clonogenic survival assay according to previous report [48]. Briefly, low density MCF-7 cells (2×10^2 cells/well) were cultivated in 2 mL media in 6-well plates in duplicates. Plates were incubated at 37 °C overnight to allow attachment. Cells were treated with either LY (100 nM), TAM (100 nM) or their combinations. Plates were incubated at 37 °C for 24 h, then medium containing compounds were aspirated, and replaced with 2 mL fresh media. Plates were checked under the microscope every 2 days, and cells forming a colony were counted. After 14 days, colonies which containing at least 50 cells were counted. Following the aspiration of media, cells were washed with cold PBS, then fixed with cold methanol for 5 min at room temperature. Cells were stained with 0.5% *v/v* methylene blue in methanol: H_2O (1:1) for 15 min. Colonies were washed with PBS and H_2O. Plates were left to dry, before counting colonies.

4.5. Apoptosis Assay Using Flow Cytometric Analysis

The ability of LY, TAM and their combinations to induce apoptosis in BC cells was quantified by flow cytometry using annexin V FITC/PI (propidium iodide) double staining assay following previous report [49,50]. MCF-7 cells (5×10^5 cells/well) were cultivated in 6 well plates for 24 h. LY (100 nM), TAM (100 nM), and their combinations were incubated with cells for further 24 h, before harvested cells were labeled by annexin V FITC/PI apoptosis detection kit (Invitrogen) according to the manufacturer's instruction. Apoptotic cells (early and late) were quantified as % by flow cytometer (FC500, Beckman Coulter, Miami, FL, USA).

4.6. Immunofluorescence Staining

The induction of apoptosis in MCF-7 cells by LY, TAM, and their combinations were confirmed by immunofluorescence staining assay to determine the co-localization of the antiapoptotic marker (Bcl-2) and the apoptotic marker (Caspase-3). MCF-7 cells were treated with LY, TAM, and their combinations for 24 h. MCF-7 cells (5 × 10^3/chamber) were seeded and incubated for 24 h. Then cells were blocked with normal donkey serum (30 min), followed by incubation with the primary mouse monoclonal and rabbit polyclonal IgG antibodies (1:200, 3 h) (Santa Cruz Biotechnology, Inc., Santa Cruz, CA, USA) for the detection of Bcl-2 and Caspase-3, respectively. Then, slides were incubated with a mixture of tagged cross-adsorbed donkey anti-mouse (Alexa Fluor 488) and anti-rabbit (Alexa Fluor 555) IgG secondary antibodies (Thermo Fisher Scientific) for 60 min. Slide sections were counterstained with ProLong Diamond Anti-fade Mountant including 4′,6-diamidino-2-phenylindole (DAPI; Thermo Fisher Scientific, Waltham, MA, USA). EVOS FL microscopy (Thermo Fisher Scientific, Waltham, MA, USA) was used for slide examination. Digital images were taken with 40× objective.

4.7. Quantitative Real-Time PCR

For more elucidation of the apoptotic effects of LY, TAM, and their combinations in BC, the RT-PCR platform (Applied Biosystems 7500 Fast Real Time PCR System, Waltham, MA, USA) was applied. RT-PCR was used to quantify the expression of the apoptosis genes: caspase-3, caspse-7, p53, p21, Bcl-2, BAX, Survivin, and Her2 in MCF-7 cells [51]. Briefly, MCF-7 cells (1 × 10^6 cells/well) were cultivated in 6 well plates for 24 h, then cells were treated with LY, TAM, and their combinations for 24 h. Total RNA was isolated according to manufactory instruction. The RT-PCR experiment was conducted with a mixture of cDNA, 2X SYBR Green I Master mix, PCR-grade water, forward and reversed human primers of selective genes, and GAPDH as housekeeping gene (Applied-Biosystems, Thermo Fisher Scientific, Waltham, MA, USA) (Table 1).

Table 1. Sequence of primers used in RT-PCR.

Gene	Sequence
Caspase-3	F: ACATGGAAGCGAATCAATGGACTC R: AAGGACTCAAATTCTGTTGCCACC
Caspase-7	F: GGACCGAGTGCCCACTTATC R: TCGCTTTGTCGAAGTTCTTGTT
p53	F: CCA CCA TAA AGC TGG GGC TT R: TCT CCC CGC CTC TTT GAC TC
p21	F: GAG TCC TGT TTG CTT CTG GGC A R: CTG CAT TGG GGC TGC CTA TGT A
BCL-2	F: CTCTCGTCGCTACCGTCGCG R: AGGCATCCCAGCCTCCGTTATCC
BAX	F: GCCCTTTTGCTTCAGGGTTT R: TCCAATGTCCAGCCCATGAT
Survivin	F: TTGCTCCTGCACCCCAGAGC R: AGGCTCAGCGTAAGGCAGCC
HER2	F: CCT CTG ACG TCC ATC GTC TC R: CGG ATC TTC TGC TGC CGT CG
GAPDH	F: AGGTCGGTGTGAACGGATTTG R: TGTAGACCATGTAGTTGAGGTCA

The RT- PCR program was run in 41 cycles of denaturation at 95 °C for 15 s followed by annealing/extension at 60 °C for 60 s ($n = 3$). Standard comparative method was used to evaluate the genes expression, where the raw Ct values were converted into relative expression levels (fold change: $2^{-\Delta\Delta Ct}$).

4.8. Cell Cycle Analysis

Cell cycle analysis was applied to explore the underlying mechanisms of cytotoxic effects of LY, TAM, and their combinations in BC. MCF-7 cells (5 × 10^5 cells/well) were treated with LY, TAM, and their combinations for 24 h. Cells were then fixed in 70% ethanol and processed for cell cycle analysis, after staining with propidium iodide (PI, Santa Cruz). FC500, Beckman Coulter, Miami, FL,

USA flow cytometer was used for analyzing a total of 20,000 single-cells, with the aid of Expo 32 software, Miami, FL, USA [52].

4.9. Western Immunoblotting

Identification of the expression change of cell cycle proteins (AKT, pAKT, CyclinD1, and GAPDH) was confirmed by immunoblotting assay. MCF7 cells (1×10^6 cells/well of 6 well plate) were treated with LY, TAM, and their combinations for 24 h. Lysis buffer was used to isolate total proteins. The Bradford Method was used to determine the concentration of total proteins, which were electrophoresed using a polyacrylamide gel and transferred to membrane. The membrane was incubated with AKT, pAKT cyclin D1 antibodies (Cell signalling) for 2 h at room temperature and secondary antibody GAPDH for 1 h. Horseradish peroxidase (HRP)-conjugated secondary antibodies were used to visualize the immunoreactivity by chemiluminescence, and images were captured by a scanner (GeneGenome, Syngene Bioimaging, Cambridge, CB4 1TF, United Kingdom) [51].

4.10. Statistics

Statistical differences were assessed by one-way ANOVA with the Tukey's post-hoc multiple comparison test. $p < 0.05$ (*), $p < 0.01$ (**), $p < 0.001$ (***), and $p < 0.0001$ (****) were taken as significant.

5. Conclusions

Our results demonstrated that the synergistic cytotoxic effect of LY and TAM is achieved by the induction of apoptosis and cell cycle distribution through cyclin D1, pAKT, caspases, and Bcl-2 signaling pathways, all which might help in reversing the resistance of MCF-7 cells to TAM and decrease the toxicity of LY. Further in vivo and genetic studies are needed to explore more information about the efficacy and molecular targeting of this combination.

Author Contributions: Conceptualization, M.E.A. and O.F.I.; Experimental part M.A.A., B.R., R.A.A., A.T.B., A.M.I., M.H.M., and S.I.; Statistical analysis and proof reading, W.H.A.; design and writing, M.E.A., M.Z.E.-R., and A.N.A. All authors have read and agreed to the published version of the manuscript.

Funding: This research received no external funding.

Conflicts of Interest: The authors declare no conflict of interest.

References

1. Bray, F.; Ferlay, J.; Soerjomataram, I.; Siegel, R.L.; Torre, L.A.; Jemal, A. Global cancer statistics 2018: GLOBOCAN estimates of incidence and mortality worldwide for 36 cancers in 185 countries. *CA Cancer J. Clin.* **2018**, *68*, 394–424. [CrossRef] [PubMed]
2. Al-Shahrani, Z.; Al-Rawaji, A.I.; Al-Madouj, A.N.; Hayder, M.S. *Cancer Incidence Report Saudi Arabia 2014*; Saudi Cancer Registry: Riyadh, Saudi Arabia, 2017; pp. 1–81.
3. Sopik, V.; Sun, P.; Narod, S.A. Predictors of time to death after distant recurrence in breast cancer patients. *Breast Cancer Res. Treat.* **2019**, *173*, 465–474. [CrossRef]
4. Alkahtani, H.M.; Alanazi, M.M.; Aleanizy, F.S.; Alqahtani, F.Y.; Alhoshani, A.; Alanazi, F.E.; Almehizia, A.A.; Abdalla, A.N.; Alanazi, M.G.; El-Azab, A.S.; et al. Synthesis, anticancer, apoptosis-inducing activities and EGFR and VEGFR2 assay mechanistic studies of 5,5-diphenylimidazolidine-2,4-dione derivatives: Molecular docking studies. *Saudi Pharm. J.* **2019**, *27*, 682–693. [CrossRef]
5. Abubakar, M.; Sung, H.; Devi, R.; Guida, J.; Tang, T.S.; Pfeiffer, R.M.; Yang, X.R. Breast cancer risk factors, survival and recurrence, and tumor molecular subtype: Analysis of 3012 women from an indigenous Asian population. *Breast Cancer Res.* **2018**, *20*, 114. [CrossRef]
6. Khalil, S.; Hatch, L.; Price, C.R.; Palakurty, S.H.; Simoneit, E.; Radisic, A.; Pargas, A.; Shetty, I.; Lyman, M.; Couchot, P.; et al. Addressing Breast Cancer Screening Disparities Among Uninsured and Insured Patients: A Student-Run Free Clinic Initiative. *J. Community Health* **2019**, *45*, 501–505. [CrossRef] [PubMed]
7. Clemons, M.; Danson, S.; Howell, A. Tamoxifen ('Nolvadex'): A review: Antitumour treatment. *Cancer Treat. Rev.* **2002**, *28*, 165–180. [CrossRef]

8. Day, C.M.; Hickey, S.M.; Song, Y.; Plush, S.E.; Garg, S. Novel Tamoxifen Nanoformulations for Improving Breast Cancer Treatment: Old Wine in New Bottles. *Molecules* **2020**, *25*, 1182. [CrossRef]
9. Silvente-Poirot, S.; de Medina, P.; Record, M.; Poirot, M. From tamoxifen to dendrogenin A: The discovery of a mammalian tumor suppressor and cholesterol metabolite. *Biochimie* **2016**, *130*, 109–114. [CrossRef]
10. Wilkes, G.M.; Barton-Burke, M. *2020–2021 Oncology Nursing Drug Handbook*; Jones & Bartlett Learning: Burlington, MA, USA, 2019.
11. Mohamed, K.E.; Elamin, A. Adherence to endocrine therapy and its relation to disease-free survival among breast cancer patients visiting an out-patient clinic at Khartoum Oncology Hospital, Sudan. *J. Eval. Clin. Pract.* **2020**, *1*, 1–13. [CrossRef]
12. Riggins, R.B.; Schrecengost, R.S.; Guerrero, M.S.; Bouton, A.H. Pathways to tamoxifen resistance. *Cancer Lett.* **2007**, *256*, 1–24. [CrossRef]
13. Liu, S.; Meng, X.; Chen, H.; Liu, W.; Miller, T.; Murph, M.; Lu, Y.; Zhang, F.; Gagea, M.; Arteaga, C.L.; et al. Targeting tyrosine-kinases and estrogen receptor abrogates resistance to endocrine therapy in breast cancer. *Oncotarget* **2014**, *5*, 9049. [CrossRef]
14. Chen, P.; Lee, N.V.; Hu, W.; Xu, M.; Ferre, R.A.; Lam, H.; Bergqvist, S.; Solowiej, J.; Diehl, W.; He, Y.-A.; et al. Spectrum and degree of CDK drug interactions predicts clinical performance. *Mol. Cancer Ther.* **2016**, *15*, 2273–2281. [CrossRef] [PubMed]
15. Maira, S.-M.; Stauffer, F.; Schnell, C.; García-Echeverría, C. *PI3K Inhibitors for Cancer Treatment: Where Do We Stand?* Portland Press Ltd.: London, UK, 2009.
16. Xing, C.-G.; Zhu, B.S.; Fan, X.Q.; Liu, H.H.; Hou, X.; Zhao, K.; Qin, Z.H. Effects of LY294002 on the invasiveness of human gastric cancer in vivo in nude mice. *World J. Gastroenterol.* **2009**, *15*, 5044. [CrossRef]
17. Zhao, W.; Qiu, Y.; Kong, D. Class I phosphatidylinositol 3-kinase inhibitors for cancer therapy. *Acta Pharm. Sin. B* **2017**, *7*, 27–37. [CrossRef] [PubMed]
18. Rahmani, F.; Ferns, G.A.; Talebian, S.; Nourbakhsh, M.; Avan, A.; Shahidsales, S. Role of regulatory miRNAs of the PI3K/AKT signaling pathway in the pathogenesis of breast cancer. *Gene* **2020**, *737*, 144459. [CrossRef] [PubMed]
19. Ortega, M.A.; Fraile-Martínez, O.; Asúnsolo, Á.; Buján, J.; García-Honduvilla, N.; Coca, S. Signal Transduction Pathways in Breast Cancer: The Important Role of PI3K/Akt/mTOR. *J. Oncol.* **2020**, *2020*, 9258396. [CrossRef] [PubMed]
20. Engelman, J.A. Targeting PI3K signalling in cancer: Opportunities, challenges and limitations. *Nat. Rev. Cancer* **2009**, *9*, 550–562. [CrossRef]
21. Miller, L.A. The National Practitioner Data Bank: A primer for clinicians. *J. Perinat. Neonatal Nurs.* **2011**, *25*, 224–225. [CrossRef]
22. Falasca, M. PI3K/Akt signalling pathway specific inhibitors: A novel strategy to sensitize cancer cells to anti-cancer drugs. *Curr. Pharm. Des.* **2010**, *16*, 1410–1416. [CrossRef]
23. McKenna, M.; McGarrigle, S.; Pidgeon, G.P. The next generation of PI3K-Akt-mTOR pathway inhibitors in breast cancer cohorts. *Biochim. Biophys. Acta Rev. Cancer* **2018**, *1870*, 185–197. [CrossRef]
24. Kanaizumi, H.; Higashi, C.; Tanaka, Y.; Hamada, M.; Shinzaki, W.; Azumi, T.; Hashimoto, Y.; Inui, H.; Houjou, T.; Komoike, Y. PI3K/Akt/mTOR signalling pathway activation in patients with ER-positive, metachronous, contralateral breast cancer treated with hormone therapy. *Oncol. Lett.* **2019**, *17*, 1962–1968. [PubMed]
25. Li, D.; Ji, H.; Niu, X.; Yin, L.; Wang, Y.; Gu, Y.; Wang, J.; Zhou, X.; Zhang, H.; Zhang, Q. Tumor-associated macrophages secrete CC-chemokine ligand 2 and induce tamoxifen resistance by activating PI3K/Akt/mTOR in breast cancer. *Cancer Sci.* **2020**, *111*, 47–58. [CrossRef]
26. Jagtap, J.C.; Parveen, D.; Shah, R.D.; Desai, A.; Bhosale, D.; Chugh, A.; Ranade, D.; Karnik, S.; Khedkar, B.; Mathur, A.; et al. Secretory prostate apoptosis response (Par)-4 sensitizes multicellular spheroids (MCS) of glioblastoma multiforme cells to tamoxifen-induced cell death. *FEBS Open Bio* **2015**, *5*, 8–19. [CrossRef] [PubMed]
27. Ko, J.C.; Chiu, H.C.; Syu, J.J.; Chen, C.Y.; Jian, Y.T.; Huang, Y.J.; Wo, T.Y.; Jian, Y.J.; Chang, P.Y.; Wang, T.J.; et al. Down-regulation of MSH2 expression by Hsp90 inhibition enhances cytotoxicity affected by tamoxifen in human lung cancer cells. *Biochem. Biophys. Res. Commun.* **2015**, *456*, 506–512. [CrossRef]

28. Ko, J.C.; Chiu, H.C.; Syu, J.J.; Jian, Y.J.; Chen, C.Y.; Jian, Y.T.; Huang, Y.J.; Wo, T.Y.; Lin, Y.W. Tamoxifen enhances erlotinib-induced cytotoxicity through down-regulating AKT-mediated thymidine phosphorylase expression in human non-small-cell lung cancer cells. *Biochem. Pharmacol.* **2014**, *88*, 119–127. [CrossRef]
29. Li, C.; Zhou, C.; Wang, S.; Feng, Y.; Lin, W.; Lin, S.; Wang, Y.; Huang, H.; Liu, P.; Mu, Y.-G.; et al. Sensitization of glioma cells to tamoxifen-induced apoptosis by Pl3-kinase inhibitor through the GSK-3beta/beta-catenin signaling pathway. *PLoS ONE* **2011**, *6*, e27053.
30. Pu, X.; Storr, S.J.; Zhang, Y.; Rakha, E.A.; Green, A.R.; Ellis, I.O.; Martin, S.G. Caspase-3 and caspase-8 expression in breast cancer: Caspase-3 is associated with survival. *Apoptosis* **2017**, *22*, 357–368. [CrossRef]
31. Nassar, A.; Lawson, D.; Cotsonis, G.; Cohen, C. Survivin and caspase-3 expression in breast cancer: Correlation with prognostic parameters, proliferation, angiogenesis, and outcome. *Appl. Immunohistochem. Mol. Morphol.* **2008**, *16*, 113–120. [CrossRef] [PubMed]
32. Cui, Q.; Yu, J.H.; Wu, J.N.; Tashiro, S.I.; Onodera, S.; Minami, M.; Ikejima, T. P53-mediated cell cycle arrest and apoptosis through a caspase-3- independent, but caspase-9-dependent pathway in oridonin-treated MCF-7 human breast cancer cells. *Acta Pharmacol. Sin.* **2007**, *28*, 1057–1066. [CrossRef]
33. O'Donovan, N.; Crown, J.; Stunell, H.; Hill, A.D.; McDermott, E.; O'Higgins, N.; Duffy, M.J. Caspase 3 in breast cancer. *Clin. Cancer Res.* **2003**, *9*, 738–742.
34. Abbas, T.; Dutta, A. p21 in cancer: Intricate networks and multiple activities. *Nat. Rev. Cancer* **2009**, *9*, 400–414. [CrossRef] [PubMed]
35. Thomadaki, H.; Scorilas, A. Molecular profile of the BCL2 family of the apoptosis related genes in breast cancer cells after treatment with cytotoxic/cytostatic drugs. *Connect. Tissue Res.* **2008**, *49*, 261–264. [CrossRef] [PubMed]
36. Luna-Vargas, M.P.A.; Chipuk, J.E. Physiological and Pharmacological Control of BAK, BAX, and Beyond. *Trends Cell Biol.* **2016**, *26*, 906–917. [CrossRef] [PubMed]
37. Da Veiga, G.L.; da Silva RD, M.; Pereira, E.C.; Azzalis, L.A.; da Costa Aguiar Alves, B.; de Sousa Gehrke, F.; Gascón, T.M.; Fonseca, F.L.A. The role of Survivin as a biomarker and potential prognostic factor for breast cancer. *Rev. Assoc. Med. Bras.* **2019**, *65*, 893–901. [CrossRef]
38. Motawi, T.M.K.; Zakhary, N.I.; Darwish, H.A.; Abdalla, H.M.; Tadros, S.A. Significance of Serum Survivin and -31G/C Gene Polymorphism in the Early Diagnosis of Breast Cancer in Egypt. *Clin. Breast Cancer* **2019**, *19*, e276–e282. [CrossRef]
39. Feng, F.F.; Zhang, D.R.; Tian, K.L.; Lou, H.Y.; Qi, X.L.; Wang, Y.C.; Duan, C.X.; Jia, L.J.; Wang, F.H.; Liu, Y.; et al. Growth inhibition and induction of apoptosis in MCF-7 breast cancer cells by oridonin nanosuspension. *Drug Deliv.* **2011**, *18*, 265–271. [CrossRef]
40. Kumar, A.; D'Souza, S.S.; Gaonkar, S.L.; Rai, K.L.; Salimath, B.P. Growth inhibition and induction of apoptosis in MCF-7 breast cancer cells by a new series of substituted-1,3,4-oxadiazole derivatives. *Investig. New Drugs* **2008**, *26*, 425–435. [CrossRef]
41. Jänicke, R.U.; Sprengart, M.L.; Wati, M.R.; Porter, A.G. Caspase-3 is required for DNA fragmentation and morphological changes associated with apoptosis. *J. Biol. Chem.* **1998**, *273*, 9357–9360. [CrossRef]
42. Jiang, H.; Fan, D.; Zhou, G.; Li, X.; Deng, H. Phosphatidylinositol 3-kinase inhibitor(LY294002) induces apoptosis of human nasopharyngeal carcinoma in vitro and in vivo. *J. Exp. Clin. Cancer Res.* **2010**, *29*, 34. [CrossRef]
43. Post, A.E.M.; Bussink, J.; Sweep, F.C.; Span, P.N. Changes in DNA Damage Repair Gene Expression and Cell Cycle Gene Expression Do Not Explain Radioresistance in Tamoxifen-Resistant Breast Cancer. *Oncol. Res.* **2020**, *28*, 33–40. [CrossRef]
44. Andre, F.; Nahta, R.; Conforti, R.; Boulet, T.; Aziz, M.; Yuan LX, H.; Meslin, F.; Spielmann, M.; Tomasic, G.; Pusztai, L.; et al. Expression patterns and predictive value of phosphorylated AKT in early-stage breast cancer. *Ann. Oncol.* **2008**, *19*, 315–320. [CrossRef] [PubMed]
45. Yang, Z.Y.; Di, M.Y.; Yuan, J.Q.; Shen, W.X.; Zheng, D.Y.; Chen, J.Z.; Mao, C.; Tang, J.L. The prognostic value of phosphorylated Akt in breast cancer: A systematic review. *Sci. Rep.* **2015**, *5*, 7758. [CrossRef] [PubMed]
46. Alkahtani, H.M.; Abdalla, A.N.; Obaidullah, A.J.; Alanazi, M.M.; Almehizia, A.A.; Alanazi, M.G.; Ahmed, A.Y.; Alwassil, O.I.; Darwish, H.W.; Abdel-Aziz, A.A.-M.; et al. Synthesis, cytotoxic evaluation, and molecular docking studies of novel quinazoline derivatives with benzenesulfonamide and anilide tails: Dual inhibitors of EGFR/HER2. *Bioorg. Chem.* **2020**, *95*, 103461. [CrossRef] [PubMed]

47. Gouda, A.M.; Abdelazeem, A.H.; Abdalla, A.N.; Ahmed, M. Pyrrolizine-5-carboxamides: Exploring the impact of various substituents on anti-inflammatory and anticancer activities. *Acta Pharm.* **2018**, *68*, 251–273. [CrossRef]
48. Fall, A.D.; Bagla VP, B.; Bassene, E.; Eloff, J.N. Phytochemical Screening, Antimicrobial and Cytotoxicity Studies of Ethanol Leaf Extract of Aphaniasenegalensis (Sapindaceae). *Afr. J. Tradit. Complement. Altern. Med.* **2017**, *14*, 135–139. [CrossRef]
49. Abdalla, A.N.; Shaheen, U.; Abdallah, Q.; Flamini, G.; Bkhaitan, M.M.; Abdelhady, M.I.; Ascrizzi, R.; Bader, A. Proapoptotic Activity of Achillea membranacea Essential Oil and Its Major Constituent 1,8-Cineole against A2780 Ovarian Cancer Cells. *Molecules* **2020**, *25*, 1582. [CrossRef]
50. Malki, W.H.; Gouda, A.M.; Ali, H.E.; Al-Rousan, R.; Samaha, D.; Abdalla, A.N.; Bustamante, J.; Elmageed, Z.Y.A.; Ali, H.I. Structural-based design, synthesis, and antitumor activity of novel alloxazine analogues with potential selective kinase inhibition. *Eur. J. Med. Chem.* **2018**, *152*, 31–52. [CrossRef]
51. Abdalla, A.N.; Abdallah, M.E.; Aslam, A.; Bader, A.; Vassallo, A.; De Tommasi, N.; Malki, W.H.; Gouda, A.M.; Mukhtar, M.H.; El-Readi, M.Z.; et al. Synergistic Anti Leukemia Effect of a Novel Hsp90 and a Pan Cyclin Dependent Kinase Inhibitors. *Molecules* **2020**, *25*, 2220. [CrossRef]
52. Shaheen, U.; Ragab, E.A.; Abdalla, A.N.; Bader, A. Triterpenoidal saponins from the fruits of Gleditsia caspica with proapoptotic properties. *Phytochemistry* **2018**, *145*, 168–178. [CrossRef]

Sample Availability: Samples of the compounds are not available.

molecules

MDPI

Article

Tacrine-Coumarin Derivatives as Topoisomerase Inhibitors with Antitumor Effects on A549 Human Lung Carcinoma Cancer Cell Lines

Eva Konkoľová [1,2], Monika Hudáčová [1], Slávka Hamuľaková [3], Rastislav Jendželovský [4], Jana Vargová [4], Juraj Ševc [4], Peter Fedoročko [4] and Mária Kožurková [1,5,*]

1 Department of Biochemistry, Institute of Chemistry, Faculty of Science, P. J. Šafárik University in Kosice, 041 80 Košice, Slovakia; eva.konkolova@upjs.sk (E.K.); monika.hudacova@student.upjs.sk (M.H.)
2 Institute of Organic Chemistry and Biochemistry AS CR, Flemingovo náměstí 2, 160 00 Prague 6, Czech Republic
3 Department of Organic Chemistry, Institute of Chemistry, Faculty of Science, P. J. Šafárik University in Košice, 041 80 Košice, Slovakia; slavka.hamulakova@upjs.sk
4 Department of Cellular Biology, Institute of Biology and Ecology, Faculty of Science, P. J. Šafárik University in Košice, 041 80 Košice, Slovakia; rastislav.jendzelovsky@upjs.sk (R.J.); jana.vargova@upjs.sk (J.V.); juraj.sevc@upjs.sk (J.Š.); peter.fedorocko@upjs.sk (P.F.)
5 Biomedical Research Center, University Hospital Hradec Kralove, 500 05 Hradec Kralove, Czech Republic
* Correspondence: maria.kozurkova@upjs.sk; Tel.: +421-9-04527704

Citation: Konkoľová, E.; Hudáčová, M.; Hamuľaková, S.; Jendželovský, R.; Vargová, J.; Ševc, J.; Fedoročko, P.; Kožurková, M. Tacrine-Coumarin Derivatives as Topoisomerase Inhibitors with Antitumor Effects on A549 Human Lung Carcinoma Cancer Cell Lines. *Molecules* **2021**, *26*, 1133. https://doi.org/10.3390/molecules26041133

Academic Editors: Marialuigia Fantacuzzi and Alessandra Ammazzalorso

Received: 27 January 2021
Accepted: 18 February 2021
Published: 20 February 2021

Publisher's Note: MDPI stays neutral with regard to jurisdictional claims in published maps and institutional affiliations.

Abstract: A549 human lung carcinoma cell lines were treated with a series of new drugs with both tacrine and coumarin pharmacophores (derivatives **1a–2c**) in order to test the compounds' ability to inhibit both cancer cell growth and topoisomerase I and II activity. The ability of human topoisomerase I (*h*TOPI) and II to relax supercoiled plasmid DNA in the presence of various concentrations of the tacrine-coumarin hybrid molecules was studied with agarose gel electrophoresis. The biological activities of the derivatives were studied using MTT assays, clonogenic assays, cell cycle analysis and quantification of cell number and viability. The content and localization of the derivatives in the cells were analysed using flow cytometry and confocal microscopy. All of the studied compounds were found to have inhibited topoisomerase I activity completely. The effect of the tacrine-coumarin hybrid compounds on cancer cells is likely to be dependent on the length of the chain between the tacrine and coumarin moieties (**1c**, **1d** = tacrine-$(CH_2)_{8-9}$-coumarin). The most active of the tested compounds, derivatives **1c** and **1d**, both display longer chains.

Keywords: tacrine-coumarin derivatives; DNA; topoisomerases I, II; cytotoxicity; lung carcinoma cells; A549

1. Introduction

Coumarins have attracted a great deal of attention due to the wide range of their biological properties [1–4]. Recent research has focused attention on the anticancer activity of coumarin and coumarin-derived compounds due to their high level of biological activity and low toxicity [5–7]. Coumarins are commonly used in the treatment of prostate cancer, colon, renal cell carcinoma and leukemia in particular [8–10]. Further research has also led to irusostat (a potent coumarin-based irreversible inhibitor) compounds entering clinical trials for possible future use in the treatment of breast cancer [11–13]. Lung cancer is one of the most commonly diagnosed malignant tumors and is the leading cause of cancer death throughout the world. The currently available therapies in the treatment of advanced lung cancer, primarily radiotherapy and chemotherapy, are still inadequate. While highly effective FDA-approved drugs such as, e.g., efitinib, erlotinib, and bevacizumab are now available for targeted therapy/chemotherapy, these drugs can cause side effects [14]. Therefore, there is an urgent need for the development of novel drugs for treating this disease. A549 human lung carcinoma cells are a well characterized cellular model for this purpose [15,16].

Different mechanisms are thought to be responsible for the anticancer activity of coumarins, including the blocking of the cell cycle, the induction of cell apoptosis, the modulation of the estrogen receptor, or the inhibition of DNA-associated enzymes such as telomerase and topoisomerase (TOP). Topoisomerase enzymes play an important role in DNA metabolism, and the search for novel enzyme inhibitors is an important target in the development of new anticancer drugs [17,18].

The relevance and significance of these compounds is obvious, and the agents have attracted considerable attention through the development of novel biologically active molecules. The approach is based on the highly effective combination principle of drug design and involves the coupling of coumarins with other bioactive molecules [19–22]. The activity of tacrine (9-amino-1,2,3,4-tetrahydroacridine) in neurological disorders such as Alzheimer's disease is now well established. Numerous studies have confirmed that the drug is an effective inhibitor of acetylcholinesterase [22–25] and it has also been reported that it is not clastogenic in mammalian cells [26]. Tacrine is a relatively weak catalytic inhibitor of TOPII (in comparison with 9-aminoacridine), which has been found to inhibit topoisomerase and DNA synthesis, thereby resulting in mitochondrial DNA depletion and apoptosis [27–29]. Hybrid molecules, formed by the combination of two or more pharmacophores, is an emerging concept in the field of medicinal chemistry and drug discovery that has attracted substantial attraction in the past few years [30].

The aim of this study is to show that these structurally novel tacrine-coumarin compounds, derivatives **1a–1d** and **2a–2c**, may exhibit anticancer properties and also to examine the antiproliferative and topoisomerase activities of the derivatives in more detail.

2. Results

2.1. *Topoisomerase Relaxation Assay*

The ability of human topoisomerase I (*h*TOPI) to relax supercoiled plasmid DNA in the presence of various concentrations of tacrine-coumarin hybrid molecules was studied with agarose gel electrophoresis and the results are shown in Figure 1. The results clearly show that supercoiled plasmid DNA (line *p*BR322) was fully relaxed under normal conditions with *h*TOPI (*h*TOPI line + *p*BR322). However, relaxation induced by *h*TOPI was inhibited when the concentration of the studied compounds (lines **1a–2c**) was gradually increased. All of the studied compounds were found to have caused partial inhibition of topoisomerase activity at a concentration of 30×10^{-6} M and complete inhibition was detected at a concentration of 60×10^{-6} M.

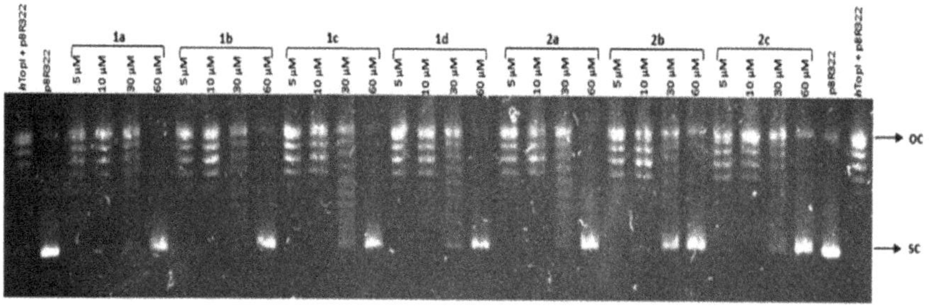

Figure 1. Electrophoresis agarose gel showing inhibitory effects of tacrine-coumarin compounds **1a–2c** on human topoisomerase I (*h*TOPI) activity. Supercoiled plasmid DNA (*p*BR322—negative control) was incubated for 30 min with 2 U of *h*TOPI in the absence (lines *h*TOPI + *p*BR322—positive control) and presence of varying concentrations of compounds **1a-2c** (lines **1a–2c**).

In order to evaluate whether the compounds can also inhibit topoisomerase IIα activity, the decatenation of catenated plasmid DNA was performed in the presence of the compounds. However, no significant inhibitory effect was detected, even at the highest concentration of 100×10^{-6} M concentration (data not shown) and therefore we suggest that compounds **1a–2c** are unable to inhibit the topoisomerase IIα enzyme.

2.2. Intracellular Localization and Cytotoxicity Assays

Flow cytometric analysis of the content of the derivatives present in A549 cells revealed the cumulative fluorescence of derivatives **1b–1d** and **2b** from the green (FL-1) to the red (FL-3) channel (Figure 2). Compound **1c** was found to display the highest level of fluorescence. The presence of compounds **1a–2c** in A549 human adherent lung carcinoma cells were analysed by observing the fluorescence of the compounds in the green channel (*Ex* = 488 nm, *Em* = 510–560 nm). This analysis was performed in order to detect the accumulation of the compounds within the cells by exploiting their natural fluorescence. This allowed us to correlate the accumulation of the derivatives with their observed effects on the cellular parameters. The accumulation of the compounds was then investigated in more detail with respect to their specific intracellular distribution using confocal microscopy.

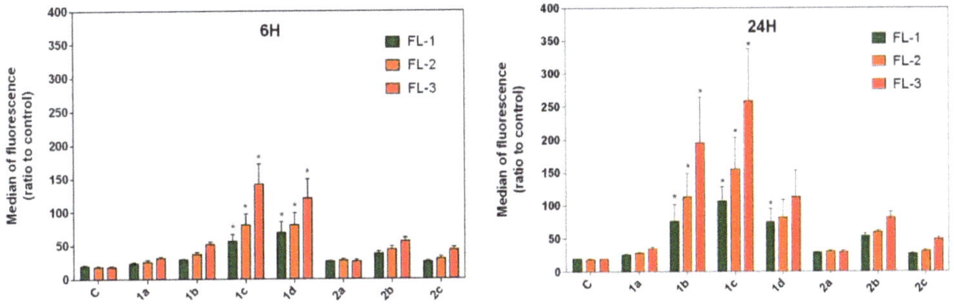

Figure 2. Flow cytometric analysis of intracellular level of derivatives **1a–2c**. Intrinsic fluorescence of compounds was detected after excitation at 488 nm and the emission was measured using a 530/30 nm band-pass filter (FL-1), 585/42 band-pass filter (FL-2) and 670 nm long-pass filter (FL-3). The results are presented as the mean values ± SD of three independent experiments; statistical significance * $p < 0.05$ for each experimental group compared to the untreated control.

According to our results (Figure 3), compound **1d** displayed the highest rate of detection in cells, with compounds **1c** and **1b** also showing weaker levels of detection. In other samples, the fluorescence of the derivatives could not be distinguished from the autofluorescence of the cancer cells. At the cellular level, the analyzed compounds were distributed in the cytoplasm with no interference with the cell nucleus. Based on mitochondrial staining and the overall distribution of the signal, we could not confirm the accumulation of the derivatives in the mitochondria or in the other organelles or membranes (data not shown).

2.3. MTT Assay

The ability of the studied compounds to inhibit the metabolic activity of A549 cancer cell lines was determined using an MTT assay. Results were obtained from three independent experiments and each experiment was carried out in triplicate. As is evident from Figure 4, the compounds were found to have inhibited metabolic activity in a time- and dose-dependent manner, and the highest efficiency was recorded in the case of the experimental group treated with compounds **1c** and **1d**.

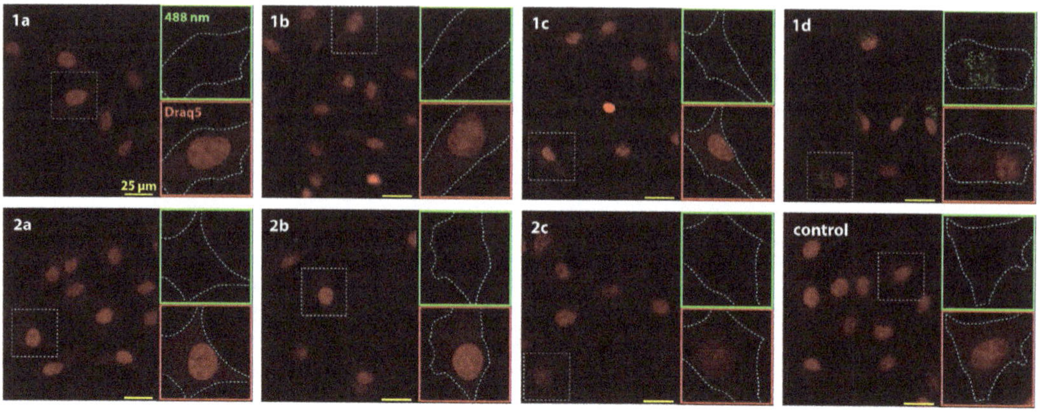

Figure 3. Confocal microscopy images of A549 cancer cell lines after 24 h incubation with compounds **1a–2c**. The microphotographs show the representative images of the samples with merged channels. Compounds **1a–2c** were visualized in cells with a 488 nm laser and the fluorescence was captured at the range of 510–560 nm (green insets). Red insets show nuclear labelling with Draq5. Scale bar = 25 µm.

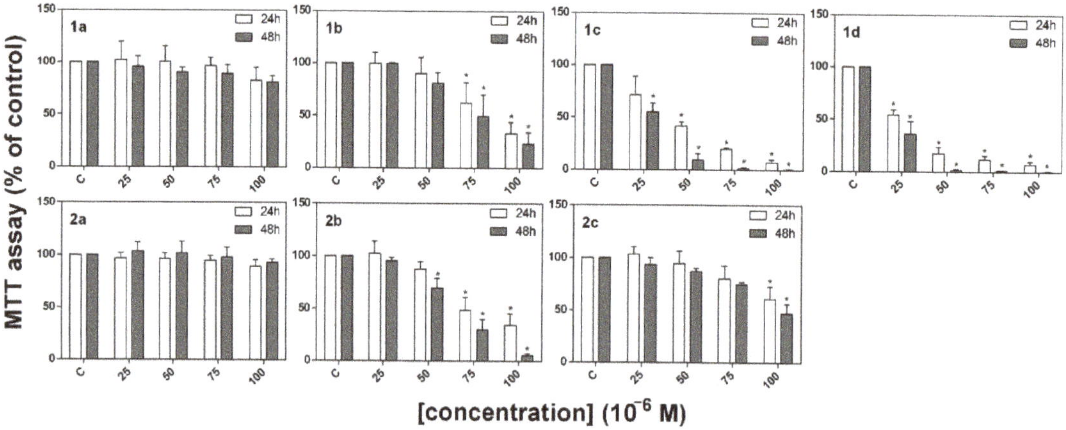

Figure 4. Effect of tacrine-coumarin hybrid compounds **1a–2c** on metabolic activity evaluated by MTT assay in A549 cancer cell lines. MTT assays are expressed as percentages of the untreated control. The results are presented as the mean values ± SD of three independent experiments; statistical significance (*): $p < 0.05$ for each experimental group compared to the untreated control.

The results obtained from the MTT assay were also used to determine IC_{50} values for each compound which are listed in Table 1. The IC_{50} values show that A549 cancer cells are more sensitive to the action of compounds **1c** and **1d** (IC_{50} = 27.04 and 21.22 × 10^{-6} M, respectively after 48 h) than to the other compounds from this series (IC_{50} > 50 × 10^{-6} M). Furthermore, these data corroborate the results obtained from the viability assay and the quantification of total cell number.

Table 1. IC_{50} values of tacrine-coumarin hybrid molecules **1a–2c** in A549 cancer cell lines.

Compound	[a] IC_{50} ($\times 10^{-6}$ M)	
	24 h	**48 h**
1a	n.d.	n.d.
1b	83.54	74.27
1c	42.36	27.04
1d	27.25	21.22
2a	n.d.	n.d.
2b	74.05	62.33
2c	n.d.	98.68

n.d.—not detected, [a] IC_{50}—the concentration of the compound at which 50% of metabolic activity is inhibited.

2.4. *Quantification of Cell Number and Viability*

The influence of the tacrine-coumarin compounds on total cell numbers was investigated after 24 h of treatment with the derivatives. As is shown in Figure 5, the total cell number decreased sharply (by more than 50%) in the case of cells treated with compounds **1c** and **1d**.

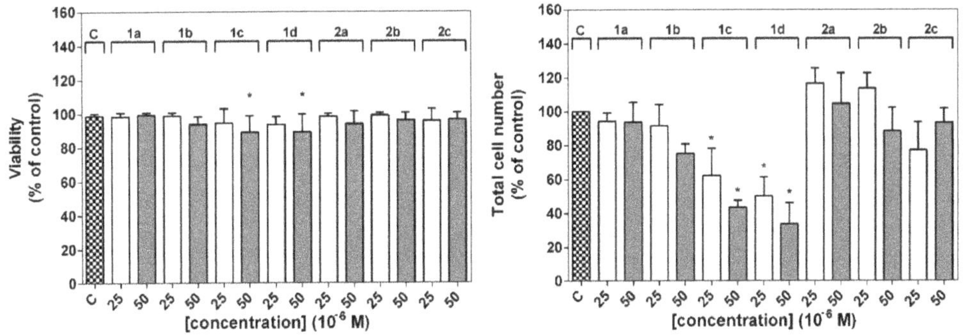

Figure 5. Effect of tacrine-coumarin hybrid compounds **1a–2c** on viability and total cell numbers in A549 cancer cell lines. The viability and total cell number were evaluated 24 h after the addition of the derivatives and are expressed as a percentage of the viable, eosin negative cells or as a percentage of the untreated control of the total cell number, respectively. The results are presented as the mean values ± SD of three independent experiments; statistical significance * $p < 0.05$ for each experimental group is compared to the untreated control.

A simultaneous analysis of viability (Figure 5) showed that higher concentrations of compounds **1c** and **1d** had a weaker but nonetheless significant effect on cell survival. These results indicate that compounds **1c** and **1d** can influence total cell numbers and viability in a concentration-dependent manner.

2.5. *Cell Cycle Distribution*

The influence of the tacrine-coumarin hybrid molecules on the cell cycle distribution of cancer cells was investigated using flow cytometry. Data were collected from three independent experiments. As is shown in Table 2, the percentage of the cells at G_0/G_1 in the control group is 53.77 ± 1.43. The A549 cells were incubated with different concentrations of the studied compounds, and after 24 h incubation, the cells treated with compounds **1b** (at a higher concentration), **1c** and **1d** displayed an increased percentage of cells at the G_0/G_1 phase.

Table 2. Effect of tacrine-coumarin hybrid compounds **1a–2c** on cell cycle distribution.

Compound	Concentration ($\times 10^{-6}$ M)	G_1	S	G_2
Control	0	53.77 ± 1.43	33.43 ± 0.71	12.81 ± 0.94
1a	25	57.03 ± 0.86	31.02 ± 0.65	11.94 ± 1.37
	50	57.88 ± 1.68	30.56 ± 0.72	11.56 ± 0.99
1b	25	59.08 ± 1.32	29.64 ± 0.22	11.29 ± 1.36
	50	71.13 ± 1.59 *	21.72 ± 1.22 *	7.15 ± 1.29 *
1c	25	79.97 ± 1.25 *	14.64 ± 1.56 *	5.39 ± 0.9 *
	50	91.86 ± 2.24 *	6.09 ± 1.98 *	2.05 ± 0.62*
1d	25	86.21 ± 1.67 *	10.73 ± 0.97 *	3.06 ± 0.85 *
	50	80.85 ± 2.30 *	12.54 ± 3.46 *	6.61 ± 1.84 *
2a	25	55.54 ± 1.43	33.00 ± 1.03	11.46 ± 1.41
	50	56.94 ±1.20	32.06 ± 0.22	11.01 ± 1.07
2b	25	58.18 ± 0.35	30.51 ± 1.20	11.30 ± 0.86
	50	56.69 ± 2.40	32.49 ± 1.56	10.83 ± 0.9
2c	25	57.03 ± 2.74	31.77 ± 1.73	11.20 ± 1.21
	50	57.68 ± 1.24	31.80 ± 0.6	10.51 ± 1.67

* Statistical significance: $p < 0.05$ for each experimental group compared to untreated control.

2.6. Clonogenic Assay

A549 cell lines were treated with two different concentrations of these derivatives. As is shown in Figure 6, no significant decrease in colony formation was observed, while a limited reduction was observed in the presence of a higher concentration of compound **1d**.

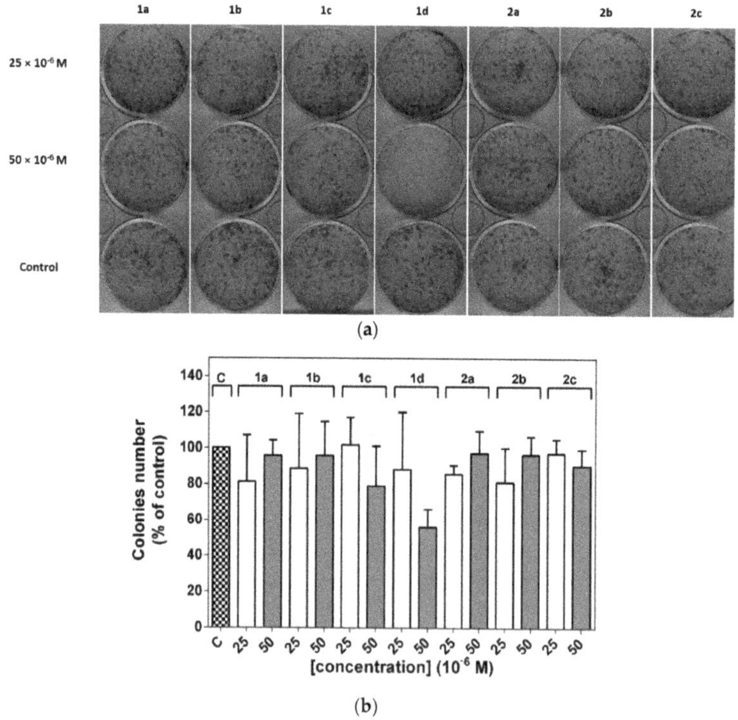

Figure 6. Clonogenic assay of A549 cancer cell lines. Cells were untreated (control) or treated with different concentrations of tacrine-coumarin hybrid derivatives **1a–2c** for 24 h. (**a**) The experimental and (**b**) graphical presentation of the results. The results of the subsequent 7-day cultivation are presented as the mean values ± SD of three independent experiments.

3. Discussion

DNA topoisomerases are crucial nuclear enzymes which control the topology of DNA by cleaving and re-joining the phosphodiester backbone of the DNA strand during various genetic processes. Clinical topoisomerase inhibitors act by generating topoisomerase-linked DNA breaks, blocking the religation of the cleavage complexes when a single drug molecule binds tightly at the interface of the topoisomerase-DNA cleavage complex [31]. As is well known, relaxed forms of supercoiled DNA migrate into a gel more slowly than non-relaxed DNA; this means that only the supercoiled band should be visible when topoisomerase activity is inhibited [32,33]. However, relaxation induced by *h*TOPI was inhibited when the concentration of the studied compounds was gradually increased, suggesting that the tacrine-coumarin compounds may cause a concentration-dependent inhibition of *h*TOPI. All of the studied compounds were found to have caused a complete inhibition at a concentration of 60×10^{-6} M. In order to evaluate whether the compounds can also inhibit topoisomerase IIα activity, the decatenation of catenated plasmid DNA was performed in the presence of the compounds. However, no significant inhibitory effect was detected, even at the highest concentration, and therefore we suggest that compounds **1a**–**2c** are unable to inhibit the topoisomerase IIα enzyme. It is important to understand that the cytotoxicity of topoisomerase inhibitors is due to the trapping of topoisomerase cleavage complexes, a process which should be distinguished from the associated topoisomerase catalytic inhibition. With the exception of molecularly defined settings, it is the topoisomerase cleavage complexes that kill the cancer cell [31]. TOPI plays an important role during the cell division process and we hypothesize that the inhibition of TOPI by tacrine-coumarin compounds can also influence cell division in A549 cell lines.

The presence of compounds **1a**–**2c** in A549 human adherent lung carcinoma cells was analysed by observing the fluorescence of the compounds in the green channel. As our results show, compound **1d** displayed the highest rate of detection in cells. In other samples, the fluorescence of derivatives was not distinguishable from the autofluorescence of the cancer cells. In cells, the compounds were distributed in the cytoplasm. Based on mitochondrial staining and the overall distribution of the signal, we were unable to confirm the accumulation of the compounds in the mitochondria or in other organelles or membranes. These observations suggest that no specific interaction through DNA binding is responsible for the observed cytotoxicity of these compounds. Flow cytometric analysis of the content of the derivatives present in the A549 cells revealed that compound **1c** was found to display the highest level of fluorescence.

The influence of the tacrine-coumarin compounds on total cell numbers was investigated after 24 h of treatment with the derivatives. The total cell number decreased sharply in the case of cells treated with compounds **1c** and **1d**. No significant changes were observed for cells treated with the other compounds from the series, but a simultaneous analysis of viability showed that higher concentrations of compounds **1c** and **1d** had a weaker but nonetheless significant effect on cell survival. These results indicate that compounds **1c** and **1d** can influence total cell numbers and viability in a concentration-dependent manner.

The ability of the studied compounds to inhibit the metabolic activity of A549 cancer cell lines was determined using an MTT assay. The compounds were found to have inhibited metabolic activity in a time- and dose-dependent manner, with the highest efficacy being recorded in the case of the experimental groups treated with compounds **1c** and **1d**. The IC_{50} values show that A549 cancer cells are more sensitive to the action of compounds **1c** and **1d** after 48 h than to the other compounds from this series. Furthermore, these data corroborate the results obtained from the viability assay and the quantification of total cell number. Tacrine was found to be a weak antiproliferative agent but we determined that the combination of tacrine and coumarin in a single molecule is more efficient against the cancer cell line.

Solarova et al. [34] have tested the cytotoxic and/or anti-cancer activities of tacrine-coumarin heterodimers **1a**–**2c** on 4T1 (mouse mammary carcinoma), MCF-7 (human breast adenocarcinoma), HCT116 (human colorectal carcinoma), A549 (human lung carcinoma),

NMuMG (normal mouse mammary gland cells) and HUVEC (human endothelial cells isolated from umbilical vein) cell lines. Based on the obtained IC_{50} values, compounds **1a–2c** showed moderate to significant activity in the µM range. The A549 tumor cells proved to be the most resistant, with a proliferation not significantly different from the other cell lines after the administration of tacrine-coumarin derivatives **1b–1d**. Among the synthesized compounds, the tacrine-coumarin heterodimer with nine methylene groups between the two amino groups in the side chain exhibited the greatest efficacy. The authors proposed that tacrine-coumarin heterodimers **1a–2c** with longer side chains (replacing some methylene groups with amine moiety) had decreased the anticancer activity. The effect of the tacrine-coumarin hybrid compounds on the cancer cells is likely dependent on the length of the chain between the tacrine and coumarin moiety (compounds **1c**, **1d** = tacrine-$(CH_2)_{8-9}$-coumarin). However, when the -CH_2 chain is interrupted by -NH groups, only a moderate inhibition effect on proliferation is recorded. Our attention was focused only on one A549 cancer cell line with the purpose of studying these compounds in more detail. According to our results, derivatives **1c** and **1d** displayed the best antiproliferative effect, a result which is similar to those reported by Solarova et al. The compounds with a greater length of chain between the tacrine and coumarin molecules showed an insignificant effect (**2a–2c**). As further evidence of the significance of hydrocarbon length, the antiproliferative activity increased in the order **1b** < **2b** < **1c** < **1d**.

A novel *bis*-tacrine and its congeners was tested for its potential as an anticancer agent by Hu et al. [35] An in-vitro cytotoxic evaluation of the compounds was carried out against a panel of 60 human cancer cell lines. Of the novel compounds, the butyl-linked *bis*-tacrine exhibited the strongest cytotoxic profile against non-small lung cancer cells. Congeners bearing a longer alkyl chain were on average 30- to 100-times less cytotoxic against these cancer cells.

We also investigated the influence of tacrine-coumarin hybrid molecules **1a–2c** on the cell cycle distribution of cancer cells. The A549 cells, which were treated with compounds **1b–1d**, displayed an increased percentage of cells at the G_0/G_1 phase. The data demonstrate that these compounds were also capable of inhibiting cells in the G_0/G_1 phase. These results are in agreement with those of Roldán-Pena et al. [36] who designed a series of tacrine-based homo- and heterodimer compounds incorporating an antioxidant tether which displayed antiproliferative activity. The compounds exhibited excellent in vitro antiproliferative activities against a panel of 6 human tumor cell lines, while cell cycle experiments indicated the accumulation of cells in the G_1 phase of the cycle. A study by Janočková et al. [37] examined the effect of 7-MEOTA tacrine urea heterodimers on HL-60 cell lines and their results clearly demonstrated a significant accumulation of cells in the G_1 phase.

In our study, the effects of derivatives **1c** and **1d** were found to be more prominent on the proliferation of cancer cells (demonstrated as a decline in total cell number) than on the viability of the cells. This agrees with the increased accumulation of cells in the G_0/G_1 phase. Finally, the inhibition of Topo I observed for the tacrine-coumarin compounds may also influence cell division in the A549 cell line. While all of these observed effects have a strong impact on the proliferation of cells (and consequently on the total cell number), this does not necessarily mean that the compounds also exert a cytotoxic effect (i.e., the compounds had not impaired cell viability to such a significant degree). Thus, the decreased cell number is primarily the result of inhibited proliferation rather than any cytotoxic effect of tacrine-coumarin hybrid compounds **1c** and **1d**.

In order to test the effect of the studied compounds on colony formation or clonogenic ability, we performed experiments with clonogenic assays. This is a simple technique which can identify biological alterations leading to irreversible losses of proliferative capacity and thus the loss of cells' ability to form new colonies [38]. The changes were accompanied by a corresponding reduction in the percentage of cells in the S and G_2/M phases. No significant decrease in colony formation was observed; a limited reduction was observed in the presence of a higher concentration of compound **1d**.

When we compare the results of all of the biological techniques used in this study, it is possible to suggest that the effect of the tacrine-coumarin hybrid compounds on cancer cells likely depends on the length of the chain between the tacrine and coumarin moiety. However, when the -CH_2 chain is interrupted by -NH groups, only a moderate inhibition effect on proliferation is recorded.

4. Materials and Methods

4.1. Compounds

All chemicals and reagents were purchased from Sigma-Aldrich Chemie (Hamburg, Germany) and used without further purification. Human topoisomerase I- hTOPI, TOPOII (Inspiralis, Ltd., Norwich, UK), Ham Nutrient Mixture (Sigma-Aldrich, St. Louis, MO, USA) foetal bovine serum (Biosera, Boussens, France) and antibiotics (Antibiotic-Antimycotic 100 × and 50 × 10^{-3} g L^{-1} gentamicin; Biosera), MitoTrackerTM Red, DRAQ5TM, ProLongTM Gold Antifade Mountant (Thermo Fisher Scientific, Waltham, MA, USA). MTT (3-[4,5-dimethylthiazol-2-yl]-2,5-diphenyltetrazolium bromide) (Sigma-Aldrich, St. Louis, MO, USA) were used in the study.

The studied tacrine-coumarin hybrids (derivatives **1a–1d** and **2a–2c**) **1a**: *N*1-{6-[(1,2,3,4-tetra-hydroacridin-9-yl)amino]hexyl}-2-(7-hydroxy-2-oxo-2*H*-chromen-4-yl)acetamide, **1b**: *N*1-{7-[(1,2,3,4-tetrahydroacridin-9-yl)amino]heptyl}-2-(7-hydroxy-2-oxo-2*H*-chromen-4-yl) acetamide, 1c: *N*1-{8-[(1,2,3,4-tetrahydroacridin-9-yl)amino]octyl}-2-(7-hydroxy-2-oxo-2*H*-chromen-4-yl)acetamide, 1d: *N*1-{9-[(1,2,3,4-tetrahydroacridin-9-yl) amino]nonyl}-2-(7-hydroxy-2-oxo-2*H*-chromen-4-yl)acetamide, **2a**: 2-(7-hydroxy-2-oxo-2*H*-chromen-4-yl)-*N*-[6-(1,2,3,4-tetrahydroacridin-9-ylamino)hexyl]acetamide, **2b:** *N*1-[3-({3-[(1,2,3,4-tetrahydroacridin -9-yl)amino]propyl}amino)propyl]-2-(7-hydroxy-2-oxo-2*H*-chromen-4-yl)acetamide, **2c:** 2-(7-hydroxy-2-oxo-2*H*-chromen-4-yl)-*N*-[3-[2-[3-(1,2,3,4-tetrahydroacridin-9-ylamino) propylamino]ethylamino]propyl]acetamide (Figure 7) [1] were dissolved in dimethyl sulfoxide (DMSO, Fluka) to a final concentration of 5 × 10^{-2} M.

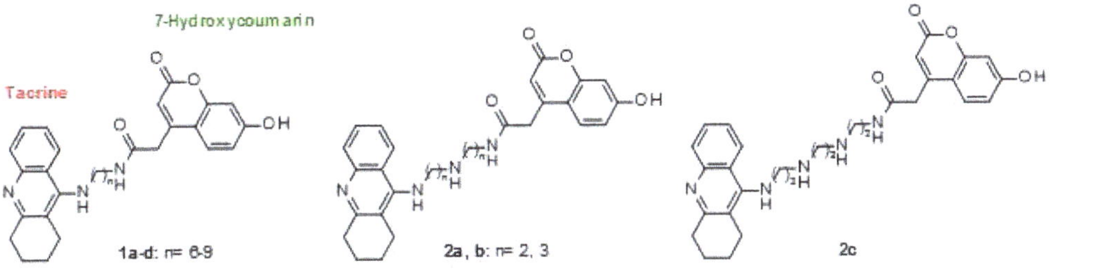

Figure 7. Structure of tacrine-coumarin hybrid molecules (derivatives **1a–1d** and **2a–2c**) [1].

4.2. Topoisomerase Relaxation Assay

The effects of compounds **1a–2c** on the relaxation of plasmid DNA with human topoisomerase I (*h*TOPI) were investigated using negatively supercoiled plasmid *p*BR322 (0.5 × 10^{-6} g) incubated for 30 min at 37 °C with 2 units of *h*TOPI (Inspiralis, Ltd., Norwich, UK) in both the presence and absence of the studied tacrine-coumarin hybrid molecules at concentrations of 5, 30 and 60 × 10^{-6} M, respectively. The method used to perform the experiment of TOPOII has been published previously [37].

4.3. Cell Culture

Human lung carcinoma cell lines A549 were purchased from the American Type Culture Collection (ATCC, Rockville, MD, USA). The cells were incubated in Kaighn's modification of F-12 Ham Nutrient Mixture supplemented with 10% fetal bovine serum (FBS) and antibiotics (1% Antibiotic-Antimycotic 100 × and 50 × 10^{-3} g L^{-1} gentamicin; Biosera) at 37 °C, 95% humidity and 5% CO_2. The cells (10,000/cm^{-2}) were seeded on

12-well μ-Chamber slides (ibidi GmbH, Martinsried, Germany) on 6, 12 and 96-well plates (TPP, Trasadingen, Switzerland) and left to settle for 24 h. This incubation method has been published previously [39].

4.4. Intracellular Localization and Cytotoxicity Assays

The derivatives were visualized in cells with an Argon Laser at 488 nm and fluorescence was captured at a range of 510–560 nm with identical exposure parameters used for all samples. Microphotographs were taken with a 100 × oil lens and were then captured and analysed using LAS AF software (Leica Microsystems, Mannheim, Germany).

Floating and adherent cells were harvested both 6 and 24 h after treatment with the derivatives, washed in PBS and resuspended in Hank's balanced salt solution (HBSS). Intracellular levels of derivatives were detected using a BD FACSCalibur flow cytometer (Becton Dickinson, San Jose, CA, USA) and determined based on fluorescence excitation at 488 nm. Fluorescence was detected via a 530/30 nm band-pass filter (FL-1), 585/42 band-pass filter (FL-2) and 670 nm long-pass filter (FL-3). The results were analyzed using FlowJo software (TreeStar Inc., Ashland, OR, USA).

MTT assays were added to the cells in a 96-well plate (at a final concentration of 0.5 g L^{-1}) 24 and 48 h after treatment with the derivatives [39]. The absorbance (λ = 584 nm) was measured using a BMG FLUOstar Optima (BMG Labtechnologies GmbH, Offenburg, Germany). The results were evaluated as percentages of the absorbance of the untreated control. IC_{50} values for each derivative were extrapolated from a sigmoidal fit to the metabolic activity data using OriginPro 8.5.0 SR1 (OriginLab Corp., Northampton, MA, USA).

For an assessment of total cell numbers and viability within individual experimental groups, floating and adherent cells were harvested 24 h after treatment with the studied derivatives and evaluated using a Bürker chamber (Paul Marienfeld GmbH&Co.KG, Lauda-Königshofen) with eosin staining. The total cell number was expressed as a percentage of the untreated control of the total cell number. Viability was expressed as a percentage of viable, eosin negative cells.

Details of the experiment with flow cytometric analysis have been published previously [38]. The DNA content was analysed using a BD FACSCalibur flow cytometer (Becton Dickinson) with a 488 nm argon-ion excitation laser, and fluorescence was detected via a 585/42 nm band-pass filter (FL-2). ModFit 3.0 software (Verity Software House, Topsham, ME, USA) was used to generate DNA content frequency histograms and to quantify the percentage of cells in the individual cell cycle phases.

4.5. Clonogenic Assay

The cells were counted using a Bürker chamber with eosin staining and 800 viable cells per well were seeded in 6-well plates. After 7 days of incubation under standard conditions, the cells in the plates were fixed and stained with 1% methylene blue dye in methanol. Visualized colonies were scanned, counted and the results were evaluated as percentages of the untreated control.

4.6. Statistical Analysis

Data were analyzed using a one-way ANOVA with Tukey´s post-test and are expressed as the mean ± standard deviation (SD) of at least three independent experiments. The experimental groups treated with the derivatives were compared with the control group: * $p < 0.05$.

5. Conclusions

This study has investigated a series of novel derivatives with both tacrine and coumarin pharmacophores, compounds **1a–2c**. Our results suggest that the novel derivatives had completely inhibited topoisomerase activity at a concentration of 60 × 10^{-6} M. The presence and content of the novel tacrine-coumarin hybrid molecules after introduction to A549 human adherent lung carcinoma cell lines were also investigated using confocal microscopy. Only compound **1d** was found to be present in the cell lines to a substantial degree. The IC_{50} values which were determined in this assay show that A549 cancer cell lines are more sensitive to the effect of compounds **1c** and **1d** (IC_{50} = 27.04 and 21.22 $\times 10^{-6}$ M, respectively after 48 h) than to the other compounds in the series. A simultaneous analysis of viability showed that higher concentrations of compounds **1c** and **1d** had a weaker but nonetheless significant effect on cell survival. These results indicate that compounds **1c** and **1d** are capable of influencing total cell numbers and viability in a concentration-dependent manner. The findings presented in this paper suggest that these tacrine-coumarin molecules exhibit promising potential as topoisomerase I inhibitors with anticancer activity against A549 human adherent lung carcinoma cells in addition to their well-known anticholinesterase effects [1] and may also serve as BSA-interacting agents [40]. These features would be of considerable use in the development of drugs with enhanced or more selective effects and greater clinical efficacy.

Author Contributions: Material preparation, data collection and analysis were performed by E.K., M.H., S.H. and M.K.; R.J., J.V., J.Š., P.F. performed and analyzed the cancer cell line experiments. The first draft of the manuscript was written by M.K. and all authors commented on earlier versions of the manuscript. All authors have read and agreed to the published version of the manuscript.

Funding: This research was funded by the Grant Project of the Ministry of Education, Science, Research and Sport of the Slovak Republic VEGA 1/0016/18, MH CZ-DRO (UHHK, 00179906) and Operational Programs Research and Innovations for the Medical University Scientific Park in Košice project (MediPark, Košice-Phase II.), ITMS2014+313011D103; Operational Program Integrated Infrastructure, project "NANOVIR", ITMS: 313011AUW7, cofinanced by the European Fund of Regional Progress.

Data Availability Statement: The data presented in this study are available on request from the corresponding author.

Acknowledgments: The authors are grateful to Gavin Cowper for assistance with the manuscript.

Conflicts of Interest: The authors declare no conflict of interest.

Sample Availability: Samples of the compounds **1c** and **1d** are available from the authors.

References

1. Hamulakova, S.; Poprac, P.; Jomova, K.; Brezova, V.; Lauro, P.; Drostinova, L.; Jun, D.; Sepsova, V.; Hrabinova, M.; Soukup, O.; et al. Targeting copper (II)-induced oxidative stress and the acetylcholinesterase system in Alzheimer's disease using multifunctional tacrine-coumarin hybrid molecules. *J. Inorg. Biochem.* **2016**, *161*, 52–62. [CrossRef] [PubMed]
2. Meng, T.; Qin, Q.P.; Wang, Z.R.; Peng, L.T.; Zou, H.H.; Gan, Z.-Y.; Tan, M.-X.; Wang, K.; Liang, F.-P. Synthesis and biological evaluation of substituted 3-(2′-benzimidazolyl) coumarin platinum (II) complexes as new telomerase inhibitors. *J. Inorg. Biochem.* **2018**, *189*, 143–150. [CrossRef] [PubMed]
3. Menezes, J.C.J.M.D.S.; Diederich, M.F. Natural dimers of coumarin; chalcones, and resveratrol and the link between structure and pharmacology. *Eur. J. Med. Chem.* **2019**, *182*, 111637. [CrossRef]
4. Akkol, K.E.; Genç, Y.; Karpuz, B.; Sobarzo-Sánchez, E.; Capasso, R. Coumarins and coumarin-related compounds in pharmacotherapy of cancer. *Cancers* **2020**, *12*, 1959. [CrossRef]
5. Carniero, A.; Matos, M.J.; Uriarte, E.; Santana, L. Trending topics on coumarin and its derivatives. *Molecules* **2021**, *26*, 501. [CrossRef]
6. Goud, N.S.; Kumar, P.; Bharath, R.W. Recent developments of target based coumarin derivatives as potential anticancer agents. *Mini-Rev. Med. Chem.* **2020**, *20*, 1754–1766. [CrossRef]
7. Al-Warhi, T.; Sabt, A.; Elkaeed, E.B.; Eldehna, W.M. Recent advancements of coumarin-based anticancer agents: An up-to-date Review. *Bioorg. Chem.* **2020**, *103*, 104163. [CrossRef]
8. Endo, S.; Oguri, H.; Segawa, J.; Kawai, M.; Hu, D.; Xia, S.; Okada, T.; Irie, K.; Fujii, S.; Gouda, H.; et al. Development of novel AKR1C3 inhibitors as new potential treatment for castration-resistant prostate cancer. *Med. Chem.* **2020**, *63*, 10396–10411. [CrossRef] [PubMed]
9. Finn, G.; Kenealy, E.; Creaven, B.; Egan, D. In vitro cytotoxic potential and mechanism of action of selected coumarins; using human renal cell lines. *Cancer Lett.* **2002**, *183*, 61–68. [CrossRef]
10. Nautiyal, J.; Banerjee, S.; Kanwar, S.S.; Yu, Y.; Patel, B.B.; Sarkar, F.H.; Majumdar, A.P. Curcumin enhances dasatinib-induced inhibition of growth and transformation of colon cancer cells. *Int. J. Cancer* **2011**, *128*, 951–961. [CrossRef] [PubMed]

11. Purohit, A.; Foster, P.A. Steroid sulfatase inhibitors for estrogen- and androgen-dependent cancers. *J. Endocrinol.* **2012**, *212*, 99–110. [CrossRef]
12. Pádua, D.; Rocha, E.; Gargiulo, D.R.; Ramos, A.A. Bioactive compounds from brown seaweeds: Phloroglucinol, Fucoxanthin and Fucoidan as promising therapeutic agents against breast cancer. *Phytochem. Lett.* **2015**, *14*, 91–98. [CrossRef]
13. Curini, M.; Cravotto, G.; Epifano, F.; Giannone, G. Chemistry and biological activity of natural and synthetic prenyloxycoumarins. *Curr. Med. Chem.* **2006**, *13*, 199–222. [CrossRef]
14. Chirieac, L.R.; Dacic, S. Target therapies in lung cancer. *Surg. Pathol. Clin.* **2010**, *3*, 71–82. [CrossRef]
15. Meng, Y.; Bai, X.; Huang, Y.; He, L.; Zhang, Z.; Li, X.; Cui, D.; Zang, X. Basic fibroblast growth factor signaling regulates cancer stem cells in lung cancer A549 cells. *J. Pharm. Pharm.* **2019**, *71*, 1412–1420. [CrossRef] [PubMed]
16. Kumar, M.; Singla, R.; Dandriyal, J.; Jaitak, V. Coumarin derivatives as anticancer agents for lung cancer therapy: A review. *Anticancer Agents Med. Chem.* **2018**, *18*, 964–984. [CrossRef] [PubMed]
17. Hueso-Falcon, I.; Amesty, A.; Anaissi-Alfonso, L.; Lozenzo-Castrillejo, I.; Machin, F.; Estevez-Braun, A. Synthesis and biological evaluation of naphtoquinone-coumarin conjugates ass topoisomerase II inhibitors. *Bioorg. Med. Chem. Lett.* **2017**, *27*, 484–489. [CrossRef] [PubMed]
18. Liang, X.; Wu, Q.; Luan, S.; Yin, Z.; He, C.; Yin, L.; He, C.; Yin, L.; Zou, Y.; Yuan, Z.; et al. A comprehensive review of topoisomerase inhibitors as anticancer agents in the past decade. *Eur. J. Med. Chem.* **2019**, *171*, 129–168. [CrossRef] [PubMed]
19. Paul, K.; Bindal, S.; Luxami, V. Synthesis of new conjugated coumarin–benzimidazole hybrids and their anticancer activity. *Bioorg. Med. Chem. Lett.* **2013**, *23*, 3667–3672. [CrossRef]
20. Chen, H.; Li, S.; Yao, Y.; Zhou, L.; Zhao, J.; Gu, Y.; Wang, K.; Li, X. Design, synthesis, and anti-tumor activities of novel triphenylethylene-coumarin hybrids, and their interactions with ct-DNA. *Bioorg. Med. Chem. Lett.* **2013**, *23*, 4785–4789. [CrossRef]
21. Musa, M.A.; Badisa, V.L.; Latinwo, L.M.; Patterson, T.A.; Owens, M.A. Coumarin-based benzopyranone derivatives induced apoptosis in human lung (A549) cancer cells. *Anticancer Res.* **2012**, *32*, 4271–4276.
22. Vijay Avin, B.R.; Thirusangu, P.; Lakshmi Ranganatha, V.; Firdouse, A.; Prabhakar, B.T.; Khanum, S.A. Synthesis and tumor inhibitory activity of novel coumarin analogs targeting angiogenesis and apoptosis. *Eur. J. Med. Chem.* **2014**, *75*, 211–221. [CrossRef] [PubMed]
23. Kozurkova, M.; Kristian, P. Biological characteristics of tacrine derivatives. In *Acridine isothiocyanates: Chemistry and Biology*; Kristian, P., Ed.; Lambert Academic Publishing: Saarbrücken, Germany, 2014; pp. 206–233.
24. Kozurkova, M.; Hamulakova, S.; Gazova, Z.; Paulikova, H.; Kristian, P. Neuroactive multifunctional tacrine congeners with cholinesterase, anti-amyloid aggregation and neuroprotective properties. *Pharmaceuticals* **2011**, *7*, 4382–4418. [CrossRef]
25. Agbo, E.N.; Gildenhuys, S.; Choong, Y.S.; Mphahlele, M.J.; More, G.K. Synthesis of furocoumarin-stilbene hybrids as potential multifunctional drugs against multiple biochemical targets associated with Alzheimer's disease. *Bioorg. Chem.* **2020**, *101*, 103997. [CrossRef]
26. Mansouri, A.; Haouzi, D.; Descatoire, V.; Demeilliers, C.H.; Sutton, A.; Vadrot, N.; Fromenty, B.; Feldman, G.; Pessayre, D.; Berson, A. Tacrine inhibits topoisomerase and DNA synthesis to cause mitochondrial DNA depletion and apoptosis in mouse liver. *Hepatology* **2003**, *38*, 715–725. [CrossRef] [PubMed]
27. Snyder, R.D.; Arone, M.R. Putative identification of functional interaction s between DNA intercalating agents and topoisomerase II using the V79 in vitro micronucleus assay. *Mutat. Res.* **2002**, *503*, 21–35. [CrossRef]
28. Krajňáková, L.; Pisarčíková, J.; Drajna, L.; Labudova, M.; Imrich, J.; Paulikova, H.; Kožurková, M. Intracellular distribution of new tacrine analogues as a potential cause of their cytotoxicity against human neuroblastoma cells SH-SY5Y. *Med. Chem. Res.* **2018**, *27*, 2353–2365. [CrossRef]
29. Sabolová, D.; Kristian, P.; Kožurková, M. Multifunctional properties of novel tacrine congeners: Cholinesterase inhibition and cytotoxic activity. *J. Appl. Tox.* **2018**, *38*, 1377–1387. [CrossRef]
30. Singh, H.; Vir Singh, J.; Bhagat, K.; Kaur Gulati, H.; Sanduja, M.; Kumar, N.; Kinarivala, N.; Sharma, S. Rational approaches, design strategies, structure activity relationship and mechanistic insights for therapeutic coumarin hybrids. *Bioorg. Med. Chem.* **2019**, *27*, 3477–3510. [CrossRef] [PubMed]
31. Thomas, A.; Bates, S.; Figg, W.D.; Pommier, Y. DNA Topoisomerase targeting drugs. *Holl. -Frei. Cancer Med.* **2017**, 1–17.
32. Shi, W.L.; Marcus, S.; Lowary, T. Cytotoxicity and topoisomerase I/II inhibition of glycosylated 2-phenyl-indoles, 2-phenyl-benzo[*b*]thiophenes and 2-phenyl-benzo[*b*] furans. *Bioorg. Med. Chem.* **2011**, *19*, 603–612. [CrossRef] [PubMed]
33. Konkoľová, E.; Janočková, J.; Perjési, P.; Vašková, J.; Kožurková, M. Selected ferrocenyl chalcones as DNA/BSA-interacting agents and inhibitors of DNA topoisomerase I and II activity. *J. Organomet. Chem.* **2018**, *861*, 1–9. [CrossRef]
34. Solárová, Z.; Kello, M.; Hamuľáková, S.; Mirossay, L.; Solár, P. Anticancer effect of tacrine-coumarin derivatives on diverse human and mouse cancer cell lines. *Acta Chim. Slov.* **2018**, *65*, 875–881. [CrossRef] [PubMed]
35. Hu, M.-K. Synthesis and in-vitro anticancer evaluation of bis-tacrine congeners. *J. Pharm. Pharm.* **2000**, *53*, 83–88. [CrossRef] [PubMed]
36. Roldan-Pena, J.M.; Alejandre-Ramos, D.; Lopez, O.; Maya, I.; Lagunes, I.; Padron, J.M.; Pena-Altamira, L.E.; Bartolini, M.; Monti, B.; Bolognesi, M.L.; et al. New tacrine dimers with antioxidant linkers as dual drugs: Anti-Alzheimer´s and antiproliferative agents. *Eur. J. Med. Chem.* **2017**, *138*, 761–773. [CrossRef]

37. Janočková, J.; Korabečný, J.; Plšíková, J.; Babková, K.; Konkoľová, E.; Kučerová, D.; Vargová, J.; Koval', J.; Jendželovský, R.; Fedoročko, P.; et al. In vitro investigating of anticancer activity of new 7-MEOTA-tacrine heterodimers. *J. Enz. Inhib. Med. Chem.* **2019**, *34*, 877–897. [CrossRef] [PubMed]
38. Brunet, C.L.; Gunby, R.H.; Benson, R.S.P.; Hickman, J.A.; Watson, A.J.M.; Brady, G. Commitment to cell death measured by loss of clonogenicity is separable from the appearance of apoptotic markers. *Cell Death Differ.* **1998**, *5*, 107–115. [CrossRef] [PubMed]
39. Janočková, J.; Plšíková, J.; Kašpárková, J.; Brabec, V.; Jendželovský, R.; Mikeš, J.; Koval', J.; Hamuľaková, S.; Fedoročko, P.; Kuča, K.; et al. Inhibition of DNA topoisomerases I and II and growth inhibition of HL-60 cells by novel acridine-based compounds. *Eur. J. Med. Chem.* **2015**, *76*, 192–202. [CrossRef]
40. Konkoľová, E.; Hudáčová, M.; Hamuľaková, S.; Kožurková, M. Spectroscopic evaluation of novel tacrine-coumarin hybrids as BSA-interacting agents. *Org. Med. Chem. Int. J.* **2019**, *8*, 1–7.

molecules

MDPI

Article

Structural Basis of Beneficial Design for Effective Nicotinamide Phosphoribosyltransferase Inhibitors

Sei-ichi Tanuma [1,2,*], Kiyotaka Katsuragi [2], Takahiro Oyama [3], Atsushi Yoshimori [4], Yuri Shibasaki [2], Yasunobu Asawa [5], Hiroaki Yamazaki [3], Kosho Makino [6], Miwa Okazawa [1], Yoko Ogino [2,7], Yoshimi Sakamoto [8], Miyuki Nomura [8], Akira Sato [2], Hideaki Abe [3], Hiroyuki Nakamura [5], Hideyo Takahashi [6], Nobuhiro Tanuma [8] and Fumiaki Uchiumi [7]

1 Department of Genomic Medicinal Science, Research Institute for Science and Technology, Organization for Research Advancement, Tokyo University of Science, Noda, Chiba 278-8510, Japan; miwa.okazawa@rs.tus.ac.jp
2 Department of Biochemistry, Faculty of Pharmaceutical Sciences, Tokyo University of Science, Noda, Chiba 278-8510, Japan; 3b12023@alumni.tus.ac.jp (K.K.); yryr.sbsk040809@gmail.com (Y.S.); ogino@rs.tus.ac.jp (Y.O.); akirasat@rs.tus.ac.jp (A.S.)
3 Hinoki Shinyaku Co., Ltd., Chiyoda-ku, Tokyo 102-0084, Japan; takahiro.oyama@hinoki.co.jp (T.O.); hymanami@gmail.com (H.Y.); hideaki.abe@hinoki.co.jp (H.A.)
4 Institute for Theoretical Medicine Inc., Fujisawa, Kanagawa 251-0012, Japan; yoshimori@itmol.com
5 Laboratory for Chemistry and Life Science, Institute of Innovative Research, Tokyo Institute of Technology, Yokohama, Kanagawa 226-8503, Japan; asawa.y.aa@m.titech.ac.jp (Y.A.); hiro@res.titech.ac.jp (H.N.)
6 Department of Medicinal Chemistry, Faculty of Pharmaceutical Sciences, Tokyo University of Science, Noda, Chiba 278-8510, Japan; kosho-maki@rs.tus.ac.jp (K.M.); hide-tak@rs.tus.ac.jp (H.T.)
7 Department of Gene Regulation, Faculty of Pharmaceutical Sciences, Tokyo University of Science, Noda, Chiba 278-8510, Japan; f_uchiumi@rs.tus.ac.jp
8 Division of Cancer Chemotherapy, Miyagi Cancer Center Research Institute, Natori, Miyagi 981-1293, Japan; yoshimi.sk.88@gmail.com (Y.S.); nomu.miyu@gmail.com (M.N.); ntanuma@med.tohoku.ac.jp (N.T.)
* Correspondence: tanuma@rs.tus.ac.jp

Academic Editors: Marialuigia Fantacuzzi and Alessandra Ammazzalorso
Received: 22 July 2020; Accepted: 6 August 2020; Published: 10 August 2020

Abstract: Inhibition of nicotinamide phosphoribosyltransferase (NAMPT) is an attractive therapeutic strategy for targeting cancer metabolism. So far, many potent NAMPT inhibitors have been developed and shown to bind to two unique tunnel-shaped cavities existing adjacent to each active site of a NAMPT homodimer. However, cytotoxicities and resistances to NAMPT inhibitors have become apparent. Therefore, there remains an urgent need to develop effective and safe NAMPT inhibitors. Thus, we designed and synthesized two close structural analogues of NAMPT inhibitors, azaindole–piperidine (**3a**)- and azaindole–piperazine (**3b**)-motif compounds, which were modified from the well-known NAMPT inhibitor FK866 (**1**). Notably, **3a** displayed considerably stronger enzyme inhibitory activity and cellular potency than did **3b** and **1**. The main reason for this phenomenon was revealed to be due to apparent electronic repulsion between the replaced nitrogen atom (N1) of piperazine in **3b** and the Nδ atom of His191 in NAMPT by our in silico binding mode analyses. Indeed, **3b** had a lower binding affinity score than did **3a** and **1**, although these inhibitors took similar stable chair conformations in the tunnel region. Taken together, these observations indicate that the electrostatic enthalpy potential rather than entropy effects inside the tunnel cavity has a significant impact on the different binding affinity of **3a** from that of **3b** in the disparate enzymatic and cellular potencies. Thus, it is better to avoid or minimize interactions with His191 in designing further effective NAMPT inhibitors.

Keywords: nicotinamide phosphoribosyltransferase; NAD^+ biosynthesis; inhibitor; azacyclohexane; anticancer drug; drug design; enthalpy effect

1. Introduction

Nicotinamide adenine dinucleotide (NAD^+) is a critical molecule in control of numerous basic cellular processes, such as ATP production and maintenance of cellular integrity and genome stability [1–4]. It not only serves as a cofactor for redox bioreactions but can also be a substrate for multiple NAD^+-consuming enzymes, such as poly(ADP-ribose) polymerases, mono-ADP-ribosyltransferases and sirtuins, participating in the epigenetic regulation of DNA transaction (transcription, replication, repair and recombination), cellular signaling processes and calcium homeostasis, and thereby in cell proliferation, differentiation and death [3–8]. Given the biological importance of this molecule, mammalian cells have evolved multiple biosynthetic pathways to produce NAD^+; it is synthesized from tryptophan, nicotinic acid and nicotinamide (NAM)/nicotinamide riboside via *de novo*, Preiss–Handler and salvage pathways, respectively [1–4,9–11].

As NAD^+ is consumed through many enzymatic processes, accelerated NAD^+ depletion is often characteristic in cancer cells [9–12]. To rapidly replenish the NAD^+ pool, cancer cells rely heavily on the NAM salvage pathway that backs NAM to NAD^+ in two steps primarily catalyzed by nicotinamide phosphoribosyltransferase (NAMPT) [13–17]. Furthermore, in various types of cancer cells, NAMPT is found to be up-regulated [8,13,16,17], although the molecular mechanisms that dictate the salvage pathway choice remain elusive. Thus, NAMPT is considered an attractive target for the development of new anticancer drugs and therapies [18–31].

NAMPT, which functions as a homodimer with two unique tunnel-shaped cavities existing adjacent to each active site at the dimer interface, catalyzes the rate-limiting primary step of the salvage pathway, the transfer of phosphoribosyl residue from 5-phosphoribosyl-1-pyrophosphate (PRPP) to NAM to produce nicotinamide mononucleotide (NMN) (Figure 1) [1–4,32–34]. Many NAMPT inhibitors, such as FK866 (**1**), CSH-828, GNE0617 and STF-11880, which bind to the tunnel cavity of NAMPT, have been reported to exert anti-tumor suppression effects and have progressed to clinical trials [18,23–25,30]. However, cytotoxicities dominated by gastrointestinal symptoms and thrombocytopenia and resistance to NAMPT inhibitors have become apparent [23,35–37]. Therefore, there remains an urgent need to develop effective and safe anticancer NAMPT inhibitors for cancer chemotherapy. Thus, detailed insights into the tunnel structure of NAMPT are required to generate effective NAMPT inhibitors with a better therapeutic index and that can overcome resistance.

In the present study, we designed and synthesized two close structural analogues of NAMPT inhibitors **3a** and **3b**, which were modified from the best explored NAMPT inhibitor 1 [18,35]. Interestingly, we showed that **3a** has a considerably stronger enzyme inhibitory activity and cellular potency than does **3b** or **1**. Furthermore, using these inhibitors as chemical probes, we characterized the inhibitor-targeting tunnel cavity of NAMPT. Importantly, our in silico binding mode analyses of these inhibitors with the tunnel cavity of NAMPT revealed that there is apparent electronic repulsion only between the nitrogen atom of piperazine in **3b** and the Nδ atom of His191 in NAMPT. These findings indicate that the electrostatic enthalpy potential inside the tunnel region has a significant impact on the different binding affinity of **3a** from **3b** in the disparate cellular potencies. Thus, these results provide new insights into the design for further effective NAMPT inhibitors for cancer chemotherapies.

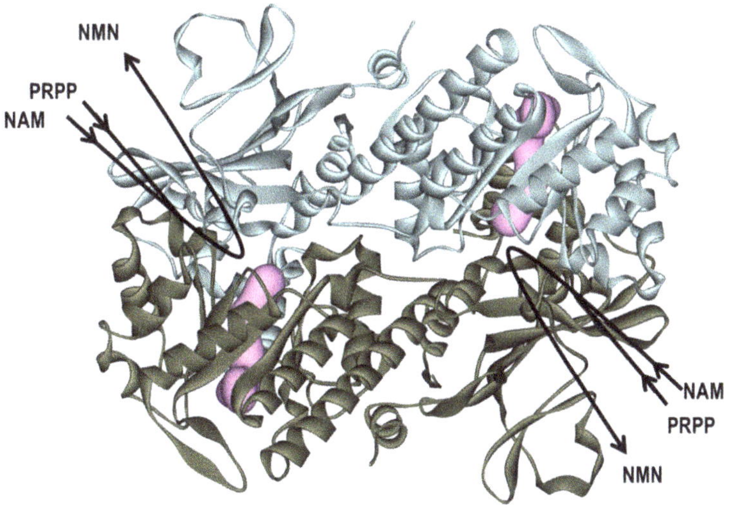

Figure 1. Overview of the human (h) nicotinamide phosphoribosyltransferase (NAMPT) as the dimer form and its enzyme reaction. The homodimer structure of hNAMPT (PDB Code: 2GVJ) [38–42] is shown in the ribbon diagram colored light blue and brown, respectively. The two tunnel-shaped cavities near the active sites in the hNAMPT molecule are shown in magenta shading. NAMPT catalyzes the conversion of nicotinamide (NAM) and phosphoribosyl pyrophosphate (PRPP) to produce nicotinamide mononucleotide (NMN).

2. Results and Discussion

2.1. Synthesis and Biochemical Properties of *3a* and *3b*

Many NAMPT inhibitors bind to the tunnel-shaped cavity of NAMPT (Figure 1), although the role of this tunnel in NAMPT function remains unknown [18–31]. These inhibitors have a unique pharmacophore consisting of three parts (Figure 2): head (a pyridine-like aromatic moiety), linker (a tunnel-interacting moiety) and tail (a solvent-exposed bulky group). To get more valuable insights into the tunnel cavity for the development of effective NAMPT inhibitors, we structure-basically designed and synthesized two close structural analogues of NAMPT inhibitors, namely azaindole–piperidine (**3a**)- and azaindole–piperazine (**3b**)-motif compounds, which were modified from the head and linker moieties of **1** (Figure 2, Scheme 1). Since the tail acts as a packing moiety against the solvent exposed tunnel exit surface, the tail structures of **3a** and **3b** were fixed as the same benzoyl group of **1**. The nitrogen-containing aromatic heads present in many NAMPT inhibitors mimic the natural NAM substrate of the enzyme [18–31]. However, the head moiety of vinylpyridine ring of **1** (Figure 2) is known to be able to non-specifically interact with proteins [43,44]. Based on this knowledge, we first replaced this head to the 5-azaindole heterocyclic ring to improve the specificity to NAMPT (Figure 2). Secondly, as the linker moiety of azacyclohexane may be considered to become a critical motif for NAMPT inhibitory activity, we synthesized a close structural set of piperidine (**3a**)- and piperazine (**3b**)-motif NAMPT inhibitors according to the methods of Bair et al. [45] and Vogel et al. [46], respectively (Scheme 1).

3a
3b
1 (FK866)

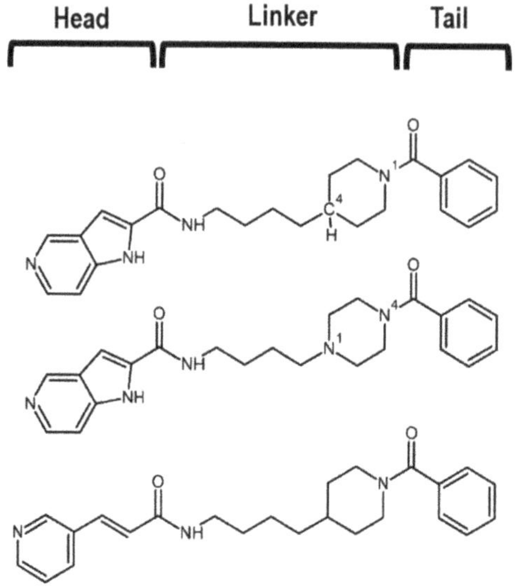

Figure 2. Chemical structures of **3a**, **3b** and **1**.

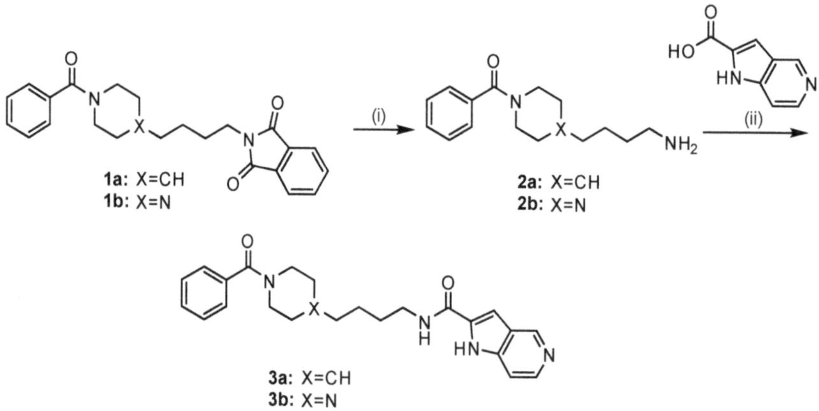

Scheme 1. Synthetic route of compounds **3a** and **3b**. Reagents and conditions: **(i)** NH_2NH_2, EtOH, r.t. to reflux, 2 h; **(ii)** 1*H*-pyrro[3,2-c]pyridine-2-carboxylic acid, EDC-HCl, DIPEA, DMF, r.t., 24 h. The targets **3a** and **3b** were prepared according to the methods of [45,46], respectively, with slight modifications.

To compare the NAMPT inhibitory activities of **3a**, **3b** and **1**, we determined the IC_{50} values by the titration curves from the standard calorimetric enzyme-cycling assay [31,36,37]. As shown in Figure 3a, the inhibitory activity of **3a** (IC_{50} = 0.11 μM) was approximately 5-fold stronger than that of **1** (IC_{50} = 0.52 μM). This result suggests that the replacement of vinylpyridine with an azaindole ring could improve anti-NAMPT activity. The binding mode analyses of these inhibitors on the NAMPT molecule support this observation, as described in the next section; a hydrogen bond formed between the N1 atom of azaindole and Asp219 of NAMPT (Figure 4b). Surprisingly, the substitution of piperidine (**3a**) with piperazine (**3b**) resulted in a dramatic loss in inhibitory activity against NAMPT; the inhibitory activity of **3b** (IC_{50} = 5.06 μM) was shown to be about 50-fold weaker than that of **3a**. The inhibition curve of **3a** was much steeper than that of **3b**, suggesting that incubation with **3a** resulted in the formation of an entity capable of extremely tight binding to the tunnel cavity of NAMPT. From these observations, we suspect that unfavorable interactions between the piperazine moiety of **3b** and the tunnel cavity of NAMPT were responsible for the considerably weak anti-NAMPT activity.

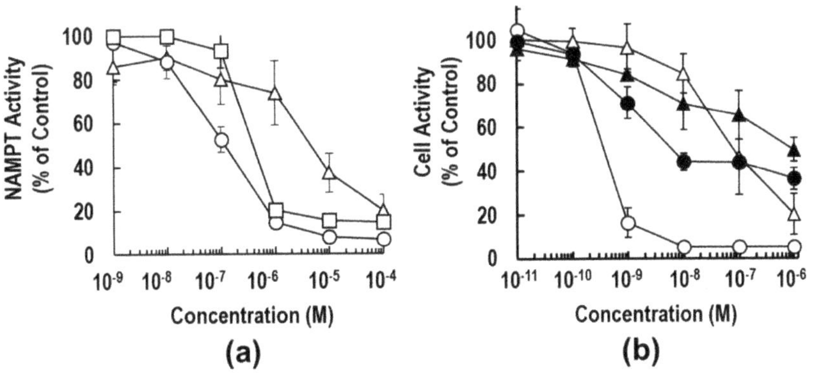

Figure 3. Biochemical properties of **3a** and **3b**. (**a**) The inhibitory activities of **3a** (open circle), **3b** (open triangle) and **1** (open square) against NAMPT enzyme were examined, as described previously [31,36,37]. NAMPT activity was measured using a coupled-enzyme reaction system (CycLex NAMPT colorimetric assay kit) in 96-well plate format using the one-step method. Data are the averages of three independent experiments, and the bars indicate the standard error (SE) values. (**b**) The anti-proliferative effects of **3a** (circle) and **3b** (triangle) on HCT116 cells were investigated as described previously [31,36,37]. HCT116 cells were treated with the indicated concentrations of each inhibitor with (closed symbol) or without (open symbol) 100 μM NMN for 72 h. The cell activity (% of control) was measured by use of the WST-8 assay. Data are presented as the means of three independent experiments ± SE, and the bars indicate the SE values.

To confirm the marked differences of anti-NAMPT activities between **3a** and **3b**, the anti-proliferation effects of these inhibitors on the human colon cancer cell line HCT116 were examined after continuous exposure for 72 h [31,36,37]. As shown in Figure 3b, compound **3b** displayed significantly weaker cell activity; the 50% effective concentration (EC_{50}) value was calculated to be 87.5 nM, which was approximately 200-fold higher than that of **3a** (EC_{50} = 0.48 nM). These results of the different inhibition degrees in cell-based assay from those in enzyme assay (Figure 3) paralleled observations by others that the degrees of potency of cell-based assessments were not always identical with those of NAMPT enzymatic inhibition [26,28,47]. In addition, there was little cytotoxicity on non-cancer cell lines, such as TIG-120, WI38 and MRC-5 cells. Both **3a** and **3b** caused more than 90% reduction of NAD^+ levels in the cancer cells after 24 h-treatment and thereby induced cell death. Furthermore, supplementation of the product of NAMPT, NMN, to the cell culture medium could significantly rescue HCT116 cells from cell death by treatment with **3a** or **3b** (Figure 3b). Additionally, the dose–response curves of **1** were similar to those of **3a**. These results confirmed that NAMPT is a target of both inhibitors. Collectively, these results indicate that the substitution of one carbon (C) atom of the piperidine moiety in **3a** for a nitrogen (N) atom (piperazine moiety in **3b**) exerts a critical effect on the anti-NAMPT activity.

2.2. *Binding Modes of **3a** and **3b** to the Tunnel Cavity of NAMPT*

To understand the different NAMPT inhibitory activities of **3a** and **3b**, we analyzed their binding modes to NAMPT (PDB Code: 2GVJ [38–42]) by our in silico binding mode analyses using RDKit [48] and LigandScout [49]. The superimpositions of these inhibitors in the tunnel cavity revealed that they adopted almost identical chair binding forms as with the case in **1** (Figure 4a). The NAMPT residues that contacted these inhibitors were observed in very similar locations in the structure. These results indicate that the binding modes of **3a** and **3b** in the tunnel cavity of NAMPT do not significantly alter as compared with that of **1**.

When observed closely, the position of the head regions of **3a** and **3b** in the tunnel cavity were nearly identical to that of **1** (Figure 4b). The subtle shifts observed in **3a** and **3b** from the position of **1** may have been introduced by their slightly different orientations of the head-azaindole bicyclic ring from the head-pyridine ring of **1** inside the tunnel cavity of NAMPT. The azaindole rings of **3a** and **3b** were sandwiched between Phe193A and Tyr18B, forming tight aromatic π–π stacks like the pyridine ring of **1**. Additionally, the nitrogen atoms (N1) in the azaindole rings of **3a** and **3b** could interact with Asp219 of NAMPT by a hydrogen bond (Figure 4b), thus suggesting that they might be involved in the tighter specific binding of **3a** and **3b** to NAMPT than that of **1**.

However, this specific contacts of the head-azaindole moiety with NAMPT could not explain the discrepancy in the considerably weaker inhibitory activity of **3b** than that of **3a** or **1**. Therefore, to better understand this phenomenon, we focused on the importance of linker-motifs for the potencies of NAMPT inhibitors. Thus, we analyzed closely the binding forms of the linker-azacyclohexane motifs of **3a** and **3b** in the tunnel cavity of NAMPT. The carbon atom (C4) of piperidine in **3a** and nitrogen atom (N1) of piperazine in **3b** were revealed to protrude approximately 1Å deeper into the NMA binding active site, as compared to the corresponding carbon atom of piperidine in **1**. Importantly, the electronic repulsion of the replaced nucleophilic N1 atom of piperazine in **3b** with the Nδ atom of the imidazole side chain of His191, located 3.82 Å away from the N1 atom, was revealed to occur (Figure 4c). In contrast, there was no electronic repulsion of the corresponding carbon atom of piperidine in **3a** with the Nδ atom as well as that of **1**. These results clearly show that the electronic repulsion interferes with the proper binding of **3b** to the tunnel cavity of NAMPT.

It is noteworthy that Zheng and colleagues have reported that the imidazole ring of His191 interacts with the linker aromatic group of GNE series inhibitors through a herringbone stacking [44,45,47]. Furthermore, NAMPT mutations, including H191R, D93del, Q388R, S165Y and G217V, have been reported to confer resistance to NAMPT inhibitors [50–52]. In addition, we have recently shown that an NAMPT mutation variant of HCT116 cells generated by continuously exposing cells to increasing concentrations of **1**, which confers cross-resistance to diverse NAMPT inhibitors, such as CHS-828, GNE-617 and STF-118804, was mapped to only H191R [36,37]. Thus, this His191 residue should be considered with higher priority in designing further effective NAMPT inhibitors. That is, it is preferable to avoid interactions with His191 in designing novel NAMPT inhibitors.

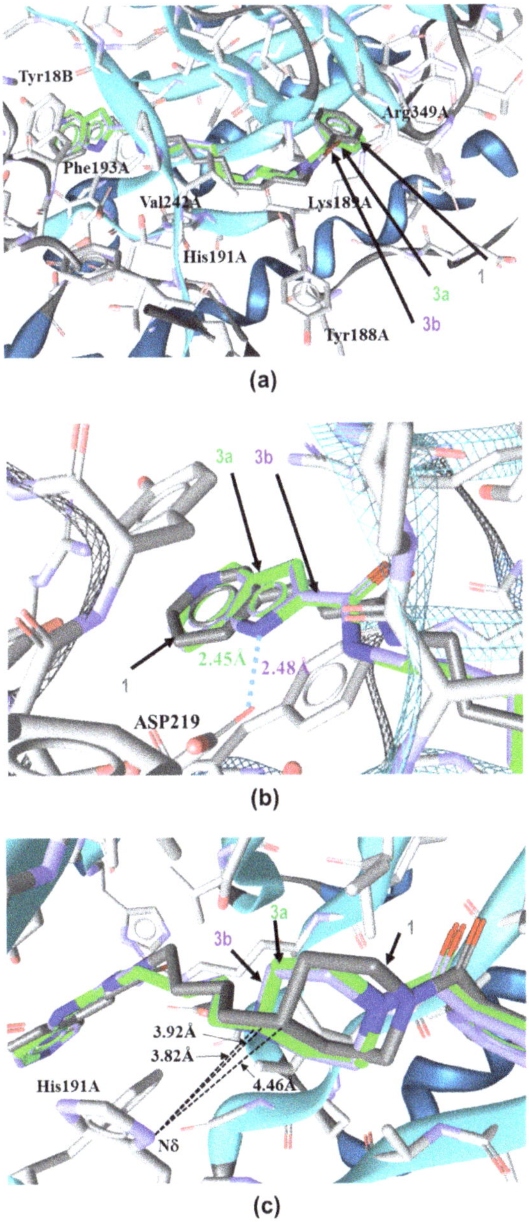

Figure 4. Binding modes of **3a**, **3b** and **1** in the tunnel cavity of NAMPT. (**a**) Binding modes of **3a, 3b** and **1** in the tunnel cavity of NAMPT were analyzed by our in silico binding mode analysis using RDKit [48] and LigandScout [49]. (**b**) Close-up view of head regions of these three NAMPT inhibitors in the tunnel cavity of NAMPT using Open3DALIGN [53]. (**c**) Close-up view of the binding interactions of azacyclohexane-linker moieties of these NAMPT inhibitors with His191A located in the tunnel cavity of NAMPT. Carbons are colored green (**3a**), magenta (**3b**) and gray (**1**). Nitrogen and oxygen are colored blue and red, respectively.

2.3. Influence of Enthalpic Effects of 3a and 3b on the Interactions with Tunnel Cavity of NAMPT

The C-to-N conversion in the azacylohexane-linker moiety was considered to be possible to introduce some entropic differences in the compounds' abilities to interact with the tunnel cavity of NAMPT. Although piperazine and piperidine rings are known to form various conformations from chairs to half-chair and skewed boat-to-boat forms in aqueous solution [54], piperazine-containing **3b** and piperidine-containing **3a** took nearly identical positions as a chair form to that occupied by **1** in the tunnel cavity analyzed by in silico binding modes and crystal structure analyses [38–42] (Figure 4). In addition, both C4 in **3a** (Figure 5a) and tertiary amine-type nitrogen (N1) containing **3b** (Figure 5b) might prefer equatorial conformations to axial ones by 1,3-diaxial hydrogen interaction [54], taking a stable chair conformation in the tunnel cavity of NAMPT. Therefore, such entropic effects in **3a** and **3b** in the tunnel space of NAMPT may not be so different from each other. Thus, it is possible to consider that the dramatic differences in enzymatic and cellular potencies between **3a** and **3b** may be due to enthalpic effects rather than entropic effects inside the tunnel cavity of NAMPT.

To prove this hypothesis, we attempted to analyze the binding affinity scores of **3a** and **3b** to NAMPT (PDB Code: 2GVJ) by our in silico binding mode analyses using RDKit [48] and LigandScout [49], as described in Materials and Methods. Remarkably, the binding affinity scores of **3a** and **3b** (non-protonation form) (Figure 5b) were calculated to be −29.07 and −22.13 kJ/mol, respectively, while that of **1** (−28.05 kJ/mol) was near to the value of **3b** (Table 1). Thus, the piperidine-motif was revealed to be beneficial for **3a** potency and has valuable influences on the interaction with the tunnel cavity of NAMPT.

The N1 and N4 atoms in **3a** and **3b**, respectively, would take an sp^2-like bond, due to the effect of the proximity of the benzoyl group (R_2) on the lone pair (Figure 5a,b). In contrast, although it is hard to know whether or not the N1 atom of piperazine in **3b**, which takes an sp^3 bond like the C4 atom in **3a**, would be protonated in the tunnel cavity of NAMPT, it is possible to be protonated in physiological conditions. Thus, the binding affinity score of **3b** in the protonation state was measured by LigandScout. Interestingly, it was calculated to be −23.85 kJ/mol and was not as good as that of the non-protonated form (Table 1). In the protonated N1 atom, the electrostatic interaction becomes attractive to the Nδ of His 191 but repulsive against the protonated Nδ. However, as the imidazole ring of His has aromaticity, the positive charge introduced by protonation does not tend to be localized on the Nδ. Thus, the repulsion may not be so strong. In addition, it seems that a hydrogen bond between the protonated Nδ of His191 and the N1 atom in **3b** could not be formed, because the angle that NδH-N1 (piperazine) takes is 106.4°. Furthermore, of course, the influence of the hydrophobic amino acids in the tunnel region on the protonated N1 in **3b** cannot be ruled out, and they may negatively influence this interaction. Accordingly, the electrostatic enthalpy effects were suggested to interfere with the proper binding of **3b** to the tunnel cavity of NAMPT. For this reason, both the non-protonated and protonated forms of **3b** are suggested to have lower binding affinities to the tunnel cavity of NAMPT than does **3a**. These outcomes indicate that the electrostatic potential (enthalpy term) inside the tunnel region of NAMPT has a significant impact on the different binding affinity of **3b** from that of **3a**.

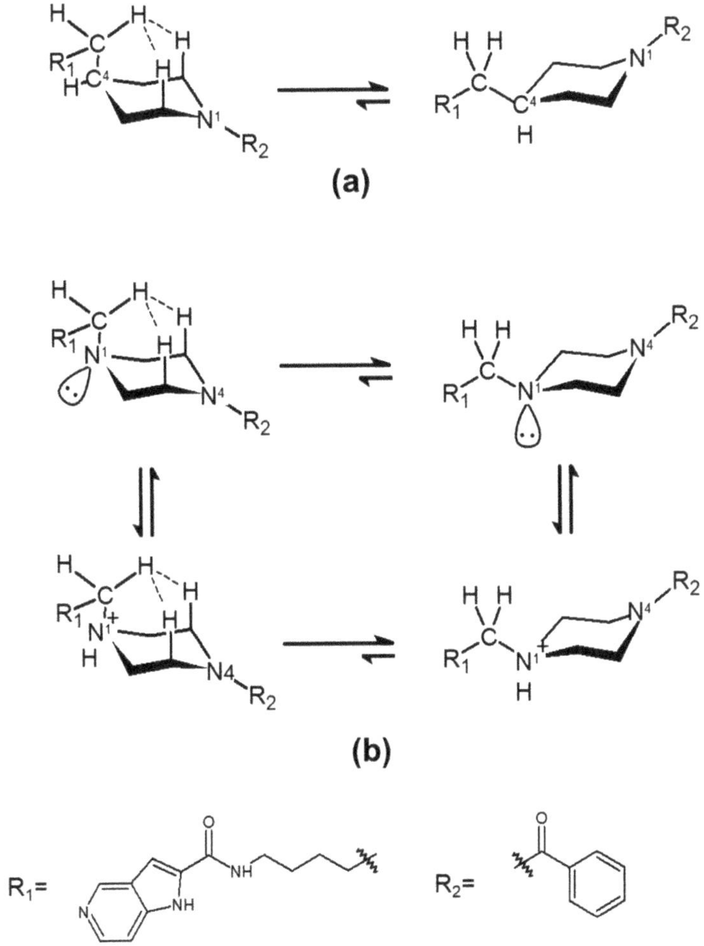

Figure 5. Stable conformers of **3a** and **3b** in the tunnel cavity of NAMPT. The conformational states of **3a** (**a**) and **3b** with its protonation form (**b**) in the tunnel cavity of NAMPT were analyzed by in silico binding mode analysis and crystal structure of **1** (PDB code: 2GVJ) [38–42]. The hydrogen interactions of axial-methylene with 1,3-diaxial hydrogens are represented by dashed lines.

Table 1. Biochemical properties and binding affinity scores of **3a** and **3b** NAMPT inhibitors.

Compound	IC_{50} [a] (μM)	Binding Affinity Score [b] (kJ/mol)	
		Non-Protonation	Protonation
3a (piperidine)	0.11	−29.07	-
3b (piperazine)	5.06	−22.13	−23.85
1 (piperidine)	0.52	−28.05	-

[a] The IC_{50} values of these three NAMPT inhibitors were determined by the titration curves in Figure 3a. [b] The binding affinity scores of these three inhibitors in the tunnel cavity of NAMPT were calculated by LigandScout [49].

3. Materials and Methods

3.1. *Enzymatic NAMPT Assay*

For the inhibitory effects of **3a** and **3b** on NAMPT activity, recombinant NAMPT activity was measured using a coupled-enzyme reaction system (CycLex NAMPT Colorimetric Assay Kit: MEDICAL & BIOLOGICAL LABORATORIES CO., LTD., Nagoya, Japan) according to the manufacturer's instructions, as described previously [31,36,37]. Briefly, NAMPT enzyme and tested compounds were put on the 96-well transparent plate. The mixture of the rest of contents (ATP, NAM, PRPP, nicotinamide nucleotide adenylyltransferase 1 (NMNAT1), water-soluble tetrazolium salts (WST-1), alcohol dehydrogenase, diaphorase and ethanol (EtOH)) were then added onto the wells. After a brief incubation, the absorbance of the samples was detected at 450 nm on every 10 min until 60 min using a SYNERGY HTX (BioTek Instruments, Inc.; Winooski, VT, USA). The inhibition rates were calculated by the initial slope of the absorbance of the tested samples divided by that of the control wells. The IC_{50} values for the samples were calculated by 4-parameter logistic regression using Image J 1.48v (https://imagej.nih.gov/ij/).

3.2. *Cells and Cell Culture*

HCT116 cell was obtained from American Type Culture Collection (ATCC) (Manassas, US) and cultured in Dulbecco's modified Eagle medium (DMEM) (FUJIFILM Wako Pure Chemical Corporation) supplemented with 10% of fetal bovine serum (Biosera Europe; Nuaillé, France), 100 Units/mL of penicillin G and 100 µg/mL of Streptomycin (FUJIFILM Wako Pure Chemical Corporation) [36,37].

3.3. *Cell Activity Assay*

One thousand HCT116 cells were inoculated into the 96-well transparent cell culture plate and cultured for 24 h. The medium was changed to new medium that contained the tested compounds and was further cultivated for 72 h. Following the culture, 1/10 volume of the WST-8 reagent (FUJIFILM Wako Pure Chemical Corporation) was added and incubated for 1 h. After the incubation, the absorbance of the samples was detected at 450 nm using a SYNERGY HTX (BioTek Instruments, Inc.). Cell activity was expressed as percentage of control cells treated with vehicle alone [31,36,37].

3.4. *In Silico Binding Mode and Binding Affinity Score Analyses*

The crystal structure of NAMPT was downloaded from the Protein Data Bank (PDB code: 2GVJ) for molecular binding mode analyses. In silico binding mode analyses were done using RDKit [48] and LigandScout [49]. First, 1000 conformations of each inhibitor were generated using the EmbedMultipleConfs and MMFFGetMoleculeForceField functions of RDKit. Second, the conformations of each inhibitor were aligned to the crystal structure of **1** using Open3DALIGN [53] implemented in RDKit. The conformation of each inhibitor, which has the highest alignment score, was selected. Third, energy minimization of the selected conformation of each inhibitor with NAMPT was performed, and then the binding affinity score of each inhibitor was calculated using LigandScout [49].

3.5. *Synthetic Procedures of the Target Compounds*

3.5.1. General Experimental Methods

^{1}H-NMR spectra were recorded at 400 MHz using a JEOL ECZ400 operating (JEOL Ltd.; Tokyo, Japan) at the indicated frequencies. Chemical shifts were expressed in ppm relative to the internal standard tetramethylsilane (ppm = 0.00). All reagents and solvents were purchased from FUJIFILM Wako Pure Chemical Corporation. The progress of all reactions was monitored by TLC using ethyl acetate/hexane, acetone/hexane, dichloromethane (CH_2Cl_2)/MeOH and CH_2Cl_2/MeOH/triethylamine (TEA) as the solvent system, and spots were visualized by irradiation with ultraviolet light (254 nm) or ninhydrin reaction. Column chromatography was performed using silica gel (200–300 mesh).

3.5.2. General Procedures for Synthesizing the Target Compounds **3a** and **3b**

Compounds 1-benzoylpiperidin-4-yl)butyl)isoindoline-1,3-dione (**1a**) and 2-(4-(4-benzoylpiperazin-1-yl)butyl)isoindoline-1,3-dione (**1b**) were synthesized according to Gilig et al. [55] with slight modifications.

3.5.3. (4-(4-aminobutyl)piperidin-1-yl)(phenyl)methanone (**2a**)

Hydrazine hydrate (0.3 mL, 6.17 mmol) was added under Ar_2 atmosphere to a solution of **1a** (1.0 g, 2.56 mmol) in EtOH at 20 °C. After stirring at 20 °C for 10 min, the mixture was heated under reflux for 2 h. After cooling to 20 °C, the white precipitate was filtered off and washed with EtOH (10 mL). The EtOH solutions were combined, and the solvent was evaporated in vacuo. The residue was taken in CH_2Cl_2 (20 mL) and a saturated aqueous solution of K_2CO_3 (20 mL). Vigorous stirring for 10 min produced two clear phases. The aqueous phase was extracted with CH_2Cl_2 (10 mL, 3 times). The combined organic phases were washed with brine (30 mL) and dried over Na_2SO_4. After solvent evaporation in vacuo, **2a** was obtained (0.530 g) as a pale-yellow oil.

3.5.4. *N*-(4-(1-benzoylpiperidin-4-yl)butyl)-1*H*-pyrrolo[3,2-c]pyridine-2-carboxamide (**3a**)

First, 1*H*-pyrro[3,2-c]pyridine-2-carboxylic acid (0.149 g, 0.918 mmol) was added to a solution of **2a** obtained above (0.239 g, 0.918 mmol) in dry DMF (8.0 mL) in a 25 mL round-bottomed flask. HOBt (0.186 g, 1.38 mmol), EDC-HCl (0.352 g, 1.84 mmol) and N, *N*-diisopropylethylamine (0.462 mL, 2.75 mmol) were added sequentially, and the suspension was allowed to stir at room temperature overnight. The reaction mixture was then poured into a separatory funnel containing water and ethyl acetate. The aqueous phase was separated and extracted three times with EtOAc. The combined organic phase was dried over Na_2SO_4, filtered and concentrated in vacuo. The resulting residue was purified by column chromatography (CH_2Cl_2/MeOH = 9/1) to afford the target product **3a** (0.215 g, yield 58%, more than 95%, as judged by ODS(C18) HPLC) as white crystals. ^{1}H-NMR (DMSO-d6) d 11.94 (s, 1H), 8.88 (s, 1H), 8.59 (t, 1H), 8.19 (d, 1H), 7.39 (m, 3H), 7.31 (m, 3H), 7.20 (s, 1H), 4.43 (m, 1H), 3.51 (m, 1H), 3.26 (m, 2H), 2.96 (m, 1H), 2.70 (m, 1H), 1.70 (m, 2H), 1.51 (m, 3H), 1.29 (m, 4H), 1.05 (m, 2H).

3.5.5. 4-(4-Aminobutyl)piperazin-1-yl)(phenyl)methanone (**2b**)

Compound **2b** was obtained from **1b** by similar synthetic processes as described in Section 3.5.3.

3.5.6. *N*-(4-(4-Benzoylpiperazin-1-yl)butyl)-1*H*-pyroro[3,2-c]pyridine-2-carboxamide (**3b**)

The procedure was the same as described above for the synthesis of **3a**. Compound **3b** was obtained as pale-yellow powder (0.104 g, yield 28%, more than 95%, as judged by ODS(C18) HPLC). ^{1}H-NMR (DMSO-d6) δ 11.97 (s, broad, 1H), 8.90 (s, 1H), 8.61 (t, 1H), 8.19 (d, 1H), 7.33–7.43 (m, 5H), 7.23 (s, 1H), 3.26–3.58 (m, 9H), 2.30–2.38 (m, 5H), 1.48–1.55 (m, 3H).

3.6. Statistical Analysis

All data were obtained from at least three independent experiments and were expressed as mean ± standard error (SE).

4. Conclusions

In this study, to understand the structural basis of beneficial design for effective NAMPT inhibitors, we designed and synthesized a close structural analogue set of potent and specific azacyclohexane-motif NAMPT inhibitors, namely **3a** (piperidine-motif) and **3b** (piperazine-motif) modified from **1**. In addition, these two compounds have 5-azaindole ring as the head structure, which is replaced by the vinylpyridine ring of **1**. Through biochemical experiments and in silico binding mode analyses using these inhibitors, we clearly showed that **3a** is the most potent NAMPT inhibitor among these inhibitors, and that the azaindole-head and piperidine-linker of NAMPT inhibitors are promising motifs that result in enthalpically higher potent inhibitory activity against NAMPT molecule and cancer cells. The main reason for this phenomenon was revealed to be due to the electronic repulsion of the piperazine-linker motif of **3b** with His191 of NAMPT. Importantly, this H191 is known to be a drug-resistance sensitive amino acid residue [36,37,50–52]. Thus, it is better to avoid interactions with His191 in designing effective NAMPT inhibitors. Further studies on the tunnel cavity of NAMPT using rigid analogues of azaindole-piperidine-motif inhibitors will allow a more definitive understanding of the inhibitor pharmacophore. Although additional confirmatory studies, such as the synthesis of novel azaindole-piperidine-motif NAMPT inhibitors and details of in vivo efficacy and resistibility are warranted, our findings provide valuable insights into the design for effective NAMPT inhibitors that offer improved therapeutic potential by making high specificity and avoiding resistance to NAMPT. Furthermore, on the basis of the characteristics of NAMPT functions and the mechanisms of action of NAMPT inhibitors, we are now trying to design additional azaindole–piperidine-motif NAMPT inhibitors available in vivo, such as the translation of a potent one into a payload for antibody–drug conjugates, which are an important therapeutic modality enabling targeted drug delivery to cancer cells [56].

Author Contributions: Conceptualization, S.-i.T. and N.T.; software, A.Y.; validation, T.O.; formal analysis, T.O. and A.Y.; investigation, K.K., Y.S. (Yuri Shibasaki), M.O., Y.O., Y.S. (Yoshimi Sakamoto) and M.N.; resources, Y.A., K.M., H.N. and H.T.; writing—original draft preparation, S.-i.T.; writing—review and editing, S.-i.T., A.Y., Y.A., H.Y., A.S., H.N., M.O., H.T., N.T. and F.U.; visualization, T.O., A.Y. and H.A.; supervision, S.-i.T.; project administration, S.-i.T.; funding acquisition, S.-i.T. and N.T. All authors have read and agreed to the published version of the manuscript.

Funding: This work was supported in part by P-CREATE for division of Pharmaceutical Research and Development from the Japan Agency for Medical Research and Development, AMED grant (18cm0106133h0001) and the Hinoki Foundation.

Acknowledgments: The authors would like to thank staffs for Science and Technology, Organization for Research Advancement, Tokyo University of Science for their assistance.

Conflicts of Interest: The authors declare no conflict of interest.

References

1. Belenky, P.; Bogan, K.L.; Brenner, C. NAD^+ metabolism in health and disease. *Trends Biochem. Sci.* **2007**, *32*, 12–19. [CrossRef] [PubMed]
2. Cantó, C.; Menzies, K.J.; Auwerx, J. NAD(+) Metabolism and the control of energy homeostasis: A balancing act between mitochondria and the nucleus. *Cell Metab.* **2015**, *22*, 31–53. [CrossRef] [PubMed]
3. Tanuma, S.; Sato, A.; Oyama, T.; Yoshimori, A.; Abe, H.; Uchiumi, F. New Insights into the roles of NAD^+-poly(ADP-ribose) metabolism and poly(ADP-ribose) glycohydrolase. *Curr. Protein Pept. Sci.* **2016**, *17*, 668–682. [CrossRef] [PubMed]
4. Liu, L.; Su, X.; Quinn, W.J., 3rd; Hui, S.; Krukenberg, K.; Frederick, D.W.; Redpath, P.; Zhan, L.; Chellappa, K.; White, E.; et al. Quantitative analysis of NAD synthesis-breakdown fluxes. *Cell Metab.* **2018**, *27*, 1067–1080.e5. [CrossRef]
5. Schreiber, V.; Dantzer, F.; Ame, J.C.; de Murcia, G. Poly(ADP-ribose): Novel functions for an old molecule. *Nat. Rev. Mol. Cell Biol.* **2006**, *7*, 517–528. [CrossRef]
6. Tanuma, S.I.; Shibui, Y.; Oyama, T.; Uchiumi, F.; Abe, H. Targeting poly(ADP-ribose) glycohydrolase to draw apoptosis codes in cancer. *Biochem. Pharmacol.* **2019**, *167*, 163–172. [CrossRef]
7. Revollo, J.R.; Grimm, A.A.; Imai, S. The NAD biosynthesis pathway mediated by nicotinamide phosphoribosyltransferase regulates Sir2 activity in mammalian cells. *J. Biol. Chem.* **2004**, *279*, 50754–50763. [CrossRef]
8. Mei, S.C.; Brenner, C. NAD as a genotype-specific drug target. *Chem. Biol.* **2013**, *20*, 1307–1308. [CrossRef]
9. Preiss, J.; Handler, P. Enzymatic synthesis of nicotinamide mononucleotide. *J. Biol. Chem.* **1957**, *225*, 759–770.
10. Bogan, K.L.; Brenner, C. Nicotinic acid, nicotinamide, and nicotinamide riboside: A molecular evaluation of NAD^+ precursor vitamins in human nutrition. *Ann. Rev. Nutr.* **2008**, *28*, 115–130. [CrossRef]
11. Chiarugi, A.; Dölle, C.; Felici, R.; Ziegler, M. The NAD metabolome—A key determinant of cancer cell biology. *Nat. Rev. Cancer* **2012**, *12*, 741–752. [CrossRef]

12. Garten, A.; Petzold, S.; Körner, A.; Imai, S.; Kiess, W. Nampt: Linking NAD biology, metabolism and cancer. *Trends Endocrinol. Metab. TEM* **2009**, *20*, 130–138. [CrossRef] [PubMed]
13. Chowdhry, S.; Zanca, C.; Rajkumar, U.; Koga, T.; Diao, Y.; Raviram, R.; Liu, F.; Turner, K.; Yang, H.; Brunk, E.; et al. NAD metabolic dependency in cancer is shaped by gene amplification and enhancer remodelling. *Nature* **2019**, *569*, 570–575. [CrossRef] [PubMed]
14. Bae, S.K.; Kim, S.R.; Kim, J.G.; Kim, J.Y.; Koo, T.H.; Jang, H.O.; Yun, I.; Yoo, M.A.; Bae, M.K. Hypoxic induction of human visfatin gene is directly mediated by hypoxia-inducible factor-1. *FEBS Lett.* **2006**, *580*, 4105–4113. [CrossRef] [PubMed]
15. Bauer, L.; Venz, S.; Junker, H.; Brandt, R.; Radons, J. Nicotinamide phosphoribosyltransferase and prostaglandin H2 synthase 2 are up-regulated in human pancreatic adenocarcinoma cells after stimulation with interleukin-1. *Int. J. Oncol.* **2009**, *35*, 97–107. [PubMed]
16. Shackelford, R.E.; Bui, M.M.; Coppola, D.; Hakam, A. Over-expression of nicotinamide phosphoribosyltransferase in ovarian cancers. *Int. J. Clin. Exp. Pathol.* **2010**, *3*, 522–527. [PubMed]
17. Wang, B.; Hasan, M.K.; Alvarado, E.; Yuan, H.; Wu, H.; Chen, W.Y. NAMPT overexpression in prostate cancer and its contribution to tumor cell survival and stress response. *Oncogene* **2011**, *30*, 907–921. [CrossRef] [PubMed]
18. Hasmann, M.; Schemainda, I. FK866, a highly specific noncompetitive inhibitor of nicotinamide phosphoribosyltransferase, represents a novel mechanism for induction of tumor cell apoptosis. *Cancer Res.* **2003**, *63*, 7436–7442.
19. Hjarnaa, P.J.; Jonsson, E.; Latini, S.; Dhar, S.; Larsson, R.; Bramm, E.; Skov, T.; Binderup, L. CHS 828, a novel pyridyl cyanoguanidine with potent antitumor activity in vitro and in vivo. *Cancer Res.* **1999**, *59*, 5751–5757.
20. Micheli, V.; Simmonds, H.A.; Sestini, S.; Ricci, C. Importance of nicotinamide as an NAD precursor in the human erythrocyte. *Arch. Biochem. Biophys.* **1990**, *283*, 40–45. [CrossRef]
21. Khan, J.A.; Tao, X.; Tong, L. Molecular basis for the inhibition of human NMPRTase, a novel target for anticancer agents. *Nat. Struct. Mol. Biol.* **2006**, *13*, 582–588. [CrossRef] [PubMed]
22. Olesen, U.H.; Christensen, M.K.; Björkling, F.; Jäättelä, M.; Jensen, P.B.; Sehested, M.; Nielsen, S.J. Anticancer agent CHS-828 inhibits cellular synthesis of NAD. *Biochem. Biophys. Res. Commun.* **2008**, *367*, 799–804. [CrossRef] [PubMed]
23. Von Heideman, A.; Berglund, A.; Larsson, R.; Nygren, P. Safety and efficacy of NAD depleting cancer drugs: Results of a phase I clinical trial of CHS 828 and overview of published data. *Cancer Chemother. Pharmacol.* **2010**, *65*, 1165–1172. [CrossRef] [PubMed]
24. Bi, T.Q.; Che, X.M. Nampt/PBEF/visfatin and cancer. *Cancer Biol. Ther.* **2010**, *10*, 119–125. [CrossRef] [PubMed]
25. Galli, U.; Travelli, C.; Massarotti, A.; Fakhfouri, G.; Rahimian, R.; Tron, G.C.; Genazzani, A.A. Medicinal chemistry of nicotinamide phosphoribosyltransferase (NAMPT) inhibitors. *J. Med. Chem.* **2013**, *56*, 6279–6296.
26. Montecucco, F.; Cea, M.; Bauer, I.; Soncini, D.; Caffa, I.; Lasiglìè, D.; Nahimana, A.; Uccelli, A.; Bruzzone, S.; Nencioni, A. Nicotinamide phosphoribosyltransferase (NAMPT) inhibitors as therapeutics: Rationales, controversies, clinical experience. *Curr. Drug Targets* **2013**, *14*, 637–643. [CrossRef]
27. Oh, A.; Ho, Y.C.; Zak, M.; Liu, Y.; Chen, X.; Yuen, P.W.; Zheng, X.; Liu, Y.; Dragovich, P.S.; Wang, W. Structural and biochemical analyses of the catalysis and potency impact of inhibitor phosphoribosylation by human nicotinamide phosphoribosyltransferase. *ChemBioChem Eur. J. Chem. Biol.* **2014**, *15*, 1121–1130. [CrossRef]
28. Adams, D.J.; Ito, D.; Rees, M.G.; Seashore-Ludlow, B.; Puyang, X.; Ramos, A.H.; Cheah, J.H.; Clemons, P.A.; Warmuth, M.; Zhu, P.; et al. NAMPT is the cellular target of STF-31-like small-molecule probes. *ACS Chem. Biol.* **2014**, *9*, 2247–2254. [CrossRef]
29. Sampath, D.; Zabka, T.S.; Misner, D.L.; O'Brien, T.; Dragovich, P.S. Inhibition of nicotinamide phosphoribosyltransferase (NAMPT) as a therapeutic strategy in cancer. *Pharmacol. Ther.* **2015**, *151*, 16–31. [CrossRef]
30. Preyat, N.; Leo, O. Complex role of nicotinamide adenine dinucleotide in the regulation of programmed cell death pathways. *Biochem. Pharmacol.* **2016**, *101*, 13–26. [CrossRef]
31. Asawa, Y.; Katsuragi, K.; Sato, A.; Yoshimori, A.; Tanuma, S.I.; Nakamura, H. Structure-based drug design of novel carborane-containing nicotinamide phosphoribosyltransferase inhibitors. *Bioorg. Med. Chem.* **2019**, *27*, 2832–2844. [CrossRef] [PubMed]

32. Wang, T.; Zhang, X.; Bheda, P.; Revollo, J.R.; Imai, S.; Wolberger, C. Structure of Nampt/PBEF/visfatin, a mammalian NAD^+ biosynthetic enzyme. *Nat. Struct. Mol. Biol.* **2006**, *13*, 661–662. [CrossRef]
33. Rongvaux, A.; Galli, M.; Denanglaire, S.; Van Gool, F.; Drèze, P.L.; Szpirer, C.; Bureau, F.; Andris, F.; Leo, O. Nicotinamide phosphoribosyl transferase/pre-B cell colony-enhancing factor/visfatin is required for lymphocyte development and cellular resistance to genotoxic stress. *J. Immunol. (Baltimore)* **2008**, *181*, 4685–4695. [CrossRef] [PubMed]
34. Zhang, L.Q.; Heruth, D.P.; Ye, S.Q. Nicotinamide phosphoribosyltransferase in human diseases. *J. Bioanal. Biomed.* **2011**, *3*, 13–25. [CrossRef] [PubMed]
35. Holen, K.; Saltz, L.B.; Hollywood, E.; Burk, K.; Hanauske, A.R. The pharmacokinetics, toxicities, and biologic effects of FK866, a nicotinamide adenine dinucleotide biosynthesis inhibitor. *Investig. N. Drugs* **2008**, *26*, 45–51. [CrossRef]
36. Ogino, Y.; Sato, A.; Uchiumi, F.; Tanuma, S.I. Cross resistance to diverse anticancer nicotinamide phosphoribosyltransferase inhibitors induced by FK866 treatment. *Oncotarget* **2018**, *9*, 16451–16461. [CrossRef]
37. Ogino, Y.; Sato, A.; Uchiumi, F.; Tanuma, S.I. Genomic and tumor biological aspects of the anticancer nicotinamide phosphoribosyltransferase inhibitor FK866 in resistant human colorectal cancer cells. *Genomics* **2019**, *111*, 1889–1895. [CrossRef]
38. Burgos, E.S. NAMPT in regulated NAD biosynthesis and its pivotal role in human metabolism. *Curr. Med. Chem.* **2011**, *18*, 1947–1961. [CrossRef]
39. Zheng, X.; Bauer, P.; Baumeister, T.; Buckmelter, A.J.; Caligiuri, M.; Clodfelter, K.H.; Han, B.; Ho, Y.C.; Kley, N.; Lin, J.; et al. Structure-based identification of ureas as novel nicotinamide phosphoribosyltransferase (Nampt) inhibitors. *J. Med. Chem.* **2013**, *56*, 4921–4937.
40. Zheng, X.; Bauer, P.; Baumeister, T.; Buckmelter, A.J.; Caligiuri, M.; Clodfelter, K.H.; Han, B.; Ho, Y.C.; Kley, N.; Lin, J.; et al. Structure-based discovery of novel amide-containing nicotinamide phosphoribosyltransferase (nampt) inhibitors. *J. Med. Chem.* **2013**, *56*, 6413–6433.
41. Gunzner-Toste, J.; Zhao, G.; Bauer, P.; Baumeister, T.; Buckmelter, A.J.; Caligiuri, M.; Clodfelter, K.H.; Fu, B.; Han, B.; Ho, Y.C.; et al. Discovery of potent and efficacious urea-containing nicotinamide phosphoribosyltransferase (NAMPT) inhibitors with reduced CYP2C9 inhibition properties. *Bioorg. Med. Chem. Lett.* **2013**, *23*, 3531–3538. [CrossRef] [PubMed]
42. Zheng, X.; Bair, K.W.; Bauer, P.; Baumeister, T.; Bowman, K.K.; Buckmelter, A.J.; Caligiuri, M.; Clodfelter, K.H.; Feng, Y.; Han, B.; et al. Identification of amides derived from 1*H*-pyrazolo[3,4-b]pyridine-5-carboxylic acid as potent inhibitors of human nicotinamide phosphoribosyltransferase (NAMPT). *Bioorg. Med. Chem. Lett.* **2013**, *23*, 5488–5497. [CrossRef] [PubMed]
43. Singh, J.; Petter, R.C.; Baillie, T.A.; Whitty, A. The resurgence of covalent drugs. *Nat. Rev. Drug Discov.* **2011**, *10*, 307–317. [CrossRef] [PubMed]
44. Backus, K.M.; Correia, B.E.; Lum, K.M.; Forli, S.; Horning, B.D.; González-Páez, G.E.; Chatterjee, S.; Lanning, B.R.; Teijaro, J.R.; Olson, A.J.; et al. Proteome-wide covalent ligand discovery in native biological systems. *Nature* **2016**, *534*, 570–574. [CrossRef] [PubMed]
45. Bair, K.W.; Baumeister, T.; Buckmelter, A.J.; Clodfelter, K.H.; Han, B.; Kuntz, J.D.; Lin, J.; Reynolds, D.J.; Smith, C.C.; Wang, Z.; et al. Piperidine Derivatives and Compositions for the Inhibition of Nicotinamide Phosphoribosyltransferase (Nampt). U.S. Patent No 9,555,039, 2017.
46. Vogel, P.; Duchosal, M.; Aimable, N.; Inmaculada, R.; Mollinedo, F.; Nencioni, A. Piperidine Derivatives for use In the Treatment of Pancreatic Cancer. U.S. Patent Application No. 16/323,473, 2019.
47. Lockman, J.W.; Murphy, B.R.; Zigar, D.F.; Judd, W.R.; Slattum, P.M.; Gao, Z.H.; Ostanin, K.; Green, J.; McKinnon, R.; Terry-Lorenzo, R.T.; et al. Analogues of 4-[(7-Bromo-2-methyl-4-oxo-3H-quinazolin-6-yl)methylprop-2-ynylamino]-N-(3-pyridylmethyl)benzamide (CB-30865) as potent inhibitors of nicotinamide phosphoribosyltransferase (Nampt). *J. Med. Chem.* **2010**, *53*, 8734–8746. [PubMed]
48. RDKit. Open-Source Cheminformatics Software. Available online: http://www.rdkit.org (accessed on 7 August 2020).
49. Wolber, G.; Langer, T. LigandScout: 3-D pharmacophores derived from protein-bound ligands and their use as virtual screening filters. *J. Chem. Inf. Model.* **2005**, *45*, 160–169. [CrossRef]

50. Watson, M.; Roulston, A.; Bélec, L.; Billot, X.; Marcellus, R.; Bédard, D.; Bernier, C.; Branchaud, S.; Chan, H.; Dairi, K.; et al. The small molecule GMX1778 is a potent inhibitor of NAD+ biosynthesis: Strategy for enhanced therapy in nicotinic acid phosphoribosyltransferase 1-deficient tumors. *Mol. Cell. Biol.* **2009**, *29*, 5872–5888. [CrossRef]
51. Olesen, U.H.; Petersen, J.G.; Garten, A.; Kiess, W.; Yoshino, J.; Imai, S.; Christensen, M.K.; Fristrup, P.; Thougaard, A.V.; Björkling, F.; et al. Target enzyme mutations are the molecular basis for resistance towards pharmacological inhibition of nicotinamide phosphoribosyltransferase. *BMC Cancer* **2010**, *10*, 677. [CrossRef]
52. Wang, W.; Elkins, K.; Oh, A.; Ho, Y.C.; Wu, J.; Li, H.; Xiao, Y.; Kwong, M.; Coons, M.; Brillantes, B.; et al. Structural basis for resistance to diverse classes of NAMPT inhibitors. *PLoS ONE* **2014**, *9*, e109366. [CrossRef]
53. Tosco, P.; Balle, T.; Shiri, F. Open3DALIGN: An open-source software aimed at unsupervised ligand alignment. *J. Comput. Aided Mol. Des.* **2011**, *25*, 777–783. [CrossRef]
54. Nelson, D.J.; Brammer, C.N. Toward consistent terminology for cyclohexane conformers in introductory organic chemistry. *J. Chem. Educ.* **2011**, *88*, 292–294. [CrossRef]
55. Gillig, A.; Majjigapu, S.R.; Sordat, B.; Vogel, P. Synthesis of a C-Iminoribofuranoside Analog of the Nicotinamide Phosphoribosyltransferase (NAMPT) Inhibitor FK866. *Helv. Chim. Acta* **2012**, *95*, 34–42. [CrossRef]
56. Neumann, C.S.; Olivas, K.C.; Anderson, M.E.; Cochran, J.H.; Jin, S.; Li, F.; Loftus, L.V.; Meyer, D.W.; Neale, J.; Nix, J.C.; et al. Targeted Delivery of Cytotoxic NAMPT Inhibitors Using Antibody-Drug Conjugates. *Mol. Cancer Ther.* **2018**, *17*, 2633–2642. [CrossRef] [PubMed]

Sample Availability: Not available.

molecules

MDPI

Article

Engineering Stem Cell Factor Ligands with Different c-Kit Agonistic Potencies

Tal Tilayov [1,†], Tal Hingaly [1,†], Yariv Greenshpan [2], Shira Cohen [3], Barak Akabayov [3], Roi Gazit [2] and Niv Papo [1,*]

1 Avram and Stella Goldstein-Goren Department of Biotechnology Engineering and the National Institute of Biotechnology in the Negev, Ben-Gurion University of the Negev, Beer-Sheva 8410501, Israel; taltil@gmail.com (T.T.); talhingaly@gmail.com (T.H.)
2 Shraga Segal Department of Microbiology, Immunology and Genetics and the National Institute of Biotechnology in the Negev, Ben-Gurion University of the Negev, Beer-Sheva 8410501, Israel; yarivg@post.bgu.ac.il (Y.G.); gazitroi@bgu.ac.il (R.G.)
3 Department of Chemistry and the National Institute for Biotechnology in the Negev (NIBN), Ben-Gurion University of the Negev, Beer-Sheva 8410501, Israel; shiracoh@post.bgu.ac.il (S.C.); akabayov@bgu.ac.il (B.A.)
* Correspondence: papo@bgu.ac.il; Tel.: +972-50-2029729
† These authors contributed equally to this work.

Academic Editors: Marialuigia Fantacuzzi and Alessandra Ammazzalorso
Received: 21 September 2020; Accepted: 19 October 2020; Published: 21 October 2020

Abstract: Receptor tyrosine kinases (RTKs) are major players in signal transduction, regulating cellular activities in both normal regeneration and malignancy. Thus, many RTKs, c-Kit among them, play key roles in the function of both normal and neoplastic cells, and as such constitute attractive targets for therapeutic intervention. We thus sought to manipulate the self-association of stem cell factor (SCF), the cognate ligand of c-Kit, and hence its suboptimal affinity and activation potency for c-Kit. To this end, we used directed evolution to engineer SCF variants having different c-Kit activation potencies. Our yeast-displayed SCF mutant (SCF_M) library screens identified altered dimerization potential and increased affinity for c-Kit by specific SCF-variants. We demonstrated the delicate balance between SCF homo-dimerization, c-Kit binding, and agonistic potencies by structural studies, in vitro binding assays and a functional angiogenesis assay. Importantly, our findings showed that a monomeric SCF variant exhibited superior agonistic potency vs. the wild-type SCF protein and vs. other high-affinity dimeric SCF variants. Our data showed that action of the monomeric ligands in binding to the RTK monomers and inducing receptor dimerization and hence activation was superior to that of the wild-type dimeric ligand, which has a higher affinity to RTK dimers but a lower activation potential. The findings of this study on the binding and c-Kit activation of engineered SCF variants thus provides insights into the structure–function dynamics of ligands and RTKs.

Keywords: receptor tyrosine kinases; protein-protein interactions; protein engineering; directed evolution; angiogenesis; binding affinity; agonistic activity

1. Introduction

Receptor tyrosine kinases (RTKs) are major players in signal transduction, regulating cellular activities according to the availability and potency of their cognate ligands. RTKs and their ligands have thus been extensively studied with the dual aims of elucidating their biochemical properties and finding the means to manipulate them for clinical purposes [1–4]. However, despite the work that has been done to date, the delicate balance of RTK-ligand interactions and functional activation is not yet fully understood. It remains difficult to predict the relationship between ligand dimerization, specific RTK-ligand affinity, and functional activation potency. It has, for example, been shown for vascular endothelial growth factor (VEGF), human growth hormone (hGH), and macrophage colony stimulating factor (M-CSF) that activation of their cognate RTKs is balanced between self-dimerization and RTK affinity [5–10]. Thus, ligand 'fitness' (optimal dimerization and binding affinity) is usually not optimal, most probably due to inherent regulatory requirements for dynamic and evolutionary tuning [11–14].

Among the early attempts to engineer the conversion of RTK agonistic ligands into antagonists were those that focused on VEGF, hGH, M-CSF and stem cell factor (SCF) [11–13]. For example, abolishing ligand dimerization aimed to generate monomers that would act as receptor antagonists [15]. However, this approach was impeded by the diminished affinity for the RTK of the monomeric ligand relative to the dimeric ligand, which limited the therapeutic usage of such monomers [11,15,16]. Current methodologies aimed at generating potent RTK antagonists and agonists are thus based on protein engineering designed to modify ligands by changing both their affinities [17] and their self-dimerization status [14]. However, since affinity and self-dimerization are not mutually exclusive, the engineering of optimized protein-based antagonists or agonists must find the delicate balance between improved binding affinity and impaired self-dimerization [18]. In practical terms, combinatorial site-directed engineering of both ligand-ligand and ligand-receptor interactions provides the means to generate improved therapeutic mediators and to gain insights into the dynamics of RTK-ligand interactions.

A prototypic RTK-ligand interaction that has been extensively studied and that has generated important milestones in the field is the c-Kit/SCF interaction [19], which plays a key role in the regulation of epithelial, endothelial, neuronal, and hematopoietic stem-progenitor cells (HSPCs) [20–22]. For example, dysregulation of c-Kit/SCF signaling and gain-of-function c-Kit mutations have been implicated in different cancers [23–28], including thyroid carcinoma, oncocytic intraductal papillary mucinous neoplasms (IPMNs) of the pancreas, and lung cancer [29–31]. To understand c-Kit/SCF signaling, it is necessary to take a brief look at the two partners and at what is currently known about them. SCF is a four-helix bundle-type small protein that forms non-covalent homo-dimers, which may be membrane-anchored or soluble, depending on alternative RNA splicing and proteolytic processing [13,32]. The functional core of SCF is the N-terminal domain, which includes the dimerization interface and the portions of the molecule that bind to c-Kit [33]. Following bivalent binding of an SCF-dimer to a c-Kit monomer, the receptor dimerizes with another c-Kit protein, thereby bringing the two intracellular kinase domains into proximity and allowing them to phosphorylate one another to promote the signal transduction cascade [34–36]. As is the case for other growth factors, such as platelet-derived growth factor (PDGF) and VEGF [37], SCF dimerization is a prerequisite for the proper activation of c-Kit [35]. Indeed, mutated SCF showed reduced c-Kit activation and reduced mitogenic activity in cells, due to impaired SCF self-dimerization, reduced c-Kit affinity, or both [13]. Although the c-Kit receptor activation process has been studied extensively using monoclonal antibodies [38], recombinant protein receptors [35,39], and small molecule kinase inhibitors [36,40–44], the correlations between SCF concentration, SCF dimerization, SCF-c-Kit binding affinity and c-Kit receptor activation are not always fully understood. A particular problem is that most studies showing that wild-type SCF (SCF_{WT}) is highly potent in activating c-Kit have been conducted with very low concentrations (low nanomolar range) of SCF_{WT}, whereas effective SCF tissue concentrations are much higher (in the micromolar range), especially when SCF is intended for use as a therapeutic. To address this problem, it is necessary to generate and study SCF-derived proteins with altered self-dimerization properties and altered affinity for c-Kit that confer, at high concentrations, a superior agonistic function in comparison to SCF_{WT}. Such engineered SCF-derived proteins will not only provide insights into the molecular mechanisms that mediate receptor activation but will also serve as a basis for further manipulations of therapeutic value.

In this study, we combined rational and combinatorial engineering approaches for transforming dimeric SCF into ligands with different agonistic potencies at high SCF concentrations. Specifically, we engineered variants with a reduced dimerization potential and an increased affinity for c-Kit. To this end, we screened random mutagenesis SCF monomer (SCF_M) libraries to identify SCF_M variants with different self-association properties and different affinities for c-Kit and hence with different degrees of activation of c-Kit. Importantly, despite the parental SCF_M being the only monomer variant that binds c-Kit and despite its lower affinity for c-Kit vs. the wild-type dimeric SCF (SCF_{WT}) and vs. the other SCF_M variants, SCF_M was superior to SCF_{WT} and to the other SCF_M variants in activating c-Kit. Our data shows that the impairment of SCF dimerization may increase the local SCF concentration near c-Kit and thereby induce enhanced dimerization and activation of the receptor. Studying a collection of SCF_M variants with optimized functions enabled us both to identify preferential agonists and also to study the relationship between ligand dimerization and c-Kit receptor activation. We suggest that potent activators for other RTKs could be generated by applying a similar structure-based library screening approach, which would, in turn, facilitate further investigation of the mechanisms underlying the activation of RTKs.

2. Results

2.1. Sorting of SCF_M Libraries for Variants with a High Affinity for c-Kit

Our strategy to generate SCF variants with different agonistic activities was based on modifying both SCF homo-dimerization and SCF binding affinity to c-Kit. We started by generating a double mutant variant, SCF_M V49L F63L, exhibiting reduced homo-dimerization [13]. We expressed this mutant on the surface of yeast, as a platform for affinity enrichment (Figure S1 in the Supplementary Material). The first yeast surface display (YSD) library based on SCF_M was then generated with an initial diversity of 4.5×10^6. By using fluorescence-activated cell sorting (FACS), this library was enriched for clones with high expression and enhanced affinity for the soluble c-Kit extracellular domain. Six rounds of sorting were performed with decreasing concentrations of c-Kit (Figure 1A). Two SCF_M clones, designated $SCF_{M,K91E}$ and $SCF_{M,S64P,F126S,V131A,E134G,V139I}$, were chosen for purification based on their high frequency in the selected population and their enhanced affinity towards soluble c-Kit in the YSD system, respectively (Figure S2A). A second-generation library, based on $SCF_{M,K91E}$, was then generated, with an initial diversity of 3×10^6. This second library was further enriched through four rounds of sorting (Figure 1B), resulting in the identification of three high-affinity variants, designated $SCF_{M,K91E,K24N}$, $SCF_{M,K91E,D97G}$ and $SCF_{M,K91E,L98R}$, with the last of these three being the most frequent mutant in the high-affinity sorting gates (Figure S2B). SCF_{WT}, SCF_M, $SCF_{M,K91E}$, $SCF_{M,K91E,L98R}$ and $SCF_{M,S64P,F126S,V131A,E134G,V139I}$ were purified in non-glycosylated form, and their purity and molecular weights were determined (Figure S3). Circular dichroism (CD) spectroscopy showed that SCF_M and $SCF_{M,K91E}$ shared the same secondary structure with SCF_{WT}, according to our measurements and in agreement with a previous publication [33] (Figure S4A). Notably, CD spectra of the glycosylated and non-glycosylated SCF_{WT} revealed that protein glycosylation did not affect the global secondary structure of the protein (Figure S4A).

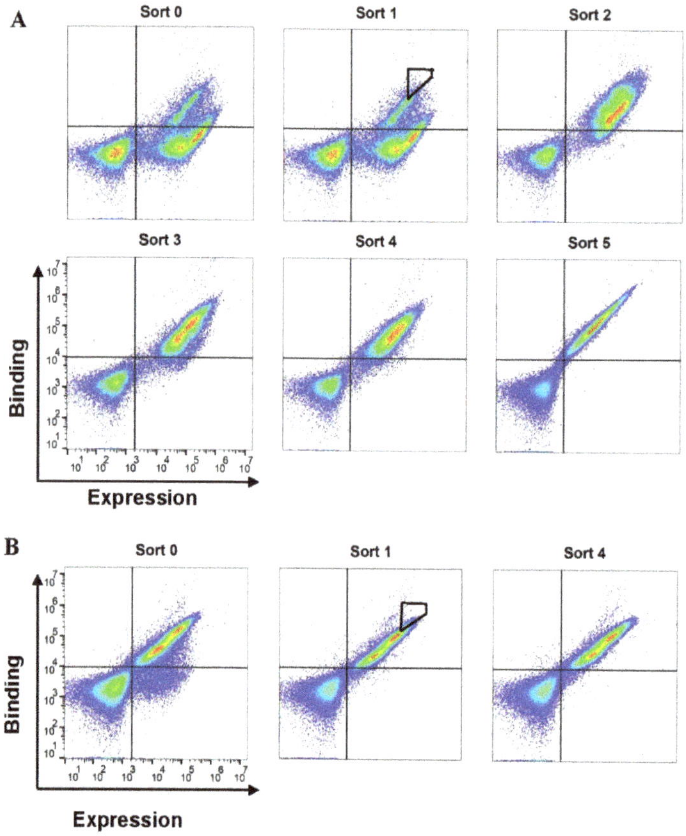

Figure 1. Flow cytometry sorting of yeast-display SCF_M library enriches the c-Kit binding population. Flow cytometry analysis of our first-generation (**A**) and second-generation (**B**) libraries. Yeast-displayed SCF was labeled with anti-c-myc antibody and secondary PE-conjugated antibodies (*x*-axis). Soluble c-Kit (added at 1 nM for analysis) was labeled with FITC (*y*-axis). Cells having variants with the highest affinities were sorted using the gates shown only for sort #1 in both panels for purposes of the illustration; the same gate was applied to all sorts.

2.2. The Dimeric State of SCF Proteins is Concentration Dependent

Biophysical experiments were then performed to determine the extent of dimerization of each SCF protein. The association of the soluble form of each protein, SCF_{WT}, SCF_M, $SCF_{M,K91E}$, $SCF_{M,K91E,L98R}$, and $SCF_{M,S64P,F126S,V131A,E134G,V139I}$, with the same SCF protein displayed on yeast was monitored (Figure 2A and Figure S1). In the concentration range of 62.5–500 nM (1×10^{-3}–8×10^{-3} mg/mL), the dimerization of SCF_{WT} and $SCF_{M,K91E,L98R}$ was stronger—by more than threefold—than that of SCF_M, $SCF_{M,K91E}$, or $SCF_{M,S64P,F126S,V131A,E134G,V139I}$. We also used dynamic light scattering (DLS) to compare the molecular sizes (hydrodynamic radii) of these purified proteins. The hydrodynamic radius of SCF_{WT} (0.5 mg/mL; 32.25 μM) of 3.39 ± 0.57 nm was larger than the hydrodynamic radii of SCFM, SCFM,K91E and SCFM,S64P,F126S,V131A,E134G,V139I, having values of 2.62 ± 0.17, 2.77 ± 0.25 and 2.65 ± 0.69 nm, respectively (Figure 2B). The hydrodynamic radius of SCFM,K91E,L98R (3.06 ± 0.2 nm) was larger than the hydrodynamic radii of the above three variants, but smaller than that of SCF_{WT}, suggesting that more SCF_{WT} and $SCF_{M,K91E,L98R}$ units are in dimeric form than those of SCF_M, $SCF_{M,K91E}$, or $SCF_{M,S64P,F126S,V131A,E134G,V139I}$ (Figure 2B). To gain additional independent information about the dimerization of soluble SCF, we calculated the radius of gyration (Rg) of SCF_{WT} and SCF_M by using small angle X-ray scattering (SAXS). The measured data indicated that both SCF_{WT} and SCF_M at concentrations of 3 or 5 mg/mL (193 or 322 μM, respectively), which are 10-fold higher than the concentrations used in DLS, are dimers (Figure 2C,D). For both proteins, the Rg value was slightly higher than the theoretical Rg of the SCF_{WT} dimer. Taken together, the above findings show that at low concentrations, SCF_{WT} forms dimers and SCF_M is monomeric, but at higher concentrations both proteins are dimers.

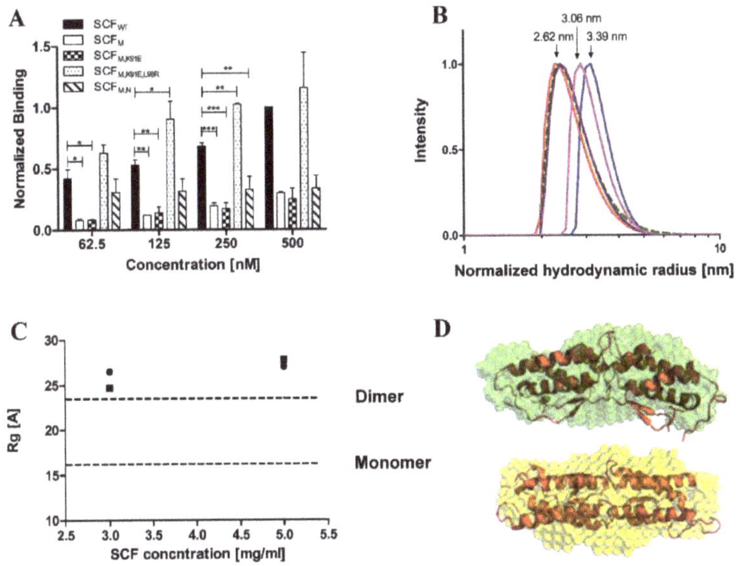

Figure 2. Mutations of SCF affect dimerization. (**A**) Homo-dimerization of soluble SCF proteins with the same yeast-surface displayed (YSD) SCF protein for: SCF_{WT} (black columns), SCF_M (white columns), $SCF_{M,K91E}$ (checkered columns), $SCF_{M,K91E,L98R}$ (dotted columns) and $SCF_{M,S64P,F126S,V131A,E134G,V139I}$ ($SCF_{M,N}$, cross-hatched columns). The values obtained for the binding of the soluble SCF proteins to YSD SCF proteins were normalized to the value that was obtained for the binding of soluble SCF_{WT} (at 500 nM) to the YSD SCF_{WT}. Values are given as means of three independent experiments ± SEM, * $p < 0.05$; ** $p < 0.01$; *** $p < 0.001$. (**B**) DLS analysis of SCF_{WT} (blue), SCF_M (red), $SCF_{M,K91E}$ (dashed green), $SCF_{M,K91E,L98R}$ (pink), and $SCF_{M,S64P,F126S,V131A,E134G,V139I}$ (purple). (**C**) SAXS results showing the radius of gyration (Rg) of SCF_{WT} (circles) and SCF_M (squares) that was measured at 3 and at 5 mg/mL. The Rg values for the theoretical SCF_{WT} monomer and dimer were calculated from the crystal structure (PDB: 1SCF) and are indicated as dashed lines. (**D**) The crystal structure of the SCF dimer was aligned with the SAXS models obtained for SCF_{WT} (green) and SCF_M (orange) using PyMOL.

2.3. $SCF_{M,K91E}$ and $SCF_{M,K91E,L98R}$ Exhibit High Affinity for c-Kit

To directly measure the affinity of each SCF protein for c-Kit, we used surface plasmon resonance (SPR) with the receptor c-Kit protein immobilized on the chip and soluble ligand concentrations of 0.62–50 nM for glycosylated and non-glycosylated SCF_{WT}, or 31.5–500 nM for SCF_M, $SCF_{M,K91E}$, $SCF_{M,K91E,L98R}$ and $SCF_{M,S64P,F126S,V131A,E134G,V139I}$ (Figure 3).

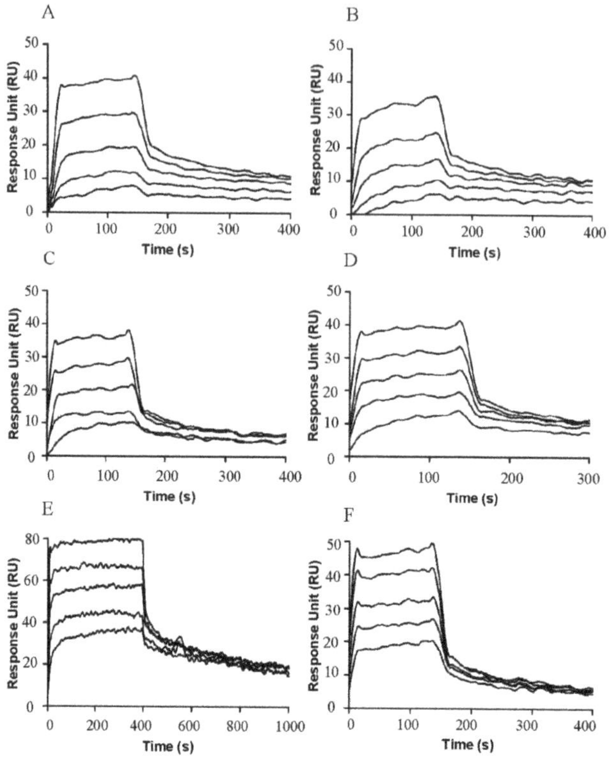

Figure 3. Affinities of SCF variants for c-Kit. The association and dissociation of the soluble SCF variants to and from surface-immobilized c-Kit. (**A**) Non-glycosylated SCF_{WT}; (**B**) Glycosylated SCF_{WT}; (**C**) SCF_{M}; (**D**) $SCF_{M,K91E}$; (**E**) $SCF_{K91E,L98R}$; and (**F**) $SCF_{M,S64P,F126S,V131A,E134G,V139I}$.

The K_D values for the glycosylated and non-glycosylated SCF_{WT} interacting with the immobilized c-Kit were very similar, namely, 5.82 ± 2.93 or 4.36 ± 1.46 nM, respectively (Table 1), with both being in the previously reported K_D range for the SCF/c-Kit interaction (0.5–65 nM) [35,45]. As expected, SCF_{M} showed a much lower affinity (K_D = 146 ± 18.3 nM) for c-Kit. The affinities of $SCF_{M,K91E}$ and $SCF_{M,S64P,F126S,V131A,E134G,V139I}$ were 88.9 ± 19.9 nM and 74.4 ± 5.09 nM, respectively. Interestingly, the affinity of $SCF_{M,K91E,L98R}$ was 40.7 ± 0.7 nM, which is higher than that for the other mutants, but still lower than that of SCF_{WT}.

Table 1. Binding affinities of SCF variants. The dissociation constant (K_D) was determined from SPR sensograms of the equilibrium-binding phase. K_D values are means ± SD of three independent experiments.

Protein	K_D (M)
SCF_{WT}	$4.36 \times 10^{-9} \pm 1.46 \times 10^{-9}$
SCF_{WT} glycosylated	$5.82 \times 10^{-9} \pm 2.93 \times 10^{-9}$
SCF_{M}	$146 \times 10^{-9} \pm 18 \times 10^{-9}$
$SCF_{M,K91E}$	$88.9 \times 10^{-9} \pm 19.9 \times 10^{-9}$
$SCF_{M,K91E,L98R}$	$40.7 \times 10^{-9} \pm 0.7 \times 10^{-9}$
$SCF_{M,S64P,F126S,V131A,E134G,V139I}$	$74.4 \times 10^{-9} \pm 5.1 \times 10^{-9}$

To further test the affinities of SCF_{WT}, SCF_{M}, $SCF_{M,K91E}$, $SCF_{M,K91E,L98R}$ and $SCF_{M,S64P,F126S,V131A,E134G,V139I}$ for c-Kit, we evaluated their binding to c-Kit in two different cell lines, namely, A172, a brain glioblastoma cell line, and murine HSPCs. In agreement with the above-mentioned YSD and SPR binding results, $SCF_{M,K91E}$ and $SCF_{M,K91E,L98R}$ exhibited a higher affinity for the A172 cells, as compared to SCF_{M}, reaching the effective binding levels of SCF_{WT}. In contrast, $SCF_{M,S64P,F126S,V131A,E134G,V139I}$ showed weaker binding to A172 cells, compared with SCF_{WT} (Figure 4A). Murine HSPCs showed high expression of the c-Kit receptor, which has 83% sequence homology with human c-Kit [35,46] (Figure 4C). These cells, too, showed $SCF_{M,K91E}$ and $SCF_{M,K91E,L98R}$ to exhibit the highest binding (Figure 4D), suggesting that $SCF_{M,K91E}$ and $SCF_{M,K91E,L98R}$ bind human or murine c-Kit with similar or even higher affinities compared to the parental SCF_{M}. The conformation that c-Kit adopts when displayed on the membrane of intact cells vs. that when it is immobilized on the SPR sensor chip may be different for the different epitopes that are exposed and available for binding $SCF_{M,S64P,F126S,V131A,E134G,V139I}$ vs. $SCF_{M,K91E,L98R}$ and/or $SCF_{M,K91E}$. These differences may result in a small discrepancy between the SPR and cell binding results.

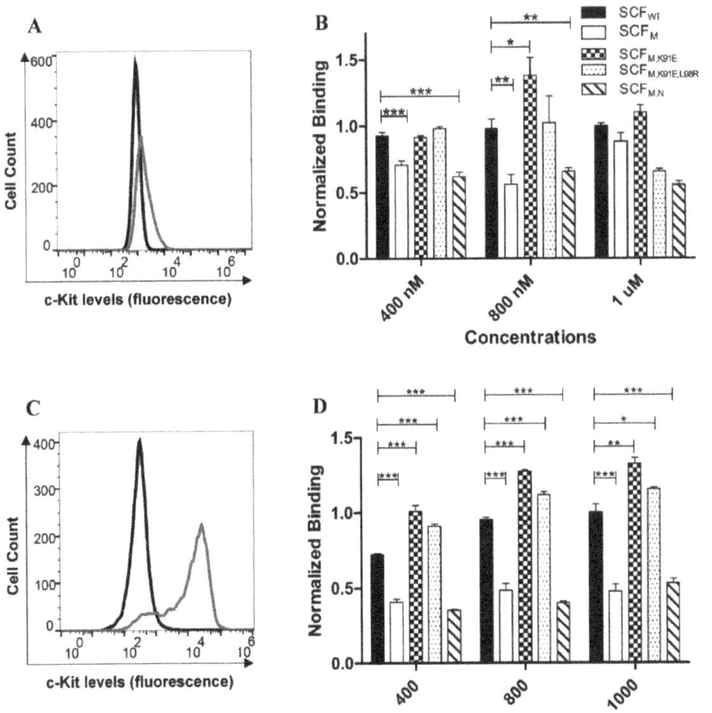

Figure 4. Improved and reduced binding of SCF variants to cell-surface c-Kit. (**A**) Expression levels of c-Kit in the A172 cell line. Grey and black lines represent c-Kit expression and background signals, respectively. (**B**) Binding of SCF variants to A172 cells expressing c-Kit. (**C**) Expression levels of c-Kit in murine HSPCs. (**D**) Binding of SCF variants to HSPCs. In panels (**B**,**D**) the columns are designated as follows: SCF_{WT} (black columns), SCF_{M} (white columns) and $SCF_{M,K91E}$ (checkered columns), $SCF_{M,K91E,L98R}$ (dotted columns) and $SCF_{M,S64P,F126S,V131A,E134G,V139I}$ (cross-hatched columns). The results were normalized to SCF_{WT} binding at the highest concentration of 1000 nM. Values are means ± SEM of independent measurements performed in triplicate. * $p < 0.05$; ** $p < 0.01$; *** $p < 0.001$.

2.4. SCF-Dimerization is the Major Determinant for c-Kit Phosphorylation in Human Umbilical Vein Endothelial Cells

Stimulation of c-Kit by SCF activates a wide array of signaling proteins and pathways, starting with c-Kit phosphorylation and followed by activation of phosphatidylinositide 3′-kinase (PI3-kinase), Scr family kinases (SFK) and Ras-Erk pathways. In human umbilical vein endothelial cells (HUVECs), these events lead to cell proliferation and the formation of capillary-like structures by the endothelial cells [47]. To test for the activation of the c-Kit receptor by the different variants, we thus performed a phosphorylation assay in HUVECs as a cell-based model of angiogenesis. For this assay, we used concentrations of the same order as those used in the above-described biophysical and biochemical assays. As shown previously, these concentrations are representative of the local concentrations of SCF in tissues rather than of global levels in serum or other body fluids [48] (even though they are substantially higher than the concentrations used in some previous studies [13]). Western blot with a specific phospho-c-Kit showed that all the proteins induced receptor activation, but to different extents. The striking—and somewhat unexpected—finding was the difference between SCF_{WT} and SCF_M: SCF_{WT} induced c-Kit activation by strongly binding to it as a dimer (Figure 5), but SCF_M bound to c-Kit as a monomer, being the only variant to do so. Furthermore, although the affinity of SCF_M for c-Kit was lower than that of SCF_{WT}, SCF_M was the only protein that increased c-Kit activation to a greater (albeit modestly) extent than SCF_{WT}. Thus, the SCF_{WT} homo-dimer and SCF_M monomer acted in a similar way as c-Kit agonists, with the latter being slightly more potent in activating c-Kit expressed in HUVECs, as shown by its ability to induce the HUVECs to assemble into tube-like structures (Figure 6). In contrast, $SCF_{M,K91E}$ and $SCF_{M,K91E,L98R}$ were inactive in this assay.

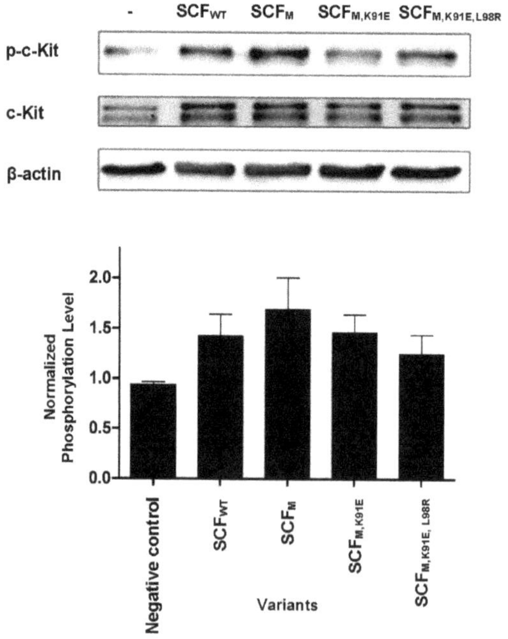

Figure 5. SCF variants activate c-Kit on primary human umbilical vein endothelial cells (HUVECs). HUVECs were incubated with SCF proteins (SCF_{WT}, SCF_M, $SCF_{M,K91E}$ or $SCF_{M,K91E,L98R}$) at a concentration of 250 nM. c-Kit phosphorylation levels were normalized to the expression levels of c-Kit (second row) and to β-actin levels (third row). Values are means ± SEM of independent measurements performed in triplicate.

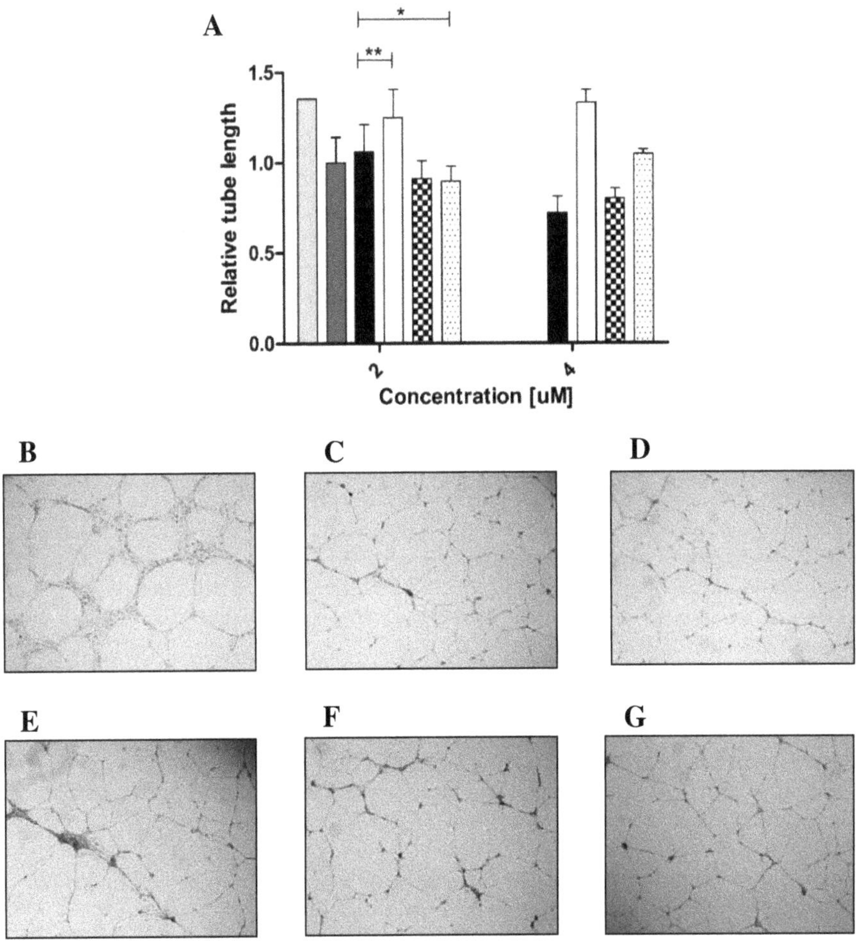

Figure 6. SCF variants with different functional effects on primary human umbilical vein endothelial cells (HUVECs). (**A**) HUVECs with 2% fetal bovine serum (FBS) as the positive control (light gray column), untreated HUVECs as negative control (dark gray column), and cells treated with 4 μM of SCF_{WT} (black columns), SCF_{M} (white columns), $SCF_{M,K91E}$ (checkered columns) and $SCF_{M,K91E,L98R}$ (dotted columns). Tube length was normalized to untreated cells, which served as a control. Values are means ± SEM of independent measurements performed in triplicate. (**B**) Positive control. (**C**) Negative control. (**D**) SCF_{WT}. (**E**) SCF_{M}. (**F**) $SCF_{M,K91E}$. (**G**) $SCF_{M,K91E,L98R}$. In panels (**B**–**G**) all proteins were added at a concentration of 4 μM. * $p < 0.05$; ** $p < 0.01$.

3. Discussion

This study of engineered SCF ligands and their interaction with c-Kit, the cognate SCF receptor, provides proof of concept that receptor-activating ligands can be modulated to confer different agonistic potencies through changes of affinity for the cognate receptor and dimerization of the ligand itself. The study also showed that enhancement of the agonistic potency of SCF was concentration dependent in that the concentration in our study was very high, being in the micromolar range vs. the nanomolar range of previous studies [13]. Currently, most studies on SCF are conducted with concentrations in the range of 3–100 ng/mL; this concentration range, which is clearly appropriate for the routine growth of cells, does not represent the actual local concentration at the cell surface. The naïve-state concentration of SCF in the circulation is 3.3 ng/mL; thus, the active concentration would certainly be higher and could reach substantially higher local concentrations at the cell surface [48]. Since it was our intention to test for robust biochemical properties of the studied mutants, we used a concentration range that would represent more faithfully the high local concentrations of SCF.

Reducing SCF dimerization while preserving or even enhancing its affinity for c-Kit will change the dynamics of binding and activation. At high concentrations, namely, at concentrations representative of tissue levels, SCF_{WT} tends to dimerize before binding to c-Kit, with the SCF_{WT} dimer, with its two binding sites, being likely to approach a single c-Kit receptor molecule. One binding site of the SCF_{WT} dimer will therefore bind to one c-Kit molecule, while the other will remain free. In such a scenario, it is likely that most or all of the c-Kit molecules are each bound to a different SCF_{WT} dimer via a single SCF monomer such that the dimerization of SCF_{WT} (bound to c-Kit) and the subsequent c-Kit dimerization and activation would be slow or unlikely. In contrast, at low (nanomolar) SCF_{WT} concentrations, as in previous studies [13], this dimeric ligand may bind two c-Kit molecules at the same time, resulting in c-Kit dimerization and activation. A different scenario is likely for the SCF_M variants. SCF_M will first bind as a monomer to c-Kit, and then dimerize with another SCF_M protein attached to another c-Kit receptor, thereby bringing two c-Kit receptors into proximity and promoting c-Kit dimerization and hence activation. This scenario may explain the increase of c-Kit activation by the monomeric SCF_M at the high concentrations tested (250 nM in the phosphorylation assay and 2 μM and 4 μM in the tube formation assay). In addition, intermediate levels of c-Kit activation could be obtained by enhancing the affinity of a mutated SCF_M ligand for its c-Kit receptor, as was the case for $SCF_{M,K91E}$ and for especially $SCF_{M,K91E,L98R}$, in order to compensate for changes in ligand dimerization, as these two characteristics are not mutually exclusive.

To identify SCF_M mutants with enhanced affinity for c-Kit, random mutations were introduced, followed by screening yeast surface displayed SCF_M libraries against c-Kit and selection of the mutants with the highest affinity in increasingly stringent sorts. The fact that during affinity maturation the SCF_M proteins were displayed as monomers on the surface of yeast was important, since it meant that mutagenesis was controlled in such a way that affinity enhancement was biased towards dimerization or a higher order of multimerization. Indeed, sequencing of various clones selected from the final sorting round for the first- and second-generation libraries yielded several unique sequences, all including V49L and F63L mutations, that conferred enhanced affinity of SCF_M variants for c-Kit. We found that the K91E mutation observed in the affinity-engineered SCF_M clones (i.e., $SCF_{M,K91E}$ and $SCF_{M,K91E,L98R}$) was near the SCF hot-spot residues related to the interaction of SCF with c-Kit and not to SCF-SCF dimerization (Supplementary Materials: Figure S5). These hot-spot residues may be involved in improving the affinity between SCF and c-Kit, either through direct binding interactions or by structural stabilization. Using SPR spectroscopy, we identified SCF variants with up to 3.7-fold higher affinity for recombinant c-Kit than the parental SCF_M, even though the variants and SCF_M possess similar receptor binding sites. SPR spectroscopy also showed that glycosylation of SCF_{WT} did not influence its affinity for c-Kit, suggesting SCF/c-Kit interactions take place through the amino-acid backbone of SCF without a direct role of post-translational modifications, such as glycosylation.

It was found that the $SCF_{M,K91E}$ and $SCF_{M,K91E,L98R}$ variants exhibited improved binding to A172 cells vs. SCF_M. Strikingly, $SCF_{M,K91E}$, and to an even greater extent $SCF_{M,K91E,L98R}$, also showed stronger binding than the dimeric SCF_{WT} to the murine primary cells. It is thus likely that the L98R mutation may be involved in improving SCF homo-dimerization such that the monomeric $SCF_{M,K91E}$ possesses only a single receptor binding site, whereas $SCF_{M,K91E,L98R}$ possesses two c-Kit receptor binding sites and thereby promotes an enhancement of SCF-c-Kit interactions. Similarly, the ability of the variants to induce c-Kit activation and to activate the formation of capillary-like structures in HUVECs to different extents could be explained by differences in both their ability to self-associate (with SCF_M and $SCF_{M,K91E}$ binding as monomers to c-Kit, and SCF_{WT} and $SCF_{M,K91E,L98R}$

binding as dimers) and in their affinity for recombinant soluble c-Kit or cell-surface-expressed c-Kit (with $SCF_{M,K91E,L98R}$ and SCF_{MK91E} having higher affinity for c-Kit than SCF_M).

Another factor contributing to the different effects of the mutant proteins may lie in their physical state: DLS measurements showed that SCF monomer self-association to a dimer was prevented for SCF_M and $SCF_{M,K91E}$, but not for SCF_{WT} and $SCF_{M,K91E,L98R}$, which did form dimers. Perhaps more importantly, SAXS measurements, which were performed to obtain low-resolution structures of SCF_{WT} and SCF_M at high concentrations in solution, demonstrated that the two proteins are similar in size and shape, both of which are compatible with a dimeric structure of SCF [49]. The mutations in the monomeric SCF_M (i.e., V49L and F63L) appeared to significantly decrease its affinity for purified and cell-expressed c-Kit relative to SCF_{WT}. This is presumably due to decreased avidity, as at low concentrations SCF_M cannot bind two c-Kit molecules. Importantly, at high concentrations (3 or 5 mg/mL), SCF_M can dimerize. In contrast, the mutation K91E in $SCF_{M,K91E}$ appears to maintain this variant in its monomeric state, while increasing its affinity for both purified and cell-expressed c-Kit relative to SCF_M. The mutation L98R in $SCF_{M,K91E,L98R}$ compensates for the V49L and F63L mutations and restores SCF homo-dimerization at low concentrations. These biophysical observations can therefore explain the order of potency in the early and late signaling biological events (i.e., phosphorylation and tube formation, respectively) of the proteins: At high concentrations, SCF_M is a monomer in solution prior to binding and becomes a dimer upon enhancement of its local concentration after binding to c-Kit expressed on cells. This makes SCF_M a strong activator of c-Kit. SCF_{WT} dimerizes better at low concentrations, such that it binds c-Kit strongly as an SCF–SCF dimer, probably capturing both binding sites (one on each monomer) on a c-Kit dimer. As a result, at the high SCF concentrations tested here, c-Kit activation following SCF_{WT} self-association and c-Kit dimerization, is weaker than that with SCF_M, but at low SCF concentrations the reverse is true, as shown in previous studies [13]. $SCF_{M,K91E,L98R}$, for example, binds c-Kit as a c-Kit dimer and thus has an effect that is similar to that of SCF_{WT}.

Our approach complements other methods for targeting SCF for therapeutic application. A recent example of that type of study was presented by a group from Novartis [50] demonstrating the potency of a c-KIT-directed ADC (a humanized anti-c-KIT antibody conjugated to a microtubule destabilizing small molecule) in models of mutant and wild-type c-KIT-positive solid tumors. In this respect, the significance of our study stems from the insight it provides into the sequence-structure–function relationships and mechanism of action of agonistic and antagonistic SCF mutants and it will therefore support engineering of further improved SCF variants as potential therapeutics. Moreover, the approach of using a natural protein ligand as a molecular scaffold for engineering high affinity agents can be applied to other ligands and to create functional protein agonists and antagonists against additional biomedical targets of interest.

4. Materials and Methods

4.1. Generating Random Mutagenesis SCF_M Libraries in Yeast

The gene encoding for SCF_M was designed on the basis of SCF_{WT} with two mutations, one at V49L and the other at F63L [13]. The gene was purchased from Integrated DNA Technologies (IDT, Coralville, IA, USA) and amplified by PCR with a Pfx50 polymerase (Life Technologies, Carlsbad, CA, USA). The PCR product and pCTCON (a generous gift from the laboratory of Dane Wittrup, MIT) [38] vector were digested with the restriction enzymes BamHI and Nhe1, ligated using T4 ligase (New England Biolabs, Ipswich, MA, USA), according to a standard protocol, and transformed into competent EBY100 *Saccharomyces cerevisiae* yeast cells using a MicroPulser electroporator (Bio-Rad, Hercules, CA, USA). The plasmid was extracted from the yeast using a Zymoprep™ yeast plasmid miniprep I kit (Zymo Research, Irvine, CA, USA). A first-generation DNA library originating from SCF_M (used as a template for error prone PCR) was constructed using error prone PCR with low fidelity Taq DNA polymerase (New England Biolabs) and 2 uM of 8-oxo dGTP and dPTP nucleotide analogs

(Jena Bioscience, Jena, Germany). The primers with pCTCON homology used for library preparation were TAAGGACAATAGCTCGACGATTGAAG and GATTTTGTTACATCTACACTGTTG. A second amplification (to generate a second-generation library) used Phusion DNA polymerase (New England Biolabs) with $SCF_{M,K91E}$ as a template DNA and the primers GTTCCAGACTACGCTCTGCAGG and CAGATCTCGAGCTATTACAAG. Cloning into pCTCON was performed according to the same protocol as that used to produce the first-generation library. These reactions allowed homologous recombination of the inserts (PCR products) and the pCTCON vector. The yeast library was grown in SDCAA medium (2% dextrose, 0.67% yeast nitrogen base, 0.5% Bacto™ Casamino acids, 1.47% sodium citrate, 0.429% citric acid monohydrate, pH 4.5) at 30 °C with shaking at 300 rpm, until the culture reached $OD_{600} = 10.0$ (10^8 cells/mL).

4.2. Screening of SCF Libraries

Yeast cells expressing each library were grown in SGCAA medium (2% galactose, 0.67% yeast nitrogen base, 0.5% Bacto Casamino acids, 1.47% sodium citrate, 0.429% citric acid monohydrate) overnight at 30 °C, with shaking at 300 rpm, until the culture reached $OD_{600} = 10$. Cells were washed with PBSA 1% [phosphate buffered saline (PBS) with 1% bovine serum albumin (BSA)]. The cells were double labeled with 1:50 anti c-myc antibody (9E10, Abcam, Cambridge, UK) and different concentrations of human recombinant c-Kit-Fc (Abcam) in PBSA 1% for 1 h at room temperature. Cells were washed with 1% PBSA and incubated with a sheep anti-mouse antibody conjugated to phycoerythrin (PE) (Sigma Aldrich, Rehovot, Israel) and a goat anti-human Fc conjugated to fluorescein isothiocyanate (FITC) (Sigma Aldrich, Rehovot, Israel), both at a 1:50 ratio for 30 min on ice in the dark. The first-generation library was sorted multiple times using SY3200 FACS (Sony Biotechnology, Bothell, WA, USA), and the second-generation library was sorted multiple times using FACS ARIA III (BD Biosciences, San Jose, CA, USA). For each sort round, the desired population was enriched by collecting the high-expressing (PE-labeled) and high c-Kit-binding (FITC-labeled) clones by using sorting gates that included 0.3–3.5% of the entire cell population. For affinity maturation of the SCF libraries, in each sort the c-Kit concentration was sequentially reduced. After each sort, the library was labeled according to the same protocol and analyzed using Accuri C6 flow cytometer (BD Biosciences) and FlowJo software (Tree star Inc., Ashland, OR, USA). SCF_M individual clones (20 to 40) from each sort were sequenced (as above) using Geneious R7 (Biomatters, Auckland, New Zealand). The binding of individual SCF variants (in their YSD format) to soluble c-Kit was analyzed (as before), and SCF_{WT}, SCF_M, $SCF_{M,K91E}$, $SCF_{M,K91E,L98R}$, and $SCF_{M,S64P,F126S,V131A,E134G,V139I}$ were chosen for production and purification as described in the Supplementary Materials.

4.3. Dimerization Assays Using Flow Cytometry

Yeast cells expressing SCF proteins (SCF_{WT}, SCF_M, $SCF_{M,K91E}$, $SCF_{M,S64P,F126S,V131A,E134G,V139I}$ and $SCF_{M,K91E,L98R}$) were induced overnight in SGCAA medium, washed with 1% PBSA, and aliquoted at 1×10^6 cells/sample. Cells displaying the SCF proteins were labeled either with anti c-myc or with different concentrations of purified proteins (SCF_{WT}, SCF_M, $SCF_{M,K91E}$, $SCF_{M,K91E,L98R}$, and $SCF_{M,S64P,F126S,V131A,E134G,V139I}$) in 1% PBSA for 2 h at 4 °C on a rotary shaker. For secondary staining, PE-conjugated sheep anti-mouse and allophycocyanin (APC)-conjugated anti-Flag (BioLegend, San Diego, CA, USA) were used. Values are presented as mean fluorescence ± SEM; statistical significance was determined using a *t*-test. p value < 0.05 was considered statistically significant.

4.4. Dynamic Light Scattering

DLS was used to determine the hydrodynamic radius of the purified proteins (SCF_{WT}, SCF_M, $SCF_{M,K91E}$, $SCF_{M,K91E,L98R}$, and $SCF_{M,S64P,F126S,V131A,E134G,V139I}$) in PBS in concentrations ranging between 0.3–0.5 mg/mL. Proteins were centrifuged for 1 h at 10,000 rpm and filtered through a 0.22-μm filter to remove contaminants. Spectra were collected with a CGS-3 goniometer (ALV, Munich, Germany). The laser power was 20 mW at the helium-neon laser line (633 nm). Correlograms were calculated by the ALV/LSE 5003 correlator, which were collected 10 times, each time over 20 s, at 25 °C. The analysis was repeated four times at the detection angles of either 90° or 60°, in independent measurements. The correlograms were fitted by the CONTIN program [51]. DLS signal intensity was transformed to number distribution based on the Stokes–Einstein equation [52].

4.5. Small Angle X-ray Scattering

SAXS data were collected on SAXLAB GANESHA 300 XL system, possessing a Genix 3D Cu-source, an integrated monochromator, three-pinhole collimation, and a two-dimensional Pilatus 300K detector. SCF_{WT} and SCF_M were measured at concentrations of 3 or 5 mg/mL. A buffer-only sample was used to set the background. The measurements were performed under vacuum at 25 °C. The scattering vector (q) ranged between 0.012 and 0.7 Å^{-1}. The magnitude of the scattering vector is described by $q = \frac{4\pi \, sin\theta}{\lambda}$, where 2θ is the scattering angle and λ is the wavelength. The values for the radius of gyration (Rg) were derived from a Guinier plot, namely, a linear small-angle part of the SAXS scattering curve ($qRg < 1.0$), in PRIMUS. In this region, the Guinier approximation is applicable:

$$I(q) = I(0)e^{\frac{-R_g^2 q^2}{3}}$$

where I is the scattering intensity and q is the scattering vector magnitude (a function of the scattering angle). Rg values were also derived using internal scripts [53] designed to perform an automatic search for the best fitting parameters using GNOM [54]. CRYSOL [55] was used to compute the artificial SAXS spectra based on the available crystal structure of SCF 1–141 (PDB: 1SCF) [49]. These spectra served as a reference for the reconstruction of the experimental SAXS data. The molecular envelope was reconstructed by GASBOR [54] based on the best GNON fit achieved from the internal script.

4.6. Surface Plasmon Resonance

The affinity constant describing the interactions between c-Kit and soluble SCF proteins was determined on a ProteOn XPR36 instrument (Bio-Rad, Hercules, CA, USA). Recombinant c-Kit (R&D Systems) was immobilized on one channel of a ProteOn GLC sensor chip using the amine coupling reagents sulfo-NHS (*N*-hydroxysuccinimide; 10 mM) and EDC (1-ethyl-3-(3 dimethylaminopropyl)-carbodiimide; 40 mM) (Bio-Rad, Hercules, CA, USA). c-Kit, 1.2 µg or 2 µg, was covalently immobilized on the chip in 10 mM sodium acetate buffer, pH 4.0, to give 3866 or 5237 response units (RU), respectively. BSA (3 µg; 4706 RU) was immobilized on the chip as a negative control on a different channel. Unbound esters were deactivated with 1 M ethanolamine HCl at pH 8.5. The temperature was set at 25 °C, and the proteins were then allowed to flow over the chip in a range of concentrations (i.e., in series of threefold dilutions from 50 nM to 0.6 nM) for the glycosylated and non-glycosylated SCF_{WT} and in a series of twofold dilutions from 500 nM to 31.25 nM for the remainder of the proteins (SCF_M, $SCF_{M,K91E}$, and $SCF_{M,S64P,F126S,V131A,E134G,V139I}$). All the proteins were dissolved in PBST solution (PBS 0.005% Tween 20) and were then allowed to flow over the SPR chip surface at 100 µL/min for 150 s, followed by a dissociation phase of 270 s in PBST. After each run, a regeneration step was conducted with 50 mM NaOH. For each protein complex, a sensogram was generated from the RUs measured during the course of the protein–protein interactions by subtracting the background response of flow cells immobilized with BSA. The dissociation constant (K_D) was determined from a sensogram of the equilibrium-binding phase. The data were analyzed with ProteOn manager 3.1.0.6 and fitted to 1:1 Langmuir binding model. To achieve statistical significance, only measurements with χ^2 values that were at least 12% or lower than the Rmax values were chosen for analysis [56].

4.7. Cell Binding Assays

The A172 glioblastoma cell line was grown in Dulbecco's modified Eagle's medium (DMEM, Biological Industries, Beit HaEmek, Israel) with 10% FBS, 1% L-glutamine (Biological Industries) and 1% penicillin streptomycin (Biological Industries, Beit-Haemek, Israel). Cells were harvested with trypsin, and distributed to give 100,000 cells/well. Volumes of 100 μL containing different concentrations of each SCF protein were incubated in the different wells for 2 h at 4 °C on a rotary shaker. Cells were washed twice and then stained with APC conjugated anti-FLAG (BioLegend, San Diego, CA, USA) for 30 min on ice in the dark. The cells were analyzed using Accuri C6, and the data was analyzed using FlowJo software.

Using the same protocol, FACS analysis was performed on murine HSPCs from bone marrow. Lineage^{-}c-Kit^{+}Sca1^{+} bone marrow primary cells were grown in BioTarget medium (Biological Industries, Beit HaEmek, Israel) with 1% L-glutamine, 1% penicillin streptomycin, 10 ng/mL SCF, thyroid peroxidase (TPO), IL-3, and FLT-3 (Peprotech, Rehovot, Israel). The cells were analyzed using Gallios flow cytometer (Beckman Coulter Inc., Carlsbad, CA, USA), and the data was analyzed by Kaluza (Beckman Coulter Inc., Carlsbad, CA, USA) and Prism software (GraphPad, San Diego, CA, USA). The results are presented as means ± SEM of triplicate measurements. Statistical significance was determined using *t*-test analysis. p value < 0.05 was considered statistically significant.

4.8. c-Kit Phosphorylation

HUVECs were grown in EGM-2 medium (Lonza, Basel, Switzerland) containing serum and growth factors[40]. Cells were grown in 6-well plates to 80% confluence and starved for 18 h by incubation in EBM-2 medium without serum and growth factors. Cells were stimulated for 7 min with 250 nM of each of the SCF proteins (i.e., SCF_{WT}, SCF_{M}, $SCF_{M,K91E}$ and $SCF_{M,K91E,L98R}$). The cells were washed twice with cold PBS and collected in 200 μL of lysis buffer [50 mM Hepes, 150 mM NaCl, 10% glycerol, 1% Triton X-100, 1.5 mM $MgCl_2$, 1 mM EDTA, 1 mM Na_3VO_4 and protease inhibitor cocktail (Roche)] for 10 min on ice. The samples were clarified by centrifugation at 15,000 rpm for 10 min at 4 °C. The quantity of total proteins in the lysed cells was determined using a BCA kit (Thermo Scientific, Waltham, MA, USA). Western blot used 20 μg of proteins per lane. After blocking the membrane with TBST (50 mM Tris-HCl, pH 7.4, 150 mM NaCl, 0.1% Tween 20) supplemented with 5% BSA, primary antibodies [i.e., rabbit-anti-phospho-c-Kit (R&D Systems, Minneapolis, MN, USA) at a dilution of 1:2500; rabbit-anti-c-Kit (R&D Systems, Minneapolis, MN, USA) at a dilution of 1:1500; or β-actin antibody (Cell Signaling Technology, Danvers, MA, USA) at a dilution of 1:1000] were added for an overnight incubation at 4 °C. The membrane was washed three times for 10 min with TBST, and then a secondary antibody, i.e., anti-rabbit IgG-HRP (Cell Signaling Technology, Danvers, MA, USA), at a dilution of 1:1000 was added for 1 h at room temperature. Blots were developed with EZ-ECL Kit (Biological Industries, Beit HaEmek, Israel). The bands were visualized by chemiluminescence with Fusion-FX7 spectra (Vilber Lourmat, Collégien, France), and the intensity of each band was measured with the image analysis ImageJ software. Values are given as means ± SEM of triplicates.

4.9. Matrigel Endothelial Tube Formation Assay

Growth factor reduced (GFR) Matrigel (Corning, New York, NY, USA) was used to coat a 96-well plate by centrifugation at 300× *g* for 10 min at 4 °C and incubation at 37 °C for 30 min. HUVEC cells (3.5×10^4 cells per well) were resuspended in EBM-2 with different concentrations of each SCF protein. After incubation of 16–18 h at 37 °C, the plate was monitored with an EVOS FL Cell Imaging System (Thermo Scientific, Waltham, MA, USA), at a ×2 magnification. The results were analyzed with ImageJ software and with Prism software (GraphPad, San Diego, CA, USA). Values are given as means ± SEM of quadruplicates.

5. Conclusions

In summary, the overall goal of this research was to use both rational and combinatorial synthetic methods to develop a new generation of SCF-derived proteins as c-Kit agonists with potential therapeutic applications and as tools to study basic ligand–receptor recognition and receptor activation during key biological processes, in this case SCF-SCF interactions and their influence on SCF/c-Kit function. We found that reduced dimerization of the SCF variants prior to receptor binding resulted in enhanced c-Kit receptor activation, whereas improved receptor binding affinity of the engineered SCF monomers resulted in a reduced receptor activation. In seeking explanations for our findings, we fully characterized the binding and biological properties of the purified variants by employing cell-based models of receptor activation. Our data shows that the impairment of SCF dimerization may increase the local SCF concentration near c-Kit and thereby induce enhanced dimerization and activation of the receptor.

Supplementary Materials: The following are available online, Figure S1: YSD; Figure S2: Binding analysis of individual SCF variants to soluble c-Kit; Figure S3: Protein production and purification; Figure S4: CD spectra of the purified proteins; Figure S5: Schematic representation showing the locations of SCF mutations in the SCF/c-Kit complex (PDB: 1SCF).

Author Contributions: T.T., T.H. and N.P. designed the research; T.T., T.H., Y.G. and S.C. performed the research; T.T., T.H., Y.G., S.C., B.A., R.G. and N.P. analyzed the data; T.T., T.H. and N.P. wrote the manuscript with assistance from R.G. All authors edited the manuscript and approved the final version. All authors have read and agreed to the published version of the manuscript.

Funding: This research was funded by the European Research Council (ERC) grant 336041 and the ISF grant 1615/19 to N.P.

Acknowledgments: We thank A. Zilka (BGU) and U. Hadad (BGU) for help with SPR and FACS experiments. The DLS and SAXS experiments were conducted at the Ilse Katz Institute for Nanoscale Science & Technology with the help of Sharon Hazan.

Conflicts of Interest: The authors declare no conflict of interest.

References

1. Baselga, J. Targeting tyrosine kinases in cancer: The second wave. *Science* **2006**, *312*, 1175–1178. [CrossRef] [PubMed]
2. Belli, S.; Esposito, D.; Servetto, A.; Pesapane, A.; Formisano, L.; Bianco, R. c-Src and EGFR Inhibition in Molecular Cancer Therapy: What Else Can We Improve? *Cancers* **2020**, *12*, 1489. [CrossRef] [PubMed]
3. Katoh, M. Fibroblast growth factor receptors as treatment targets in clinical oncology. *Nat. Rev. Clin. Oncol.* **2019**, *16*, 105–122. [CrossRef] [PubMed]
4. Sangwan, V.; Park, M. Receptor tyrosine kinases: Role in cancer progression. *Curr. Oncol.* **2006**, *13*, 191–193. [PubMed]
5. Bocharov, E.V.; Sharonov, G.V.; Bocharova, O.V.; Pavlov, K.V. Conformational transitions and interactions underlying the function of membrane embedded receptor protein kinases. *Biochim. Biophys. Acta Biomembr.* **2017**, *1859 Pt A*, 1417–1429. [CrossRef]
6. Changeux, J.P.; Christopoulos, A. Allosteric modulation as a unifying mechanism for receptor function and regulation. *Diabetes Obes. Metab.* **2017**, *19* (Suppl. 1), 4–21. [CrossRef] [PubMed]
7. Ferguson, K.M.; Hu, C.; Lemmon, M.A. Insulin and epidermal growth factor receptor family members share parallel activation mechanisms. *Protein Sci.* **2020**, *29*, 1331–1344. [CrossRef]
8. Kazi, J.U.; Ronnstrand, L. FMS-like Tyrosine Kinase 3/FLT3: From Basic Science to Clinical Implications. *Physiol. Rev.* **2019**, *99*, 1433–1466. [CrossRef]
9. Paul, M.D.; Hristova, K. The transition model of RTK activation: A quantitative framework for understanding RTK signaling and RTK modulator activity. *Cytokine Growth Factor Rev.* **2019**, *49*, 23–31. [CrossRef]
10. Purba, E.R.; Saita, E.I.; Maruyama, I.N. Activation of the EGF Receptor by Ligand Binding and Oncogenic Mutations: The "Rotation Model". *Cells* **2017**, *6*, 13. [CrossRef]
11. Boesen, T.P.; Soni, B.; Schwartz, T.W.; Halkier, T. Single-chain vascular endothelial growth factor variant with antagonistic activity. *J. Biol. Chem.* **2002**, *277*, 40335–40341. [CrossRef]
12. Fuh, G.; Li, B.; Crowley, C.; Cunningham, B.; Wells, J.A. Requirements for binding and signaling of the kinase domain receptor for vascular endothelial growth factor. *J. Biol. Chem.* **1998**, *273*, 11197–11204. [CrossRef] [PubMed]
13. Hsu, Y.R.; Wu, G.M.; Mendiaz, E.A.; Syed, R.; Wypych, J.; Toso, R.; Mann, M.B.; Boone, T.C.; Narhi, L.O.; Lu, H.S.; et al. The majority of stem cell factor exists as monomer under physiological conditions. Implications for dimerization mediating biological activity. *J. Biol. Chem.* **1997**, *272*, 6406–6415. [CrossRef] [PubMed]

14. Zur, Y.; Rosenfeld, L.; Keshelman, C.A.; Dalal, N.; Guterman-Ram, G.; Orenbuch, A.; Einav, Y.; Levaot, N.; Papo, N. A dual-specific macrophage colony-stimulating factor antagonist of c-FMS and alphavbeta3 integrin for osteoporosis therapy. *PLoS Biol.* **2018**, *16*, e2002979. [CrossRef] [PubMed]
15. Deng, P.; Wang, Y.L.; Pattengale, P.K.; Rettenmier, C.W. The role of individual cysteine residues in the processing, structure, and function of human macrophage colony-stimulating factor. *Biochem. Biophys. Res. Commun.* **1996**, *228*, 557–566. [CrossRef] [PubMed]
16. Rosenfeld, L.; Shirian, J.; Zur, Y.; Levaot, N.; Shifman, J.M.; Papo, N. Combinatorial and Computational Approaches to Identify Interactions of Macrophage Colony-stimulating Factor (M-CSF) and Its Receptor c-FMS. *J. Biol. Chem.* **2015**, *290*, 26180–26193. [CrossRef] [PubMed]
17. Spiess, K.; Jeppesen, M.G.; Malmgaard-Clausen, M.; Krzywkowski, K.; Dulal, K.; Cheng, T.; Hjorto, G.M.; Larsen, O.; Burg, J.S.; Jarvis, M.A.; et al. Rationally designed chemokine-based toxin targeting the viral G protein-coupled receptor US28 potently inhibits cytomegalovirus infection in vivo. *Proc. Natl. Acad. Sci. USA* **2015**, *112*, 8427–8432. [CrossRef]
18. Shlamkovich, T.; Aharon, L.; Barton, W.A.; Papo, N. Utilizing combinatorial engineering to develop Tie2 targeting antagonistic angiopoetin-2 ligands as candidates for anti-angiogenesis therapy. *Oncotarget* **2017**, *8*, 33571–33585. [CrossRef]
19. Yuzawa, S.; Opatowsky, Y.; Zhang, Z.; Mandiyan, V.; Lax, I.; Schlessinger, J. Structural basis for activation of the receptor tyrosine kinase KIT by stem cell factor. *Cell* **2007**, *130*, 323–334. [CrossRef]
20. Ahmad, I.; Das, A.V.; James, J.; Bhattacharya, S.; Zhao, X. Neural stem cells in the mammalian eye: Types and regulation. *Semin Cell Dev. Biol.* **2004**, *15*, 53–62. [CrossRef]
21. Das, A.V.; James, J.; Zhao, X.; Rahnenfuhrer, J.; Ahmad, I. Identification of c-Kit receptor as a regulator of adult neural stem cells in the mammalian eye: Interactions with Notch signaling. *Dev. Biol.* **2004**, *273*, 87–105. [CrossRef] [PubMed]
22. Matsui, J.; Wakabayashi, T.; Asada, M.; Yoshimatsu, K.; Okada, M. Stem cell factor/c-kit signaling promotes the survival, migration, and capillary tube formation of human umbilical vein endothelial cells. *J. Biol. Chem.* **2004**, *279*, 18600–18607. [CrossRef] [PubMed]
23. Broudy, V.C.; Smith, F.O.; Lin, N.; Zsebo, K.M.; Egrie, J.; Bernstein, I.D. Blasts from patients with acute myelogenous leukemia express functional receptors for stem cell factor. *Blood* **1992**, *80*, 60–67. [CrossRef]
24. D'Amato, G.; Steinert, D.M.; McAuliffe, J.C.; Trent, J.C. Update on the biology and therapy of gastrointestinal stromal tumors. *Cancer Control* **2005**, *12*, 44–56. [CrossRef]
25. Heinrich, M.C.; Blanke, C.D.; Druker, B.J.; Corless, C.L. Inhibition of KIT tyrosine kinase activity: A novel molecular approach to the treatment of KIT-positive malignancies. *J. Clin. Oncol.* **2002**, *20*, 1692–1703. [CrossRef] [PubMed]
26. Heinrich, M.C.; Griffith, D.J.; Druker, B.J.; Wait, C.L.; Ott, K.A.; Zigler, A.J. Inhibition of c-kit receptor tyrosine kinase activity by STI 571, a selective tyrosine kinase inhibitor. *Blood* **2000**, *96*, 925–932. [CrossRef]
27. Hongyo, T.; Li, T.; Syaifudin, M.; Baskar, R.; Ikeda, H.; Kanakura, Y.; Aozasa, K.; Nomura, T. Specific c-kit mutations in sinonasal natural killer/T-cell lymphoma in China and Japan. *Cancer Res.* **2000**, *60*, 2345–2347. [PubMed]
28. Ikeda, H.; Kanakura, Y.; Tamaki, T.; Kuriu, A.; Kitayama, H.; Ishikawa, J.; Kanayama, Y.; Yonezawa, T.; Tarui, S.; Griffin, J.D. Expression and functional role of the proto-oncogene c-kit in acute myeloblastic leukemia cells. *Blood* **1991**, *78*, 2962–2968. [CrossRef] [PubMed]
29. Guo, Y.N.; Liang, L.; Ren, S.; Wu, M.; Shi, D.C.; Mo, W.J.; Chen, G. Cd117 Expression is Correlated with Poor Survival of Patients and Progression of Lung Carcinoma: A Meta-Analysis with a Panel of 2645 Patients. *Pol. J. Pathol.* **2019**, *70*, 63–78. [CrossRef]
30. Makhlouf, A.M.; Chitikova, Z.; Pusztaszeri, M.; Berczy, M.; Delucinge-Vivier, C.; Triponez, F.; Meyer, P.; Philippe, J.; Dibner, C. Identification of CHEK1, SLC26A4, c-KIT, TPO and TG as new biomarkers for human follicular thyroid carcinoma. *Oncotarget* **2016**, *7*, 45776–45788. [CrossRef]
31. Mattiolo, P.; Hong, S.M.; Paolino, G.; Rusev, B.C.; Marchegiani, G.; Salvia, R.; Andrianello, S.; Capelli, P.; Piccoli, P.; Parolini, C.; et al. CD117 Is a Specific Marker of Intraductal Papillary Mucinous Neoplasms (IPMN) of the Pancreas, Oncocytic Subtype. *Int. J. Mol. Sci.* **2020**, *21*, 5794. [CrossRef] [PubMed]
32. Opatowsky, Y.; Lax, I.; Tome, F.; Bleichert, F.; Unger, V.M.; Schlessinger, J. Structure, domain organization, and different conformational states of stem cell factor-induced intact KIT dimers. *Proc. Natl. Acad. Sci. USA* **2014**, *111*, 1772–1777. [CrossRef] [PubMed]

33. Zhang, Z.; Zhang, R.; Joachimiak, A.; Schlessinger, J.; Kong, X.P. Crystal structure of human stem cell factor: Implication for stem cell factor receptor dimerization and activation. *Proc. Natl. Acad. Sci. USA* **2000**, *97*, 7732–7737. [CrossRef]
34. Blume-Jensen, P.; Wernstedt, C.; Heldin, C.H.; Ronnstrand, L. Identification of the major phosphorylation sites for protein kinase C in kit/stem cell factor receptor in vitro and in intact cells. *J. Biol. Chem.* **1995**, *270*, 14192–14200. [CrossRef] [PubMed]
35. Lev, S.; Yarden, Y.; Givol, D. Dimerization and activation of the kit receptor by monovalent and bivalent binding of the stem cell factor. *J. Biol. Chem.* **1992**, *267*, 15970–15977.
36. Philo, J.S.; Wen, J.; Wypych, J.; Schwartz, M.G.; Mendiaz, E.A.; Langley, K.E. Human stem cell factor dimer forms a complex with two molecules of the extracellular domain of its receptor, Kit. *J. Biol. Chem.* **1996**, *271*, 6895–6902. [CrossRef]
37. Potgens, A.J.; Lubsen, N.H.; van Altena, M.C.; Vermeulen, R.; Bakker, A.; Schoenmakers, J.G.; Ruiter, D.J.; de Waal, R.M. Covalent dimerization of vascular permeability factor/vascular endothelial growth factor is essential for its biological activity. Evidence from Cys to Ser mutations. *J. Biol. Chem.* **1994**, *269*, 32879–32885.
38. Colby, D.W.; Kellogg, B.A.; Graff, C.P.; Yeung, Y.A.; Swers, J.S.; Wittrup, K.D. Engineering antibody affinity by yeast surface display. *Methods Enzymol.* **2004**, *388*, 348–358.
39. Liu, Y.C.; Kawagishi, M.; Kameda, R.; Ohashi, H. Characterization of a fusion protein composed of the extracellular domain of c-kit and the Fc region of human IgG expressed in a baculovirus system. *Biochem. Biophys. Res. Commun.* **1993**, *197*, 1094–1102. [CrossRef]
40. Fratto, M.E.; Imperatori, M.; Vincenzi, B.; Tomao, F.; Santini, D.; Tonini, G. New perspectives: Role of Sunitinib in Breast Cancer. *Clin. Ter.* **2011**, *162*, 251–257.
41. London, C.A.; Malpas, P.B.; Wood-Follis, S.L.; Boucher, J.F.; Rusk, A.W.; Rosenberg, M.P.; Henry, C.J.; Mitchener, K.L.; Klein, M.K.; Hintermeister, J.G.; et al. Multi-center, placebo-controlled, double-blind, randomized study of oral toceranib phosphate (SU11654), a receptor tyrosine kinase inhibitor, for the treatment of dogs with recurrent (either local or distant) mast cell tumor following surgical excision. *Clin. Cancer Res.* **2009**, *15*, 3856–3865. [CrossRef] [PubMed]
42. Thanopoulou, E.; Judson, I. The safety profile of imatinib in CML and GIST: Long-term considerations. *Arch. Toxicol.* **2012**, *86*, 1–12. [CrossRef] [PubMed]
43. Weigel, M.T.; Dahmke, L.; Schem, C.; Bauerschlag, D.O.; Weber, K.; Niehoff, P.; Bauer, M.; Strauss, A.; Jonat, W.; Maass, N.; et al. In vitro effects of imatinib mesylate on radiosensitivity and chemosensitivity of breast cancer cells. *BMC Cancer* **2010**, *10*, 412. [CrossRef] [PubMed]
44. Wilmes, L.J.; Pallavicini, M.G.; Fleming, L.M.; Gibbs, J.; Wang, D.; Li, K.L.; Partridge, S.C.; Henry, R.G.; Shalinsky, D.R.; Hu-Lowe, D.; et al. AG-013736, a novel inhibitor of VEGF receptor tyrosine kinases, inhibits breast cancer growth and decreases vascular permeability as detected by dynamic contrast-enhanced magnetic resonance imaging. *Magn. Reason. Imaging* **2007**, *25*, 319–327. [CrossRef]
45. Lev, S.; Yarden, Y.; Givol, D. A recombinant ectodomain of the receptor for the stem cell factor (SCF) retains ligand-induced receptor dimerization and antagonizes SCF-stimulated cellular responses. *J. Biol. Chem.* **1992**, *267*, 10866–10873.
46. Fleischman, R.A. From white spots to stem cells: The role of the Kit receptor in mammalian development. *Trends Genet.* **1993**, *9*, 285–290. [CrossRef]
47. Babaei, M.A.; Kamalidehghan, B.; Saleem, M.; Huri, H.Z.; Ahmadipour, F. Receptor tyrosine kinase (c-Kit) inhibitors: A potential therapeutic target in cancer cells. *Drug Des. Dev. Ther.* **2016**, *10*, 2443–2459. [CrossRef]
48. Ho, C.C.M.; Chhabra, A.; Starkl, P.; Schnorr, P.J.; Wilmes, S.; Moraga, I.; Kwon, H.S.; Gaudenzio, N.; Sibilano, R.; Wehrman, T.S.; et al. Decoupling the Functional Pleiotropy of Stem Cell Factor by Tuning c-Kit Signaling. *Cell* **2017**, *168*, 1041–1052. [CrossRef]
49. Weng, Y.P.; Ku, W.Y.; Wu, M.H.; Tsai, Y.L.; Chen, C.Y.; Kuo, C.A.; Huang, L.L. Full-length recombinant human SCF1-165 is more thermostable than the truncated SCF1-141 form. *PLoS ONE* **2014**, *9*, e103251. [CrossRef]
50. Abrams, T.; Connor, A.; Fanton, C.; Cohen, S.B.; Huber, T.; Miller, K.; Hong, E.E.; Niu, X.H.; Kline, J.; Ison-Dugenny, M.; et al. Preclinical Antitumor Activity of a Novel Anti-c-KIT Antibody-Drug Conjugate against Mutant and Wild-type c-KIT-Positive Solid Tumors. *Clin. Cancer Res.* **2018**, *24*, 4297–4308. [CrossRef] [PubMed]

51. Bobba, A.; Cavatorta, P.; Attimonelli, M.; Riccio, P.; Masotti, L.; Quagliariello, E. Estimation of protein secondary structure from circular dichroism spectra: A critical examination of the CONTIN program. *Protein Seq. Data Anal.* **1990**, *3*, 7–10. [PubMed]
52. Aliyu, A.; Kariim, I.; Abdulkareem, S.A. Effects of aspect ratio of multi-walled carbon nanotubes on coal washery waste water treatment. *J. Environ. Manag.* **2017**, *202 Pt 1*, 84–93. [CrossRef]
53. Akabayov, B.; Akabayov, S.R.; Lee, S.J.; Tabor, S.; Kulczyk, A.W.; Richardson, C.C. Conformational dynamics of bacteriophage T7 DNA polymerase and its processivity factor, Escherichia coli thioredoxin. *Proc. Natl. Acad. Sci. USA* **2010**, *107*, 15033–15038. [CrossRef] [PubMed]
54. Svergun, D.I.; Petoukhov, M.V.; Koch, M.H. Determination of domain structure of proteins from X-ray solution scattering. *Biophys. J.* **2001**, *80*, 2946–2953. [CrossRef]
55. Joubert, A.M.; Byrd, A.S.; LiCata, V.J. Global conformations, hydrodynamics, and X-ray scattering properties of Taq and Escherichia coli DNA polymerases in solution. *J. Biol. Chem.* **2003**, *278*, 25341–25347. [CrossRef] [PubMed]
56. Ramyadevi, J.; Jeyasubramanian, K.; Marikani, A.; Rajakumar, G.; Rahuman, A.A.; Santhoshkumar, T.; Kirthi, A.V.; Jayaseelan, C.; Marimuthu, S. Copper nanoparticles synthesized by polyol process used to control hematophagous parasites. *Parasitol. Res.* **2011**, *109*, 1403–1415. [CrossRef] [PubMed]

Sample Availability: Samples of the compounds SCF_{WT}, SCF_{M}, $SCF_{M,K91E}$, $SCF_{M,K91E,L98R}$, and $SCF_{M,S64P,F126S,V131A,E134G,V139I}$ are available from the authors.

molecules

Article

The Potential Role of Cathepsin K in Non-Small Cell Lung Cancer

Hui Yang [1], Jasmine Heyer [2], Hui Zhao [1], Shengxian Liang [1], Rui Guo [1,*] and Li Zhong [1,2,*]

1 Institute of Life Science and Green Development, College of Life Sciences, Hebei University, Baoding 071000, China; huiyanglucky@163.com (H.Y.); huizhaols@yahoo.com (H.Z.); liangshengxiansr@163.com (S.L.)
2 College of Osteopathic Medicine of the Pacific, Western University of Health Sciences, Pomona, CA 91766, USA; jheyer44@gmail.com
* Correspondence: rguo@hbu.edu.cn (R.G.); lzhong@westernu.edu (L.Z.)

Academic Editors: Marialuigia Fantacuzzi and Alessandra Ammazzalorso
Received: 19 August 2020; Accepted: 8 September 2020; Published: 10 September 2020

Abstract: (1) Background: Cathepsin K has been found overexpressed in several malignant tumors. However, there is little information regarding the involvement of Cathepsin K in non-small cell lung cancer (NSCLC). (2) Methods: Cathepsin K expression was tested in human NSCLC cell lines A549 and human embryo lung fibroblast MRC-5 cells using Western blot and immunofluorescence assay. Cathepsin K was transiently overexpressed or knocked down using transfection with a recombinant plasmid and siRNA, respectively, to test the effects on cell proliferation, migration, invasion, and on the mammalian target of rapamycin (mTOR) signaling pathway. (3) Results: Expression of Cathepsin K was increased significantly in A549 cells and diffused within the cytoplasm compared to the MRC-5 cells used as control. Cathepsin K overexpression promoted the proliferation, migration, and invasion of A549 cells, accompanied by mTOR activation. Cathepsin K knockdown reversed the above malignant behavior and inhibited the mTOR signaling activation, suggesting that Cathepsin K may promote the progression of NSCLC by activating the mTOR signaling pathway. (4) Conclusion: Cathepsin K may potentially represent a viable drug target for NSCLC treatment.

Keywords: NSCLC; Cathepsin K; cell proliferation; cell migration; cell invasion; mTOR

1. Introduction

Non-small cell lung cancer (NSCLC) is the leading cause of cancer death among men and women worldwide, with an incidence rate of 1.3 million cases per year [1]. Since NSCLC remains asymptomatic during early stages, about 80% of patients are already in metastatic stages when they are diagnosed, and their 5-year survival rates are below 15% [2]. Despite recent progress in the development of novel medications and immunotherapies in treating NSCLC, the therapeutic efficacies still remain unsatisfactory [3]. Therefore, finding new therapeutic targets for the treatment of NSCLC has become a prioritized task [4].

Cathepsin K is a type of lysosomal cysteine protease which belongs to the papain-like cysteine peptidase family; other members include Cathepsin B, Cathepsin D and Cathepsin L etc. Physiologically, Cathepsin K functions in mediating cellular protein turnover, collagen degradation, and remodeling of the extracellular matrix, which plays an important role in pulmonary fibrosis [5–8]. Deficiency of Cathepsin K can lead to severe bone abnormalities, as it is the main peptidase involved in bone remodeling in osteoclasts [9,10]. In addition, increased expression and activity of Cathepsin K have been reported in patients diagnosed with breast cancer [11], bone cancer [12], prostate cancer [13], and many other types of epithelial-derived cell cancers [14–16]. Similar to the dysregulated Cathepsin B expression in the tumor microenvironment inducing tumor progression [17], Cathepsin K over-expression is associated with cancer metastatic disease, indicating its potential diagnostic and prognostic value. Distinct expression patterns of Cathepsin K have been identified in lung cancer cells and stromal cells, which provide further supporting evidence for this protease's significant prognostic value [18]. However, the specific role and mechanism of Cathepsin K in NSCLC is still unknown.

In this study, we revealed the effect of Cathepsin K expression on NSCLC cells in terms of cell proliferation, migration, and invasion in vitro. In order to understand the mechanisms, we also investigated the mammalian target of rapamycin (mTOR) signaling pathway. The mTOR signaling pathway plays an important role in maintaining cell growth, proliferation, motility, and survival [19]. Upregulation of the mTOR pathway has also been reported in a large number of NSCLC tumors, with increased p-mTOR expression in up to 90% of patients with adenocarcinoma, 60% of patients with large cell carcinoma, and 40% of patients with squamous cell carcinoma [20–22]. mTOR activation may also be associated with poor prognosis in early NSCLC [23,24]. Thus, mTOR inhibitors have been widely studied and employed clinically in order to suppress tumor growth and sensitize cells to anticancer drugs. Previous studies have demonstrated that inhibition of Cathepsin K can significantly reduced the phosphorylation of mTOR at S2448 in Caki cells [25]. Therefore, Cathepsin K may mediate activation of the mTOR signaling pathway in NSCLC. Our findings indicate that Cathepsin K has the potential in developing as a therapeutic target for NSCLC.

2. Results

2.1. *Cathepsin K Was Highly Expressed in A549 Cells and Diffused in the Cytoplasm*

Endogenous expression of Cathepsin K was detected in human embryonic lung fibroblasts MRC-5 and NSCLC cells A549 using a Western blot (WB) analysis and immunofluorescence (IF) assay. As shown in Figure 1a,b of WB results, compared to MRC-5 cells, the expression levels of Cathepsin K in A549 cells were significantly increased. An IF assay revealed that Cathepsin K was slightly expressed in MRC-5 cells, while Cathepsin K in A549 cells was largely expressed and diffused in the cytoplasm (Figure 1c), the cell fluorescence intensity was significantly increased (Figure 1d).

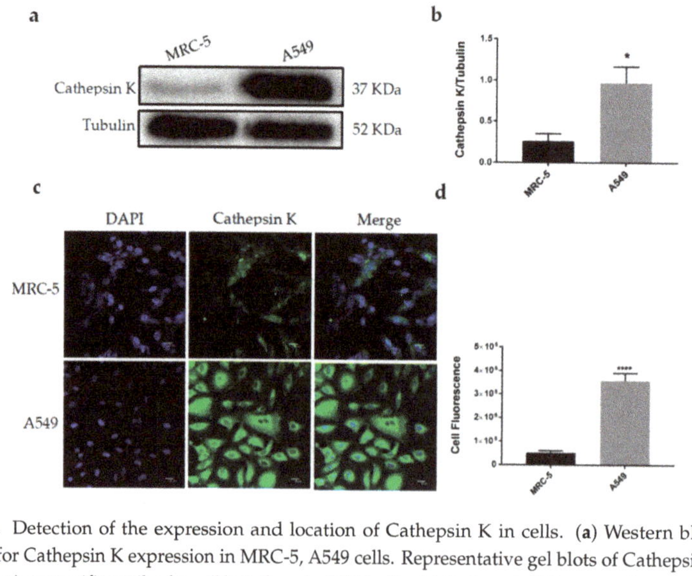

Figure 1. Detection of the expression and location of Cathepsin K in cells. (**a**) Western blot (WB) analysis for Cathepsin K expression in MRC-5, A549 cells. Representative gel blots of Cathepsin K and Tubulin using specific antibodies. (**b**) Cathepsin K/Tubulin; (**c**) Cathepsin K immunofluorescence (IF) staining in MRC-5 and A549 cells. (**d**) The cell fluorescence intensity was calculated using Image J software (mean ± SEM, $n \geq 3$, * $p \leq 0.05$, ** $p \leq 0.01$, *** $p \leq 0.001$).

2.2. *Cathepsin K Overexpression and Silence Models Were Successfully Reconstructed In Vitro*

In order to observe the phenotypic variations mediated by Cathepsin K, it was transiently overexpressed or knocked down using transfection with a recombinant plasmid and siRNA into A549 cells respectively. As shown in Figure 2a, Cathepsin K mRNA expression levels were significantly increased in the Cathepsin K overexpression cells (*CTSK*-OE) compared to control A549 cells. The protein levels of Cathepsin K were also increased 1.5 times compared to A549 cells, and increased 1.6 times compared to the vector group (Figure 2b,c). Three Cathepsin K siRNA sequences were constructed for transfection, and the optimal sequence was selected according to its silencing efficiency. The results revealed that both siRNA 2# and siRNA 3# can effectively and markedly silence Cathepsin K expression (Figure 2d,e). The 3# sequence was selected to construct the Cathepsin K knock down (*CTSK*-KD) model.

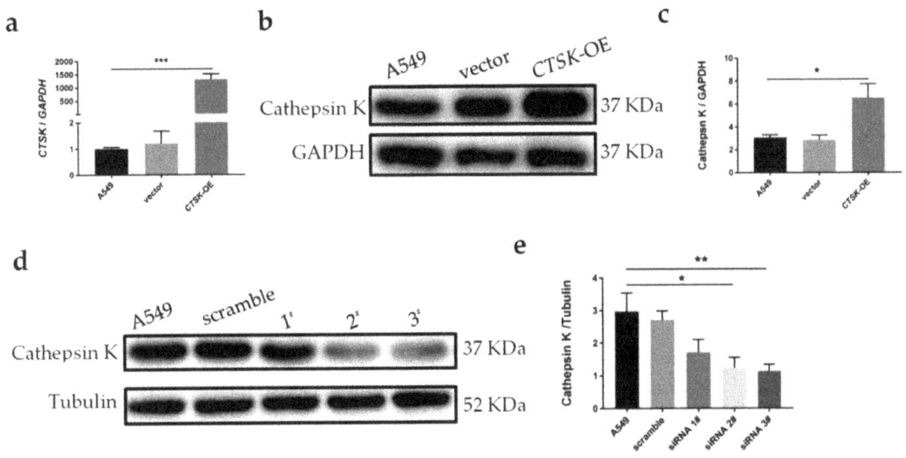

Figure 2. Construction of the Cathepsin K overexpression and knockdown models in vitro. (**a**) qRT-PCR analysis for *CTSK* expression in cells. *CTSK/GAPDH*; (**b**) WB analysis for Cathepsin K expression in cells. Representative gel blots of Cathepsin K and Tubulin using specific antibodies. (**c**) Cathepsin K/Tubulin; (**d**) WB analysis for Cathepsin K expression in cells. Representative gel blots of Cathepsin K and Tubulin using specific antibodies. (**e**) Cathepsin K/Tubulin (mean ± SEM, $n \geq 3$, * $p \leq 0.05$, ** $p \leq 0.01$, *** $p \leq 0.001$).

2.3. *CTSK-OE Promoted the Proliferation, Migration and Invasion and CTSK-KD Inhibited the Proliferation, Migration, and Invasion of A549 Cells*

In order to understand whether *CTSK*-OE and *CTSK*-KD could have a significant effect on the proliferation, migration, and invasiveness of A549 cells, cell proliferation, cell scratch repair, and Transwell assays were conducted in A549 cells as shown in Figure 3. *CTSK*-OE significantly promoted the proliferation of A549 cells from the time point 48 onward (Figure 3a), significantly promoting cell migration and invasion (Figure 3b,c). In contrast, *CTSK*-KD inhibited the proliferation of A549 cells from the time point 72 onward (Figure 3a), significantly inhibiting cell migration and invasion (Figure 3b,c).

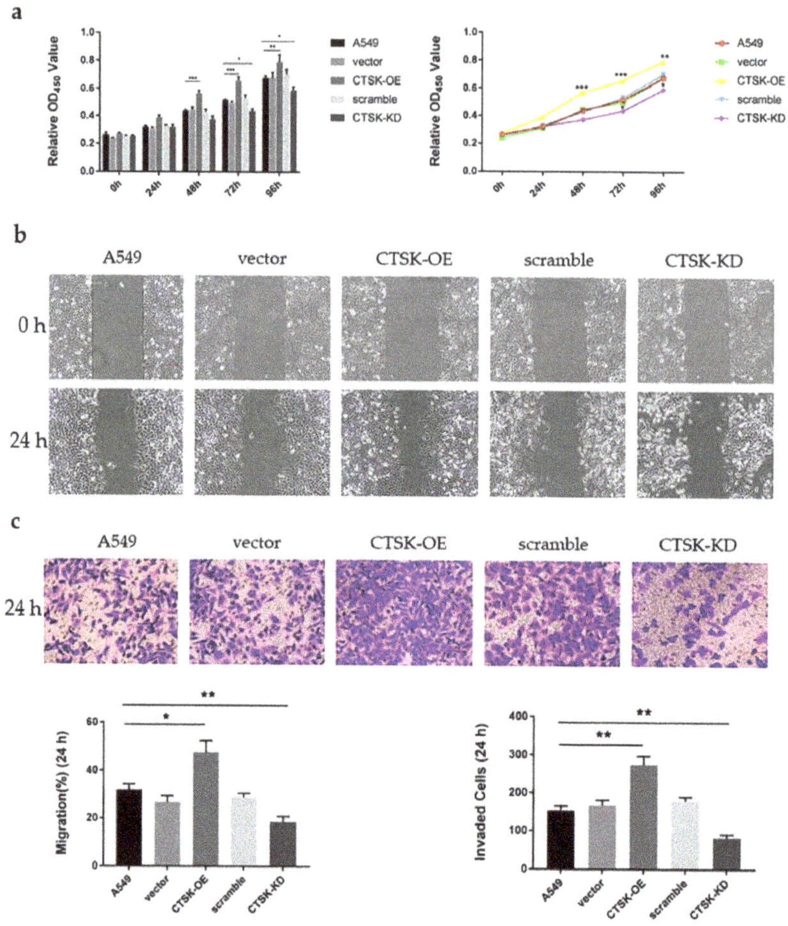

Figure 3. Detection of cell behavior in vitro. (**a**) Cell Counting Kit-8 (CCK-8) analysis for A549 cell proliferation. (**b**) Cell scratch repair analysis for A549 cell migration. (**c**) Invasion experiment analysis for A549 cell invasion (mean ± SEM, $n \geq 3$, * $p \leq 0.05$, ** $p \leq 0.01$, *** $p \leq 0.001$).

2.4. CTSK-OE Promoted While CTSK-KD Inhibited the Activation of the mTOR Signaling in A549 Cells.

In order to understand the mechanism of Cathepsin K in NSCLC, we detected mTOR and p-mTOR expression. The results are shown in Figure 4a. With a change in Cathepsin K expression levels (Figure 4b), *CTSK*-OE significantly increased level of p-mTOR and p-mTOR/mTOR, which promoted over-activation of the mTOR signaling pathway (Figure 4c,d). In contrast, *CTSK*-KD significantly decreased levels of p-mTOR and p-mTOR/mTOR, which inhibited activation of the mTOR signaling pathway (Figure 4c,d). No significant differences were found in the mTOR/Tubulin ratio among the groups (Figure 4e).

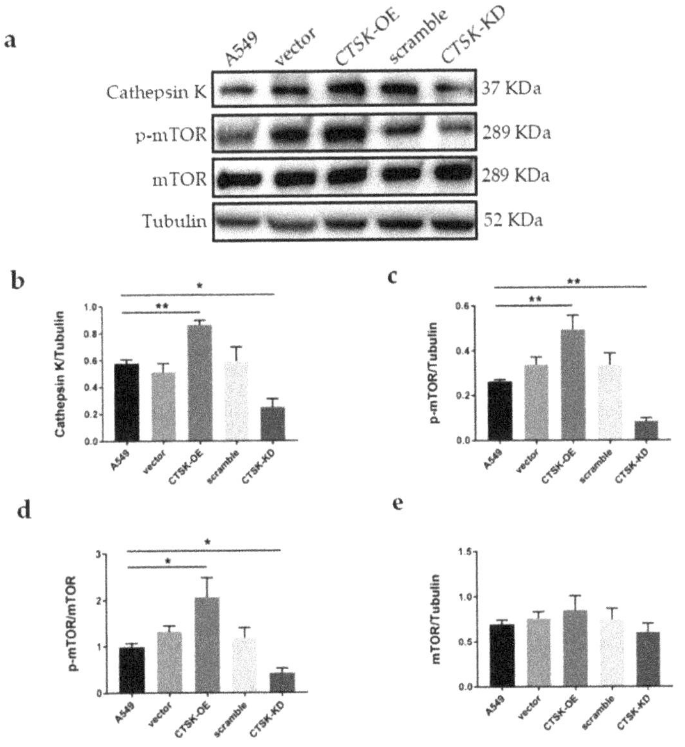

Figure 4. WB analysis for mTOR signaling protein expression in A549 cells. (**a**) Representative gel blots of Cathepsin K, p-mTOR, mTOR and Tubulin using specific antibodies. (**b**) Cathepsin K/Tubulin; (**c**) p-mTOR/Tubulin; (**d**) p-mTOR/mTOR; (**e**) mTOR/Tubulin. (mean ± SEM, $n \geq 3$, * $p \leq 0.05$, ** $p \leq 0.01$, *** $p \leq 0.001$).

3. Discussion

In addition to normal physiological functions [26–28], Cathepsin K also exhibits deleterious effects on the body, as evidenced by its role in the progression of a variety of tumors. Over the past few years, accumulated data have shown overexpression of Cathepsin K in multiple cancer types, indicating its role in tumor progression and its potential diagnostic and prognostic values. For example, strong expression of Cathepsin K has been observed in primary melanoma and melanoma metastases [29]. Colorectal cancer is associated with high LPS secretion and overexpression of Cathepsin K [30]. In order to study the expression of Cathepsin K in NSCLC, human NSCLC cell lines A549 were selected in this experiment, and human embryo lung fibroblast MRC-5 cells were used as controls. WB and IF assays showed that the expression level of Cathepsin K in A549 was higher than that in MRC-5, which is consistent with the conclusion that Cathepsin K is highly expressed in cancer tissues and cells in the literature. Compared with MRC-5 cells in which Cathepsin K was slightly expressed in cells, Cathepsin K was largely expressed in A549 cells and diffused into the cytoplasm. Cathepsin K is isolated into lysosomes through the endosome, and it can also be secreted into the other compartments of the cell and extracellular environment [31,32], which is essential for its role in promoting the development of cancer cells in tumors. It is worth noting that Cathepsin K seems to also be distributed in the nucleus of MRC-5 cells. In general, the pathway for Cathepsin proteins entering the nucleus without nuclear localization sequence (NLS) has been a controversial issue. A recent study demonstrated that Cathepsin proteins could be "chaperoned" into the nucleus from a cytoplasmic source following possible leakages from the lysosome [33]. The mechanism of Cathepsin positioning to the nucleus and its role in the nucleus are also matters for further exploration.

Proteases play important roles in cancer initiation, development and metastasis. Cathepsin K–shRNA transfection has been demonstrated to downregulate Cathepsin K, inhibiting the proliferation and metastasis of breast cancer cells [34]. In squamous cell carcinoma, mesenchymal fibroblasts expressing Cathepsin K are secreted by tumor cells through interleukin-1 stimulation and are associated with tumor aggressiveness [35]. In vitro, Cathepsin K knockdown has been shown to inhibit migration and invasiveness of the OV-2008 cell line in epithelial ovarian cancer [36]. In order to explore the effects of Cathepsin K on the proliferation, migration, and invasion of NSCLC, this experiment used a transfection method to introduce a Cathepsin K recombinant plasmid and *CTSK*-siRNA into A549 cells to construct *CTSK*-OE and *CTSK*-KD experimental models. This research employed a two-way crossover study in order to investigate the role of Cathepsin K in A549 cells. In CCK-8 detection at 48 h, the results showed that cell proliferation in the *CTSK*-OE was significantly increased. At 72 h, *CTSK*-KD significantly decreased in the cell proliferation. From the time course prospective, it is likely because siRNA displays characteristics that are distinct from the recombinant plasmid [37,38], it plays a role at a longer time point in the experiment compared to the recombinant plasmid. This phenomenon was not observed in cell migration and invasion experiments, which might be due to the researchers' selection of a specific time point for cellular detection.

In the cell scratch repair experiment, considering the damage of the transfection reagent to the cells, 1% fetal bovine serum was added to the culture medium. The cell proliferation cycle is generally 24 h in length. In order to exclude the effect of serum on migration experiments, the time point of 24 h was selected for the detection. In the same manner that the invasion experiment was conducted, no serum was present in the upper chamber of Transwell, but the medium in the lower chamber contained a serum concentration of 20%. The large concentration gradient between the upper and lower chambers resulted in a tendency for the A549 cells to be preferentially located in the lower chamber. The time point at 24 h was selected in order to avoid the potential proliferation of cells after penetration of the polycarbonate membrane, a factor that could influence the accuracy of the experiment. The results of the migration and invasion experiments were consistent with the results of the cell proliferation experiments. *CTSK*-OE significantly enhanced the migration and invasion ability of A549 cells. In contrast, the migration and invasion ability of *CTSK*-KD was significantly reduced. This is consistent with the conclusion that Cathepsin K is highly expressed during tumor invasion and metastasis [39] and has a stimulating effect on the aggressive phenotype of various types of cancer. Soond et al. [40] reported that the findings of use of utilizes combined chemotherapeutic treatment such as with Tocilizumab or Rituximab inhibited signaling transduction pathways which up-regulate the intracellular Cathepsins look very encouraging for targeting cancer. In the gastric metastasis model, the use of the pharmaceutical agent Odanacatib significantly inhibited the metastases of cancer cells, suggesting that Cathepsin K inhibition may be employed as a new therapeutic strategy to prevent tumor metastasis [41–43].

In addition to its well-known role in extracellular matrix degradation and remodeling, Cathepsin K may mediate activation of the mTOR signaling pathway. mTOR promotes anabolism and protein synthesis by phosphorylating its substrates S6 and EIF4E1 [44–46], as shown in Figure 5. It can further activate downstream products of the eIF4 complex to promote tumor development, regulate the cell cycle, and inhibit autophagy and apoptosis [19]. Seo et al. [25] demonstrated that inhibition of mTOR enhanced the chemosensitivity of cancer cells. They also revealed that treatment with mTOR inhibitors reduced tumor size and increased apoptosis in a xenograft model. Evimus, an inhibitor of mTOR, selectively inhibits mTOR signaling. It has been comprehensively evaluated in several phase I trials of previously treated advanced NSCLC [47].

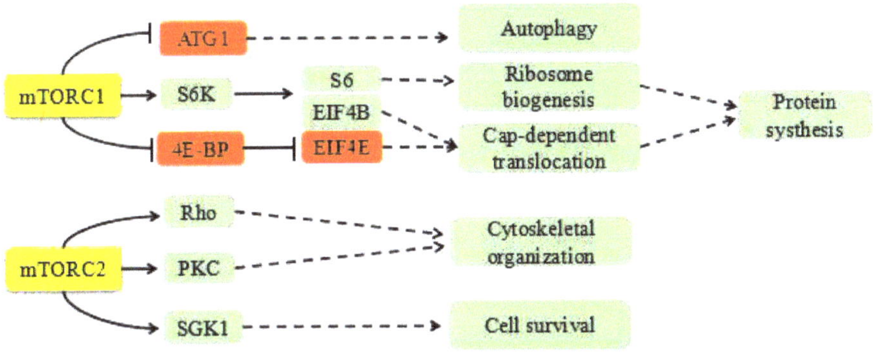

Figure 5. The role of mTOR in vivo. mTOR promotes protein synthesis by phosphorylating its substrates S6 and EIF4E1. It can further activate downstream products of eIF4 complex to promote tumor development, regulate the cell cycle, and inhibit autophagy and apoptosis.

In this experiment, *CTSK*-OE significantly increased levels of p-mTOR and p-mTOR/mTOR, which promoted over-activation of the mTOR signaling pathway. In contrast, *CTSK*-KD significantly decreased levels of p-mTOR and p-mTOR/mTOR, which inhibited activation of the mTOR signaling pathway. Previous studies have demonstrated that inhibition of Cathepsin K can induce proteasomal degradation of proteins associated with regulatory mechanisms on the target of rapamycin [25]. This conclusion is inconsistent with our experiment, which suggests that Cathepsin K may play a role in NSCLC through regulation of the mTOR signaling pathway. However, the mechanism of action by which Cathepsin K promotes the proliferation, migration, invasion, and other malignant behavior of NSCLC cells is unclear. Potential mediators involved in the effects of Cathepsin K could include a certain molecule's unique and powerful hydrolytic activity or its role in the mTOR signaling pathway. In addition, whether the changes of Cathepsin K in NSCLC cells are related to the levels of p-mTOR remains unclear. Therefore, it is necessary to supplement the Cathepsin K activity detection and mTOR signaling pathway inhibitor experiments in further research.

In summary, our results demonstrated that Cathepsin K was overexpressed in NSCLC cells and permeated the cytoplasm. Through the detection of cell biological functions, it was found that increased expression of Cathepsin K promoted the proliferation, migration, invasion, and activation of the mTOR signaling pathway of NSCLC cells, while silencing Cathepsin K expression reversed the above behavior. These findings suggest that Cathepsin K may potentially represent a new therapeutic target for NSCLC.

4. Materials and Methods

4.1. Cell Culture and Transfection

The MRC-5 and A549 cells were maintained in Dulbecco's modified Eagle's medium (DMEM) (Sangon Biotech, Shanghai, China) supplemented with 10% fetal bovine serum (FBS) (ExCell Bio, Beijing, China) and cultured in 5% CO_2 at 37 °C. The A549 cells were stably upregulated and downregulated for Cathepsin K expression using the Cathepsin K plasmid and siRNA (Genepharma, Shanghai, China), respectively. DNA transfection was performed using Lipofectamine-3000 (Thermo Fisher, Waltham, MA, USA), and siRNA was transfected at a final concentration of 50 nM using Lipofectamin-3000.

4.2. qRT-PCR

Total RNA was isolated using RNAiso Plus (TaKaRa, Kusatsu-shi, Japan), and RNAs were quantified using a NanoDropTM 2000 spectrophotometer (Thermo Fisher Scientific, Waltham, MA,

USA). Synthesis of cDNA and reverse transcription was performed using 1 μg of total RNA in a 25 μL system following the instructions of a FastQuant RT Kit (Tiangen, Beijing, China). *CTSK* and *GAPDH* primers for qPCR were designed by PrimerPremier5 software. The sequences were *CTSK*-F: 5′-CCTTGAGGCTTCTCTTGG-3′ *CTSK*-R: 5′-AGGGTGTCATTACTGCGG-3′; *GAPDH-F*: 5′-AGAAGGCTGGGGCTCATTTG-3′ *GAPDH-F*: 5′-AGGGGCCATCCACAGTCTTC-3′. Quantitative real-time PCR was performed for *CTSK* and *GAPDH* (housekeeping gene) using a C1000 Touch Thermal Cycler CFX96TM Real-Time System (Bio-Rad, Shanghai, China) per the Universal SYBR Green qPCR Supermix (UE, Suzhou, China) instructions. Real-time PCR was triplicated for each cDNA sample.

4.3. *Western Blot Analysis*

Total protein was isolated using radio immunoprecipitation assay (RIPA) lysate (strong) (Solarbio, Beijing, China), and the whole process was performed on ice. Proteins were quantified using a Microplate reader (Molecular Devices, Silicon Valley, CA, USA) following the instructions of a bicinchoninic acid (BCA) protein quantification kit (Solarbio, Beijing, China). Protein samples were then separated onto SDS-polyacrylamide gels and transferred electrophoretically to polyvinylidene fluoride (PVDF) membranes. The membranes were blocked with 5% milk and incubated overnight at 4 °C with anti-CathepsinK (1:1000; ab19027), anti-mTOR (1:1000; CST2983), anti-p-mTOR (1:1000; CST5536), anti-GAPDH (1:10,000; Proteintech10494-1-p), and anti-Tubulin (1:1000; CST2144). Blots were incubated with a horseradish peroxidase (HRP)-conjugated secondary antibody (1:3000; CST7074). Antigens were detected using a luminescence method. Band densities were determined using Image Lab software (version 5.1, Bio-Rad).

4.4. *Immunofluorescence Assays*

The cells were incubated successively for fixation and permeation with 4% paraformaldehyde (Leagene Biotechnology, Anhui, China) and 0.1% TritonX-100 (Leagene Biotechnology, Anhui, China). After successively incubating the cells with the configured PBST (phosphate buffer saline (PBS) (Sangon Biotech, Shanghai, China) + 0.1% Tween 20 + 1% BSA + 22.52 mg/mL Glycine) to block the non-specific binding of the antibody, the slides were rinsed and incubated with the appropriate primary antibody for Cathepsin K (1:100) overnight at 4 °C. The following day, the slides used for IF staining were incubated with fluorescein-conjugated goat anti-rabbit IgG and subsequently stained with nuclear dye 4′,6-diamidino-2-phenylindole (DAPI). Finally, the slides were then examined and imaged using an Olympus fluorescence microscope (fv3000), and the fluorescence intensity was calculated using Image J software (version 1.48v). In this experiment, 3 images were collected in each group, and each image outlines 10 cells for fluorescence intensity analysis.

4.5. *Proliferation Assays*

A Cell Counting Kit (APE×BIO, Houston, TX, USA) was used to evaluate the variation in cell proliferation, which is based on the dehydrogenase activity detected in viable cells. The formazan dye generated by dehydrogenases absorbs light at a wavelength of 450 nm. The amount of formazan dye present in cells is directly proportional to the number of living cells. In brief, 100 μL of cell suspension (1×10^3) was incubated in 96-well culture plates, and 10 μL of CCK-8 solution was added at the time set by the experiment. Cells were incubated at 37 °C for 2 h. Absorbance was analyzed at 450 nm using a microplate reader.

4.6. *Migration Assays*

A migration assay was used to detect the variation in cell migration. A549 cells were plated in 6-well plates at a certain amount (1×10^6) and allowed to form a confluent monolayer for 24 h. The monolayer was scratched with a sterile pipette tip (10 μL), followed by a wash with PBS to remove floating and detached cells. The cells were then imaged (at time 0 h and 24 h) by fluorescent inversion fluorescence microscopy (Olympus, Tokyo, Japan). Image J software was used to measure the scratch area and length of each image at 0 h and 24 h. According to the formula area/length, calculate the scratch width of the two periods and make the difference of the corresponding image, and the scratch width difference/corresponding initial width is the respective migration of each group.

4.7. Invasion Assays

The invasion assay was performed using a Transwell 24-well dish with a pore size of 8 μm (Costar, NY, USA). Mix the serum-free DMEM medium and Matrigel (Corning, Corning, NY, USA) at a ratio of 6:1 on ice, and added 60 μL to the Transwell chamber. 100 μL of DMEM serum-free medium cell suspension (5×10^4) was placed in the upper chamber, and 500 μL of DMEM medium containing 20% serum was placed in the lower chamber. The cells were incubated for 24 h at 37 °C in 5% CO_2, then fixed in 4% methanol and stained with 0.1% crystal violet. Cells on the upper side of the filters were removed with cotton-tipped swabs and the filters were then washed with PBS. Cells on the underside of the filters were examined and counted under a microscope.

4.8. Statistical Analysis

Results were representative of at least three independent experiments, and all values were expressed as mean ± SEM. Statistical significance ($p < 0.05$) for each variable was estimated by an unpaired t-test (two-tailed) or a one-way analysis of variance (ANOVA) followed by a Tukey's post hoc analysis.

Author Contributions: Conceptualization, L.Z. and R.G.; methodology, H.Y. and H.Z; validation, J.H., H.Y. and S.L.; formal analysis, H.Y. and S.L.; writing—original draft preparation, H.Y.; writing—review and editing, L.Z., R.G. and H.Y. All authors have read and agreed to the published version of the manuscript.

Funding: This research was supported in part by an NSFC grant (81773178, L.Z.), the Hebei Natural Science Foundation (#C2019201349, R.G.), and the National Natural Science Foundation of China (#31900534, R.G.).

Acknowledgments: The authors gratefully acknowledge Guo-ping Shi, from Harvard Medical School, Brigham and Women's Hospital, for kindly providing us with the *CTSK* plasmid.

Conflicts of Interest: The authors declare no conflict of interest. The funders had no role in the design of the study; in the collection, analyses, or interpretation of data; in the writing of the manuscript, or in the decision to publish the results.

References

1. Bray, F.; Ferlay, J.; Soerjomataram, I.; Siegel, R.L.; Torre, L.A.; Jemal, A. Global cancer statistics 2018: GLOBOCAN estimates of incidence and mortality worldwide for 36 cancers in 185 countries. *CA Cancer J. Clin.* **2018**, *68*, 394–424. [CrossRef] [PubMed]
2. Goldstraw, P.; Chansky, K.; Crowley, J.; Rami-Porta, R.; Asamura, H.; Eberhardt, W.E.; Nicholson, A.G.; Groome, P.; Mitchell, A.; Bolejack, V. The IASLC Lung Cancer Staging Project: Proposals for Revision of the TNM Stage Groupings in the Forthcoming (Eighth) Edition of the TNM Classification for Lung Cancer. *J. Thorac. Oncol. Off. Publ. Int. Assoc. Study Lung Cancer* **2016**, *11*, 39–51. [CrossRef] [PubMed]
3. Facchinetti, F.; Marabelle, A.; Rossi, G.; Soria, J.C.; Besse, B.; Tiseo, M. Moving Immune Checkpoint Blockade in Thoracic Tumors beyond NSCLC. *J. Thorac. Oncol. Off. Publ. Int. Assoc. Study Lung Cancer* **2016**, *11*, 1819–1836. [CrossRef] [PubMed]
4. Herbst, R.S.; Morgensztern, D.; Boshoff, C. The biology and management of non-small cell lung cancer. *Nature* **2018**, *553*, 446–454. [CrossRef]
5. Abdel-Magid, A.F. Inhibition of Cathepsin K: A Novel and Promising Treatment for Osteoporosis. *ACS Med. Chem. Lett.* **2015**, *6*, 628–629. [CrossRef]
6. Turk, V.; Stoka, V.; Vasiljeva, O.; Renko, M.; Sun, T.; Turk, B.; Turk, D. Cysteine cathepsins: From structure, function and regulation to new frontiers. *Biochim. Biophys. Acta* **2012**, *1824*, 68–88. [CrossRef]
7. Bühling, F.; Gerber, A.; Häckel, C.; Krüger, S.; Köhnlein, T.; Brömme, D.; Reinhold, D.; Ansorge, S.; Welte, T. Expression of Cathepsin K in lung epithelial cells. *Am. J. Respir. Cell Mol. Biol.* **1999**, *20*, 612–619. [CrossRef]
8. Bühling, F.; Röcken, C.; Brasch, F.; Hartig, R.; Yasuda, Y.; Saftig, P.; Brömme, D.; Welte, T. Pivotal role of Cathepsin K in lung fibrosis. *Am. J. Pathol.* **2004**, *164*, 2203–2216. [CrossRef]

9. Gelb, B.D.; Shi, G.P.; Chapman, H.A.; Desnick, R.J. Pycnodysostosis, a lysosomal disease caused by Cathepsin K deficiency. *Science* **1996**, *273*, 1236–1238. [CrossRef]
10. Garnero, P.; Borel, O.; Byrjalsen, I.; Ferreras, M.; Drake, F.H.; McQueney, M.S.; Foged, N.T.; Delmas, P.D.; Delaissé, J.M. The collagenolytic activity of cathepsin K is unique among mammalian proteinases. *J. Biol. Chem.* **1998**, *273*, 32347–32352. [CrossRef]
11. Littlewood-Evans, A.J.; Bilbe, G.; Bowler, W.B.; Farley, D.; Wlodarski, B.; Kokubo, T.; Inaoka, T.; Sloane, J.; Evans, D.B.; Gallagher, J.A. The osteoclast-associated protease cathepsin K is expressed in human breast carcinoma. *Cancer Res.* **1997**, *57*, 5386–5390. [PubMed]
12. Bühling, F.; Waldburg, N.; Gerber, A.; Häckel, C.; Krüger, S.; Reinhold, D.; Brömme, D.; Weber, E.; Ansorge, S.; Welte, T. Cathepsin K expression in human lung. *Adv. Exp. Med. Biol.* **2000**, *477*, 281–286. [PubMed]
13. Brubaker, K.D.; Vessella, R.L.; True, L.D.; Thomas, R.; Corey, E. Cathepsin K mRNA and protein expression in prostate cancer progression. *J. Bone Miner. Res. Off. J. Am. Soc. Bone Miner. Res.* **2003**, *18*, 222–230. [CrossRef] [PubMed]
14. Joyce, J.A.; Baruch, A.; Chehade, K.; Meyer-Morse, N.; Giraudo, E.; Tsai, F.Y.; Greenbaum, D.C.; Hager, J.H.; Bogyo, M.; Hanahan, D. Cathepsin cysteine proteases are effectors of invasive growth and angiogenesis during multistage tumorigenesis. *Cancer Cell* **2004**, *5*, 443–453. [CrossRef]
15. Kleer, C.G.; Bloushtain-Qimron, N.; Chen, Y.H.; Carrasco, D.; Hu, M.; Yao, J.; Kraeft, S.K.; Collins, L.C.; Sabel, M.S.; Argani, P.; et al. Epithelial and stromal cathepsin K and CXCL14 expression in breast tumor progression. *Clin. Cancer Res. Off. J. Am. Assoc. Cancer Res.* **2008**, *14*, 5357–5367. [CrossRef]
16. Boutté, A.M.; Friedman, D.B.; Bogyo, M.; Min, Y.; Yang, L.; Lin, P.C. Identification of a myeloid-derived suppressor cell cystatin-like protein that inhibits metastasis. *FASEB J. Off. Publ. Fed. Am. Soc. Exp. Biol.* **2011**, *25*, 2626–2637.
17. Li, Y.; Mei, T.; Han, S.; Han, T.; Sun, Y.; Zhang, H.; An, F. Cathepsin B-responsive nanodrug delivery systems for precise diagnosis and targeted therapy of malignant tumors. *Chin. Chem. Lett.* **2020**, 1–14.
18. Cordes, C.; Bartling, B.; Simm, A.; Afar, D.; Lautenschläger, C.; Hansen, G.; Silber, R.E.; Burdach, S.; Hofmann, H.S. Simultaneous expression of Cathepsins B and K in pulmonary adenocarcinomas and squamous cell carcinomas predicts poor recurrence-free and overall survival. *Lung Cancer (Amst. Neth.)* **2009**, *64*, 79–85. [CrossRef]
19. Guri, Y.; Hall, M.N. mTOR Signaling Confers Resistance to Targeted Cancer Drugs. *Trends Cancer* **2016**, *2*, 688–697. [CrossRef]
20. Dobashi, Y.; Suzuki, S.; Matsubara, H.; Kimura, M.; Endo, S.; Ooi, A. Critical and diverse involvement of Akt/mammalian target of rapamycin signaling in human lung carcinomas. *Cancer* **2009**, *115*, 107–118. [CrossRef]
21. Dobashi, Y.; Suzuki, S.; Kimura, M.; Matsubara, H.; Tsubochi, H.; Imoto, I.; Ooi, A. Paradigm of kinase-driven pathway downstream of epidermal growth factor receptor/Akt in human lung carcinomas. *Hum. Pathol.* **2011**, *42*, 214–226. [CrossRef] [PubMed]
22. Hiramatsu, M.; Ninomiya, H.; Inamura, K.; Nomura, K.; Takeuchi, K.; Satoh, Y.; Okumura, S.; Nakagawa, K.; Yamori, T.; Matsuura, M.; et al. Activation status of receptor tyrosine kinase downstream pathways in primary lung adenocarcinoma with reference of KRAS and EGFR mutations. *Lung Cancer (Amst. Neth.)* **2010**, *70*, 94–102. [CrossRef] [PubMed]
23. Obenauf, A.C.; Zou, Y.; Ji, A.L.; Vanharanta, S.; Shu, W.; Shi, H.; Kong, X.; Bosenberg, M.C.; Wiesner, T.; Rosen, N.; et al. Therapy-induced tumour secretomes promote resistance and tumour progression. *Nature* **2015**, *520*, 368–372. [CrossRef] [PubMed]
24. Lastwika, K.J.; Wilson, W., 3rd; Li, Q.K.; Norris, J.; Xu, H.; Ghazarian, S.R.; Kitagawa, H.; Kawabata, S.; Taube, J.M.; Yao, S.; et al. Control of PD-L1 Expression by Oncogenic Activation of the AKT-mTOR Pathway in Non-Small Cell Lung Cancer. *Cancer Res.* **2016**, *76*, 227–238. [CrossRef] [PubMed]
25. Seo, S.U.; Woo, S.M.; Kim, M.W.; Lee, H.S.; Kim, S.H.; Kang, S.C.; Lee, E.W.; Min, K.J.; Kwon, T.K. Cathepsin K inhibition-induced mitochondrial ROS enhances sensitivity of cancer cells to anti-cancer drugs through USP27x-mediated Bim protein stabilization. *Redox Biol.* **2020**, *30*, 101422. [CrossRef] [PubMed]
26. Aits, S.; Jäättelä, M. Lysosomal cell death at a glance. *J. Cell Sci.* **2013**, *126*, 1905–1912. [CrossRef]
27. Mason, S.D.; Joyce, J.A. Proteolytic networks in cancer. *Trends Cell Biol.* **2011**, *21*, 228–237. [CrossRef]

28. He, S.W.; Du, X.; Wang, G.H.; Wang, J.J.; Xie, B.; Gu, Q.Q.; Zhang, M.; Gu, H.J. Identification and characterization of a cathepsin K homologue that interacts with pathogen bacteria in black rockfish, Sebastes schlegelii. *Fish. Shellfish Immunol.* **2020**, *98*, 499–507. [CrossRef]
29. Xie, L.; Moroi, Y.; Hayashida, S.; Tsuji, G.; Takeuchi, S.; Shan, B.; Nakahara, T.; Uchi, H.; Takahara, M.; Furue, M. Cathepsin K-upregulation in fibroblasts promotes matrigel invasive ability of squamous cell carcinoma cells via tumor-derived IL-1α. *J. Dermatol. Sci.* **2011**, *61*, 45–50. [CrossRef]
30. Li, R.; Zhou, R.; Wang, H.; Li, W.; Pan, M.; Yao, X.; Zhan, W.; Yang, S.; Xu, L.; Ding, Y.; et al. Gut microbiota-stimulated cathepsin K secretion mediates TLR4-dependent M2 macrophage polarization and promotes tumor metastasis in colorectal cancer. *Cell Death Differ.* **2019**, *26*, 2447–2463.
31. Mohamed, M.M.; Sloane, B.F. Cysteine cathepsins: Multifunctional enzymes in cancer. *Nat. Rev. Cancer* **2006**, *6*, 764–775. [CrossRef] [PubMed]
32. Droga-Mazovec, G.; Bojic, L.; Petelin, A.; Ivanova, S.; Romih, R.; Repnik, U.; Salvesen, G.S.; Stoka, V.; Turk, V.; Turk, B. Cysteine cathepsins trigger caspase-dependent cell death through cleavage of bid and antiapoptotic Bcl-2 homologues. *J. Biol. Chem.* **2008**, *283*, 19140–19150. [CrossRef] [PubMed]
33. Soond, S.M.; Kozhevnikova, M.V.; Frolova, A.S.; Savvateeva, L.V.; Plotnikov, E.Y.; Townsend, P.A.; Han, Y.P.; Zamyatnin, A.A., Jr. Lost or Forgotten: The nuclear cathepsin protein isoforms in cancer. *Cancer Lett.* **2019**, *462*, 43–50. [CrossRef] [PubMed]
34. Gu, X.; Peng, Y.; Zhao, Y.; Liang, X.; Tang, Y.; Liu, J. A novel derivative of artemisinin inhibits cell proliferation and metastasis via down-regulation of cathepsin K in breast cancer. *Eur. J. Pharmacol.* **2019**, *858*, 172382. [CrossRef]
35. Yan, X.; Takahara, M.; Xie, L.; Oda, Y.; Nakahara, T.; Uchi, H.; Takeuchi, S.; Tu, Y.; Moroi, Y.; Furue, M. Stromal expression of cathepsin K in squamous cell carcinoma. *J. Eur. Acad. Dermatol. Venereol.* **2011**, *25*, 362–365. [CrossRef]
36. Fan, X.; Wang, C.; Song, X.; Liu, H.; Li, X.; Zhang, Y. Elevated Cathepsin K potentiates metastasis of epithelial ovarian cancer. *Histol. Histopathol.* **2018**, *33*, 673–680.
37. Singh, A.; Trivedi, P.; Jain, N.K. Advances in siRNA delivery in cancer therapy. *Artif. Cells Nanomed. Biotechnol.* **2018**, *46*, 274–283. [CrossRef]
38. Xu, H.; Ma, Y.; Zhang, Y.; Pan, Z.; Lu, Y.; Liu, P.; Lu, B. Identification of Cathepsin K in the Peritoneal Metastasis of Ovarian Carcinoma Using in-silico, Gene Expression Analysis. *J. Cancer* **2016**, *7*, 722–729. [CrossRef]
39. Soond, S.M.; Kozhevnikova, M.V.; Zamyatnin, A.A., Jr. 'Patchiness' and basic cancer research: Unravelling the proteases. *Cell Cycle* **2019**, *18*, 1687–1701. [CrossRef]
40. Soond, S.M.; Kozhevnikova, M.V.; Townsend, P.A.; Zamyatnin, A.A., Jr. Cysteine Cathepsin Protease Inhibition: An update on its Diagnostic, Prognostic and Therapeutic Potential in Cancer. *Pharmaceuticals* **2019**, *12*, 87. [CrossRef]
41. Duong, L.T.; Wesolowski, G.A.; Leung, P.; Oballa, R.; Pickarski, M. Efficacy of a cathepsin K inhibitor in a preclinical model for prevention and treatment of breast cancer bone metastasis. *Mol. Cancer Ther.* **2014**, *13*, 2898–2909. [CrossRef]
42. Chapurlat, R.D. Odanacatib: A review of its potential in the management of osteoporosis in postmenopausal women. *Ther. Adv. Musculoskelet. Dis.* **2015**, *7*, 103–109. [CrossRef] [PubMed]
43. Husmann, K.; Muff, R.; Bolander, M.E.; Sarkar, G.; Born, W.; Fuchs, B. Cathepsins and osteosarcoma: Expression analysis identifies cathepsin K as an indicator of metastasis. *Mol. Carcinog.* **2008**, *47*, 66–73. [CrossRef] [PubMed]
44. Laplante, M.; Sabatini, D.M. mTOR signaling in growth control and disease. *Cell* **2012**, *149*, 274–293. [CrossRef]
45. Thoreen, C.C.; Chantranupong, L.; Keys, H.R.; Wang, T.; Gray, N.S.; Sabatini, D.M. A unifying model for mTORC1-mediated regulation of mRNA translation. *Nature* **2012**, *485*, 109–113. [CrossRef] [PubMed]
46. Perluigi, M.; Di Domenico, F.; Butterfield, D.A. mTOR signaling in aging and neurodegeneration: At the crossroad between metabolism dysfunction and impairment of autophagy. *Neurobiol. Dis.* **2015**, *84*, 39–49. [CrossRef]

47. Vansteenkiste, J.; Solomon, B.; Boyer, M.; Wolf, J.; Miller, N.; Di Scala, L.; Pylvaenaeinen, I.; Petrovic, K.; Dimitrijevic, S.; Anrys, B.; et al. Everolimus in combination with pemetrexed in patients with advanced non-small cell lung cancer previously treated with chemotherapy: A phase I study using a novel, adaptive Bayesian dose-escalation model. *J. Thorac. Oncol. Off. Publ. Int. Assoc. Study Lung Cancer* **2011**, *6*, 2120–2129. [CrossRef]

Sample Availability: Not available.

molecules MDPI

Review

Regulation of ZMYND8 to Treat Cancer

Yun Chen [1,2], Ya-Hui Tsai [1,2,*] and Sheng-Hong Tseng [1,3,*]

1 Department of Surgery, Far Eastern Memorial Hospital, Pan-Chiao, New Taipei 220, Taiwan; ychen@mail.femh.org.tw
2 Department of Chemical Engineering and Materials Science, Yuan Ze University, Chung-Li, Taoyuan 320, Taiwan
3 Department of Surgery, National Taiwan University Hospital, Taipei 100, Taiwan
* Correspondence: yahuitsi@gmail.com (Y.-H.T.); shenghongtseng@gmail.com (S.-H.T.); Tel.: +886-2-89-667-000 (ext. 2923) (Y.-H.T.); +886-2-23-123-456 (ext. 65110) (S.-H.T.)

Abstract: Zinc finger myeloid, nervy, and deformed epidermal autoregulatory factor 1-type containing 8 (Zinc finger MYND-type containing 8, ZMYND8) is a transcription factor, a histone H3-interacting protein, and a putative chromatin reader/effector that plays an essential role in regulating transcription during normal cellular growth. Mutations and altered expression of ZMYND8 are associated with the development and progression of cancer. Increased expression of ZMYND8 is linked to breast, prostate, colorectal, and cervical cancers. It exerts pro-oncogenic effects in breast and prostate cancers, and it promotes angiogenesis in zebrafish, as well as in breast and prostate cancers. In contrast, downregulation of ZMYND8 is also reported in breast, prostate, and nasopharyngeal cancers. ZMYND8 acts as a tumor suppressor in breast and prostate cancers, and it inhibits tumor growth by promoting differentiation; inhibiting proliferation, cell-cycle progression, invasiveness, and metastasis; and maintaining the epithelial phenotype in various types of cancers. These data together suggest that ZMYND8 is important in tumorigenesis; however, the existing data are contradictory. More studies are necessary to clarify the exact role of ZMYND8 in tumorigenesis. In the future, regulation of expression/activity of ZMYND8 and/or its binding partners may become useful in treating cancer.

Keywords: ZMYND8; tumorigenesis; epigenetic regulation; pro-oncogenic effects; tumor suppression

Citation: Chen, Y.; Tsai, Y.-H.; Tseng, S.-H. Regulation of ZMYND8 to Treat Cancer. *Molecules* **2021**, *26*, 1083. https://doi.org/10.3390/molecules26041083

Academic Editor: Marialuigia Fantacuzzi

Received: 18 January 2021
Accepted: 15 February 2021
Published: 18 February 2021

1. Characteristics and Functions of ZMYND8

Zinc finger myeloid, nervy, and deformed epidermal autoregulatory factor 1-type containing 8 (Zinc finger MYND-type containing 8, ZMYND8) is a multifunctional transcription factor harboring conserved chromatin-binding module with affinity for chromatin [1]. It was initially identified as activated protein-kinase-C (PKC)-binding protein and is a member of the receptor for activated C-kinase (RACK) family proteins that anchor activated PKC and increase its phosphorylation and duration of inactivation; it is also called RACK7 [2,3]. ZMYND8 contains a Pro-Trp-Trp-Pro (PWWP) chromatin-binding domain, a bromodomain (BRD), a plant homeodomain (PHD) type zinc finger, and a MYND domain for protein–protein interaction (Figure 1) [3,4]. The PHD–BRD–PWWP (PBP) domains are histone readers, and the proteins containing PBP domains have various chromatin-related functions [5].

ZMYND8 is a core chromatin reader/effector, with distinct affinity for histone H3 and H4 [2,4–6]. The N-terminal PHD–BRD–PWWP domains of ZMYND8 can read several acetyl and methyl lysine residues on histones, including acetyl lysine 14 of H3 (H3K14ac), H4K16ac, and di- and tri-methyl lysine 36 of H3 (H3K36me2, H3K36me3) [6,7]. The PHD–BRD–PWWP domains of ZMYND8 form a stable structural reader ensemble and simultaneously engage histones and DNA, and then ZMYND8 is recruited to the transcriptional sites of the chromatin [7]. Mutation of the reader ensemble may affect the binding of ZMYND8 to histones by disrupting the interaction interface or destabilizing the domain topology [7]. ZMYND8 has been found to regulate gene expression by recognizing dual histone marks [8]. It regulates the expression of all-trans retinoic acid (ATRA)-responsive genes through specific recognition of H3K36me2/H4K16ac [9,10]. It also recognizes H3K4me1/H3K14ac in DU154 and CWR22Rv1 prostate cancer cells [8], as well as H3K36me2/H4K16ac in SH-SY5Y neuroblastoma cells [4,9]. The dual recognition of two different histone modification by ZMYND8 suggests that the two separate conserved domains PWWP and BRD have different affinities towards their cognate histone binding partners [11]. When both H3K36me2 and H4K16ac exist in same histone octamer, the initial binding and recognition of the ZMYND8 to chromatin is considered through H3K36me2 because of its higher association rate, and the stability of the ZMYND8–nucleosome complex relies more on the binding to H4K16ac, due to its lower association rate [11].

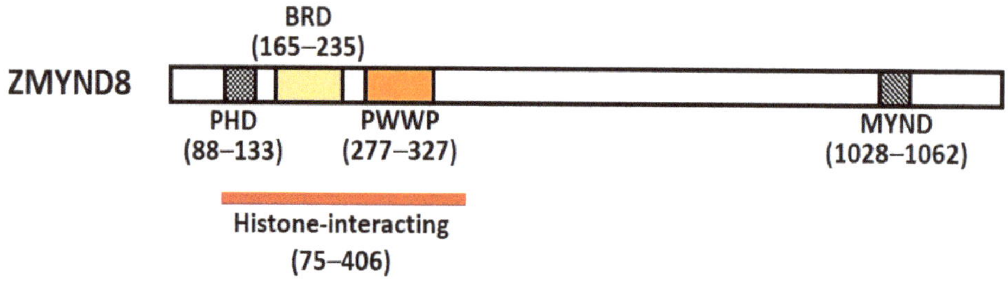

Figure 1. Schematic representation of ZMYND8. ZMYND8 domains include the N-terminal PHD/BRD/PWWP reader cassette and a C-terminal MYND interacting domain. MYND: Myeloid, nervy, and deformed epidermal autoregulatory factor 1; ZMYND8: Zinc finger MYND-type containing 8; PHD: Plant homeodomain; BRD: Bromodomain; PWWP: Pro-Trp-Trp-Pro.

ZMYND8 is involved in transcription activation and in regulating transcription initiation through its interaction with the RNA polymerase II complex [4,12]. Through its putative coiled-coil domain, ZMYND8 forms a homodimer that preferentially associates with positive transcription elongation factor b (P-TEFb) complex, whereas the monomer associates with the chromodomain helicase DNA-binding protein 4 (CHD4) subunit of repressor nucleosome remodeling and deacetylase (NuRD) complex [4,12,13]. ZMYND8 and NuRD share a large number of genome-wide binding sites, mostly in active promoters and enhancers [14]. Both ZMYND8 and CHD4 modulate the expression of many genes and maintain genome integrity; silencing any one of them can alter global gene expression [4,12]. Silencing of ZMYND8 in HeLa cells increases the expression of 331 genes and decreases that of 438 genes [4]. ZMYND8 is important in modulating chromatin integrity and DNA repair [6,15,16]. Upon DNA double-strand break (DSB), histone modifications are altered to accommodate the DNA-damage signaling and the repair [6,15], and BRD2 protein and ZMYND8 are recruited to the DNA damages sites [17]. BRD2 occupies a spatially restricted region extending 2 kb either side of the DSB, and ZMYND8 spreads along the flanking chromatin [17]. The hyperacetylated chromatin domain is required for DBS repair, and the binding of BRD2 to H4ac protects the underlying acetylated chromatin from attack by histone deacetylases, whereas ZMYND8 is a repressor factor which limits transcription during DSB repair [17]. This creates a spatially restricted H4ac/BRD domain which facilitates DSB repair [17]. ZMYND8 interacts with various chromatin-remodeling complexes, histone demethylases/deacetylases, and acetyl transferases, including lysine demethylase 1A (KDM1A), KDM5A, KDM5C, and KDM5D, as well as histone acetyltransferase Tat-interactive protein-60KDa (TIP60) [4,6,8,12,16,18]. KDM5A-dependent demethylation is crucial for the binding of the ZMYND8–NuRD complex to chromatin and its recruitment to the locations of DNA damage (Figure 2) [15]. KDM5A causes H3K4me3 demethylation within chromatin, near the sites of DSB, while ZMYND8, NuRD complex, and KDM5A interact to repress transcription upon DNA damage [6,15]. KDM5A deficiency impairs the transcriptional silencing and the repair of DSBs by homologous recombination [15]. ZMYND8 also interacts with the NuRD complex and TIP60, to mediate DNA repair through homologous recombination [6,16]. In Xenopus embryos, ZMYND8 interacts with RE1-silencing transcription factor corepressor 2 (RCOR2), and together they function as transcriptional repressors in regulating neural differentiation [19]. Both ZMYND8 and p53 play a role in DSB repair [6,15,16]. In several breast cancer cells with distinct p53 genotypes, ZMYND8 loss induced consistent micronucleus formation and DNA-damage response [20]. Additionally, in ZMYND8-depleted human U2OS osteosarcoma cells, laser micro-irradiation induced sustained p53 phosphorylation, which is a DSB marker; in contrast, there was no sustained p53 phosphorylation in control cells [6]. These results imply ZMYND8 and p53 may function independently for repair of DNA damage.

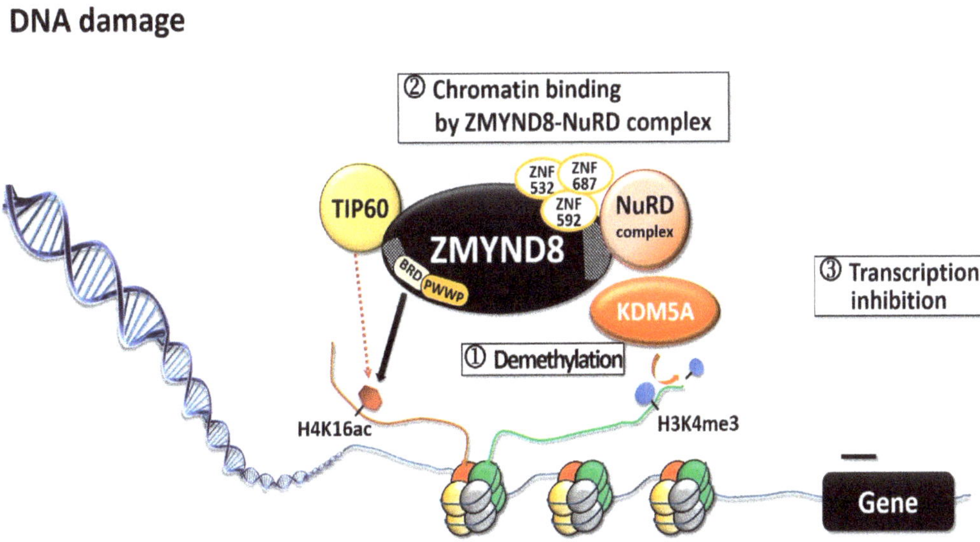

Figure 2. Diagram showing the KDM5A–ZMYND8–NuRD pathway during DNA damage. Upon DNA damage, the hisTable 5. A. ZMYND8 interacts with the NuRD complex and recognizes the TIP60-dependent acetylation. Then ZMYND8–NuRD complex binds to the DNA damaged site, inhibits transcription, and promotes DNA repair. TIP60: Histone acetyltransferase Tat-interactive protein-60KDa; NuRD: Nucleosome remodeling and deacetylase; KDM5A: Lysine demethylase 5A; H4K16ac: Acetyl lysine 16 of H4; H3K4me3: Tri-methyl lysine 4 of H3.

As ZMYND8 is important for transcriptional regulation and chromatin integrity, it may have a role in oncogenesis. However, the reports regarding the influence of ZMYND8 on cancers are ambiguous [2,8,9,21–25]. In this review, we summarize the evidence for both pro-oncogenic and tumor-suppressive effects of ZMYND8 in various types of cancer. We conducted a PubMed literature search, using a combination of the following keywords and their variants: ZMYND8, RACK7, cancers, neoplasms, oncogenesis, carcinogenesis, and epigenetic regulation (up to November 30, 2020). The search covered all English articles listed in PubMed. The titles and abstracts of the identified articles concerning ZMYND8, RACK7, cancer, angiogenesis, proliferation, invasiveness, metastasis, and tumor growth were included. The selected articles were read in full, and further articles that were identified from their reference lists were also reviewed, to include studies that may have been missed in the initial search. A total of 39 references were thus included in the present review.

2. Association of ZMYND8 and Cancers

Many epigenetic effectors, including ZMYND8, contain structurally conserved domains of PHD fingers, and alterations in the PHD finger-containing proteins are linked to cancer [4,6,26,27]. ZMYND8 is essential for regulating transcription during normal cellular growth and DNA repair, the perturbation of which may promote cancer initiation and progression [6,15,16]. In fact, ZMYND8 is a cutaneous T-cell lymphoma-associated antigen [28]. In addition, the ZMYND8-v-rel reticuloendotheliosis viral oncogene homolog A (avian) (RELA) chimeric transcripts were reported in a four-month-old patient with acute erythroid leukemia, a type of acute myeloid leukemia (AML) [29]. This fusion gene was thought to be a possible cause of constitutive activation of nuclear factor-kB in AML cells, since the RELA gene was under the control of the ZMYND8 promoter [29]. In breast cancer cells, ZMYND8 may be present as a fusion protein with centrosomal protein 250 (CEP250), which is required for centriole–centriole cohesion during interphase [3,30]. However, the ZMYND8-CEP250 fusion mRNA was not reported in the 111 breast cancer specimens studied [3]. Mutation frequency of *ZMYND8* was 19% in mismatch repair-deficient colorectal cancers [31]. In high-grade serous ovarian cancer, the *ZMYND8* gene is located within a region with recurrent alterations of somatic copy number [32]. An increased copy number (two to six copies) of *ZMYND8* is also found in DU-145, PC-3, LNCaP-FGC, BPH-1, and 22RV1 prostate cancer cells [2]. All of these findings indicate that ZMYND8 may be involved in development and progression of cancer.

3. ZMYND8 and Histone Modification in Cancer Cells

The function of ZMYND8 in cancer cells is mainly through modulation of histone methylation and acetylation [4,9,11,25,32]. It selectively recognizes H3K36me2/H4K16ac and regulates all-trans retinoic acid (ATRA)-responsive genes in SH-SY5Y neuroblastoma cells [4]. In MDA-MB-231 breast cancer cells, ZMYND8 is recruited to its target genes by binding to H3K36me2 and H4K16Ac (Figure 3A) [11]. Furthermore, in HeLa and MCF7 breast cancer cells, ATRA induces an H3K27me3 to H3K27ac switch and upregulates ZMYND8 expression [9]. Modulation of histone methylation and acetylation in the enhancer regions by ZMYND8 is particularly important, as the dysregulation of this process may cause over-activation of transcription and contribute to tumorigenesis [25]. ZMYND8 and the KDM5 family cooperatively act on super-enhancer regions and are crucial regulators of expression and repression of oncogenes and tumor-suppressor genes in various types of cancer [8,12,16,18,25,33–35]. In ZR-75-30 breast cancer cells, ZMYND8 promotes the recruitment of KDM5C to the super-enhancer region, shown by the co-binding of ZMYND8 and KDM5C to 88.7% super-enhancers (Figure 3B) [25]. Ablation of either ZMYND8 or KDM5C in ZR-75-30 breast cancer cells results in over-activation of their target enhancers, characterized by the deposition of H3K4me3 and H3K27ac, decreased H3K4me1, and increased transcription of enhancer RNAs (eRNAs) and nearby genes [25]. In DU145 prostate cancer cells, in addition to KDM5C, ZMYND8 interacts with KDM5D, to act as transcriptional co-repressors, involved in regulating metastasis-linked genes (Figure 3C) [8]. ZMYND8 and KDM5D act as general negative regulators of enhancers in prostate cancer cells, and they antagonize the expression of these genes by recognizing the gene-activation-related dual-histone marker H3K4me1-H3K14ac [8].

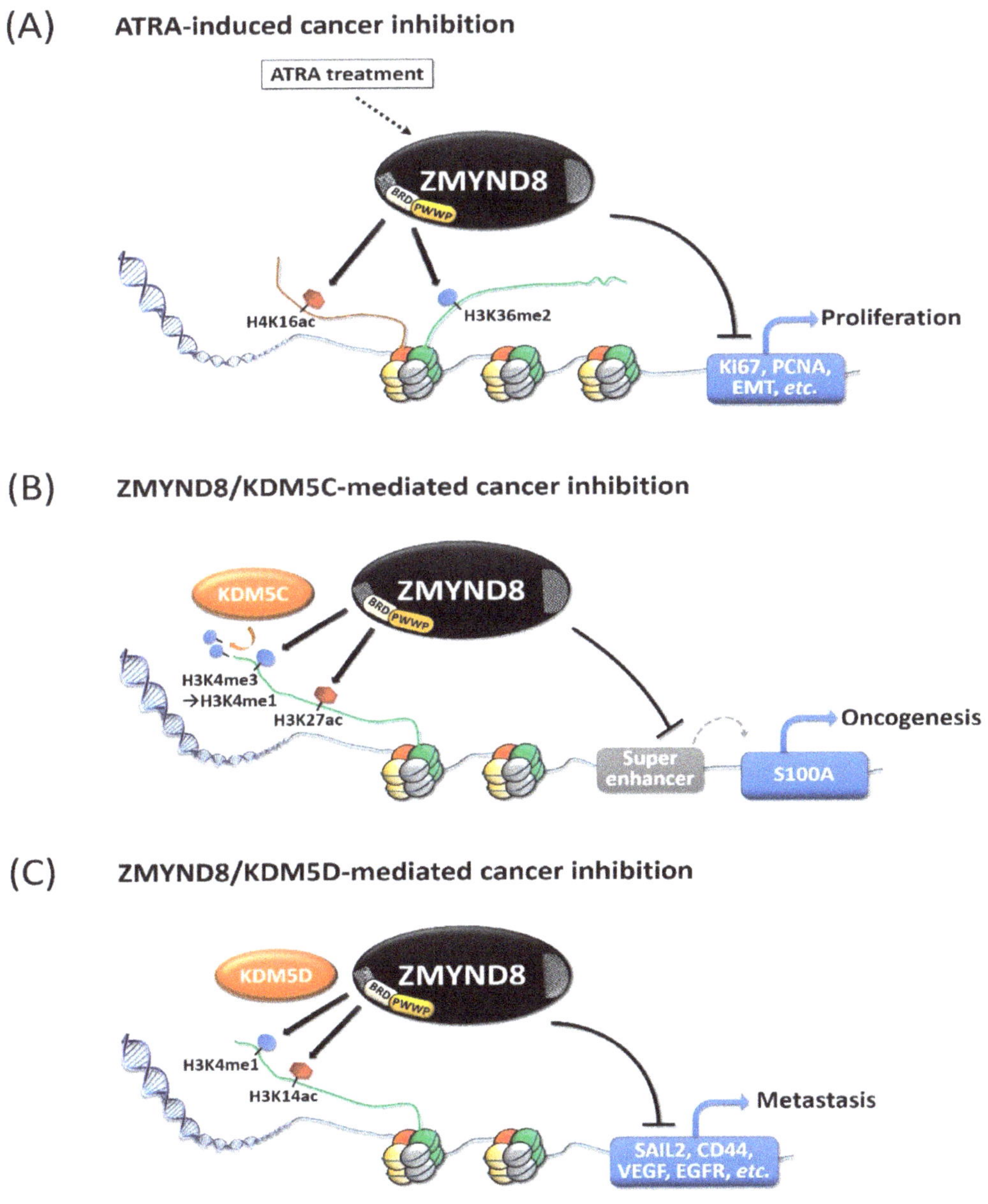

Figure 3. Diagrams showing the mechanisms of the tumor-suppression effects of ZMYND8 and demethylases. The tumor-suppression effects may involve recognition of dual histone marks. (**A**) The all-trans retinoic acid (ATRA)-induced inhibition of transcription of proliferation genes and epithelial–mesenchymal transition (EMT). (**B**) ZMYND8 cooperates with KDM5C to suppress super-enhancer and transcription of oncogenes in breast cancer. (**C**) ZMYND8 cooperates with KDM5D to suppress transcription of metastasis genes in prostate cancer. PCNA: Proliferating cell nuclear antigen; VEGF: Vascular endothelial growth factor; EGFR: Epidermal growth factor receptor.

4. Tumor Suppression by ZMYND8

The expression of ZMYND8 decreases in some cancers [10,25,36]. It is downregulated in invasive ductal and lobular breast cancer tissues, compared with normal tissues [10]. In addition, ZMYND8 expression is lower in breast cancer patients with invasive ductal carcinoma than in ductal carcinoma in situ [25]. In 190 patients with nasopharyngeal carcinoma, low ZMYND8 expression was correlated with late T stage, presence of lymph node metastasis, advanced stage, and poor overall patient survival [36]. ZMYND8 is a retinoic acid–inducible gene, and ATRA, a differentiation-inducing drug, can reprogram the epigenetic features of the upstream regulatory region of ZMYND8 and promote its expression [4,9]. On the other hand, ZMYND8 can facilitate the regulation of ATRA-responsive genes in SH-SY5Y neuroblastoma cells [4]. Differentiation of neuronal precursor cells induced by ATRA also requires transcriptional regulation, mediated by the ZMYND8–P-TEFb complex [13]. In MDA-MB-231 breast cancer cells, ZMYND8 upregulates differentiation genes and induces cellular differentiation [11]. The induction of breast cancer cell differentiation by ZMYND8 was noted through the H3K36me2/H4K16ac reader function of ZMYND8 [11]. Microarray analysis of breast cancer cells with ZMYND8 knockout by siRNA revealed that depletion of ZMYND8 reduces the expression of terminal differentiation markers, such as epithelial cell adhesion molecule (EPCAM) and cytokeratin 18 (CK18), by 80% and 86%, respectively [11]. In contrast, overexpression of ZMYND8 induces a 1.5-fold increase in EPCAM and CK18 levels [11]. In addition, ZMYND8 knockdown downregulates the stemness-related genes, prevents tumor cell differentiation, and maintains cancer cells in an undifferentiated state [11]. An in vivo study also showed that ZMYND8 overexpression significantly reduces the subcutaneous 4T1 murine breast cancer growth and increases the expression of differentiation-related genes, including *CK5*, *CK18*, *CK19*, and *EPCAM* in Balb/c mice [11]. All of these results suggest that, in cancer cells, ZMYND8 positively regulates the expression of differentiation-promoting genes and induces differentiation [11].

ZMYND8 also influences cancer cell proliferation. In HeLa and MCF7 breast cancer cells, knocking down ZMYND8 increases the proliferation by about two folds, whereas ZMYND8 overexpression reduces it by about 2.5 to 3 folds [10]. ZMYND8 can be directly recruited to proliferation-promoting genes, including *Ki67* and proliferating cell nuclear antigen (*PCNA*), and affect their expression [10,11]. ZMYND8 knockdown increases the expression of *Ki67* and *PCNA* by about 14 and 4 folds, respectively, in HeLa cells; about 8 and 3 folds in MCF7 breast cancer cells; and about 9 and 2.5 folds in T47D metastatic breast cancer cells [10]. In contrast, overexpression of ZMYND8 reduces the expression of *Ki67* and *PCNA* to 0.1–0.4 fold in these cells [10], and reduces the uptake of bromodeoxyuridine (BrdU) in HeLa cells [10]. However, deletion of ZMYND8 by short hairpin RNA (shRNA) does not affect the proliferation of DU145 prostate cancer cells significantly [8]. Knocking out ZMYND8 can enhance the tumor growth in a mammary fat pad xenograft model of ZR-75-30 breast cancer cells [25]. In contrast, invasive MCF-7 or 4T1 breast cancer cells overexpressing ZMYND8 show a reduction in the tumor size and tumor weight in mice, compared with the control [10,11]. ZMYND8 modulates cell-cycle progression, and its overexpression reduces the *Cyclin* genes, including *G1/S-specific cyclin-E1 (CCNE1)*, *CCNA2*, and *G2/mitotic-specific cyclin-B1 (CCNB1)* in HeLa cells; meanwhile, the inhibition of ZMYND8 by siRNA upregulates their expression [10]. However, in breast cancer cells, the expression of CDKN1A mRNA was upregulated by ZMYND8 loss, which suggests ZMYND8 depletion can increase the p21, which is an inhibitor of cell-cycle progression [20].

In addition to the suppression of cell proliferation, ZMYND8 also affects the tumor cell migration and invasion [8,10]. It can repress the expression of genes that promote metastasis and invasion, and enhance the transcription of epithelial genes [8,10]. In the wound-healing assay, ZMYND8 silencing causes faster wound closure, and its overexpression inhibits this process [10]. In a three-dimension-based assay, ZMYND8-null ZR-75-30 breast cancer cells show increased anchorage-independent growth, migration, and invasion, which can be reversed by restoration of ZMYND8 [25]. In the Matrigel invasion assay, ZMYND8 knockout results in a 1.6-2-fold increase in the invasiveness of HeLa and MCF7 breast cancer cells, and its overexpression reduces the invasiveness by 1.3–1.5 folds in these two cells [10]. Suppression of migration and invasion by ZMYND8 in breast cancer cells is through cooperation with KDM5C and modulation of SA100, as knockout of ZMYND8 or KDM5C can de-repress S100A [25].

The influence of ZMYND8 on cancer cell invasion and metastasis is related to the interaction between ZMYND8, TROJAN, and ZNF592 in breast cancer [24]. Both TROJAN and ZNF592 are the binding partners of ZMYND8, and the function of ZMYND8 is affected by the competitive binding of TROJAN and NF152 with it [24]. TROJAN, an endogenous retrovirus-derived long noncoding RNA, is upregulated in multiple cancer cell lines and is highly expressed in human triple-negative breast cancer [24]. ZNF592 can prevent ZMYND8 degradation, and TROJAN interferes with its ability to bind ZMYND8 [24]. In MDA-MB-231 LM2 breast cancer cells, TROJAN binds to ZMYND8, and increases its degradation through the ubiquitin-proteasome pathway, by repelling ZNF592 [24]. TROJAN knockdown increases ZMYND8 protein, while overexpression of TROJAN or knockdown of ZNF592 decreases it in MDA-MB231 LM2 cells [24]. Both TROJAN and ZMYND8 occupy epidermal growth factor receptor (EGFR), vascular endothelial growth factor-A (VEGF-A), and mouse double minute 2 homolog (MDM2) promoters, suggesting that they co-regulate these metastasis- and angiogenesis-related genes [24]. In an in vivo study, mice intravenously injected with MB-231 LM2 cells with TROJAN knockdown showed fewer metastatic lung nodules, as compared with the control, whereas mice injected with ZMYND8-inactivated cells showed more of them [24]. Increased metastatic ability of MDA-MB-231 LM2 breast cancer cells, induced by ZMYND8 knockdown, can be partially reversed by simultaneous knockdown of TROJAN [24]. In human breast cancer tissues, the expression of TROJAN negatively correlates with ZMYND8 expression, and it positively correlates with EGFR, VEGF-A, and MDM2 expression [24]. In addition, the TROJAN–ZMYND8 combined expression signature can be used to predict the relapse-free survival and overall survival of patients with triple-negative breast cancers (TNBCs); those with high TROJAN and low ZMYND8 expression have worse prognosis, and the ones with low TROJAN and high ZMYND8 levels survive better [24].

ZMYND8 also prevents metastasis of prostate cancer cells [8]. Knockdown of ZMYND8 increases the invasiveness of DU145 and CWR22Rv1 human prostate cancer cells in vitro, and this was also noted in an intravenous mouse xenograft model [8]. In mice injected with luciferase-expressing DU145 prostate cancer cells with ZMYND8 silencing by shRNA (shZMYND8), the luciferase signals were about five-fold higher than in those treated with the control shRNA, eight weeks after injection [8]. Histological examination of the lungs confirmed tumor development in the shZMYND8 group [8]. These results suggest that ZMYND8 suppresses invasiveness and metastasis of prostate cancer cells, both in vitro and in vivo [8]. The ZMYND8-induced suppression of invasiveness and metastasis in prostate cancer cells was demonstrated to be through cooperating with its transcriptional corepressor KDM5D [8]. They co-occupy multiple metastasis-linked genes, such as *SAIL2, CD44, VEGF*, and *EGFR*, and hinder the expression of these genes by interacting with the gene-activation-related dual-histone mark H3K4me1-H3K14ac [8]. Knockdown of either ZMYND8 or KDM5D can upregulate these metastasis-related genes [8]. KDM5D levels are significantly reduced in metastatic prostate tumors (100%, 6/6) and primary prostate tumors (41%, 28/68), as compared with normal tissues (10%, 2/21) [37]. These observations suggest that cooperation between ZMYND8-mediated recognition of H3K4me1-H3K14ac and KDM5D-catalyzed H3K4 demethylation can hamper the expression of metastasis-linked genes [8,37]. H3K4me1-H3K14ac may act as a poised epigenetic signature, and it is converted to active dual marker H3K4me3-H3K14ac during cancer metastasis [8]. Therefore, the epigenetic switch is critical for regulating the expression of metastasis-linked factors, including Slug, CD44, VEGFA, and EGFR, which, in turn, modulate the invasiveness of prostate cancer cells [8].

ZMYND8 can regulate the epithelial–mesenchymal transition (EMT), which is important for cellular invasion [10]. It regulates EMT genes through recognizing H3K36me2/H4K16ac on respective genes [10]. The epithelial phenotype of cancer cells is governed by claudin-1 *(CLDN1)*, claudin-7 *(CLDN7)*, and E-cadherin *(CDH1)* genes, while the mesenchymal phenotype is regulated by *ZEB1*, *SNAI1*, *SNAI2*, and Vimentin *(VIM)* genes [10,38]. In MDA-MB-231 breast cancer cells, ZMYND8 is directly recruited to metastasis-linked genes *SNAI2* and *TWIST1*, to regulate EMT [11]. Overexpression of ZMYND8 reduces the expression of *VIM*, *SNAI1*, and *ZEB1* and increases that of *CLDN1* and *CDH1* in MCF7, HeLa, and T47D cells [10]. ZMYND8 knockdown reduces the expression of *CLDN1/7* and *CDH1* genes in MCF7 and HeLa cells, and that of *CDH1* and *CLDN7* in T47D cells, while it increases the expression of *VIM*, *SNAI1*, and *ZEB1* in MCF7, HeLa, and T47D cells [10]. These observations suggest that ZMYND8 is involved in maintaining the epithelial cell phenotype, and the deletion of ZMYND8 enhances the mesenchymal transition [10].

Overall, ZMYND8 appears to act as a tumor suppressor in breast, prostate, and nasopharyngeal cancers [8,9,24,25]. It can induce differentiation; inhibit cell proliferation, cell-cycle progression, invasiveness, and metastasis; and maintain the epithelial phenotype in these cells [8,9,24,25].

5. Pro-Oncogenic Effects of ZMYND8

The level of ZMYND8 expression is crucial for proliferation and invasiveness of cancer cells, and increased ZMYND8 expression is reported in colorectal, cervical, breast, and prostate cancers [2,21,23,36]. Analyses of the Cancer Genome Atlas (TCGA) and Gene Expression Omnibus (GEO) database suggested that high expression of ZMYND8 was closely correlated with poor overall and disease-free survival in 174 colorectal cancer patients [23]. Increased ZMYND8 expression was linked to the high-grade cervical intraepithelial neoplasia and cervical carcinoma [21], zebrafish prostate cancer DU145 xenografts, and prostate cancer tissues from patients [2]. In addition, ZMYND8 expression is inversely correlated with metastasis-free survival in breast cancer patients, with high ZMYND8 expression being associated with shorter survival of patients with breast cancer [22,27]. However, increased ZMYND8 expression is associated with high mortality in patients with different subtypes and stages of breast cancer, but not with different grades of tumor [22]. ZMYND8 is a downstream target of estrogen receptor α (ERα), and it is involved in a positive feedback circuit of the ER pathway [27]. It is highly expressed in ER-positive and triple-negative breast cancers [22,27]. Amplification and overexpression of ZMYND8 are more frequent in luminal B breast cancer subtypes [22,27]. Tissue microarray analysis of 160 human TNBC specimens and 91 paired adjacent normal breast tissues revealed that 80% of tumors showed an increased expression of ZMYND8, with 50% showing moderate expression and 30% showing high expression [22]. In contrast, only 18% of the normal tissues had moderate ZMYND8 expression and none showed high expression [22]. An in vitro study also showed that ZMYND8 knockdown by small interfering RNA (siRNA) suppressed colony formation and reduced the number of MCF-7 breast cancer cell colonies; however, ZMYND8 knockdown did not affect the proliferation rate of the breast cancer cells [22]. In vivo experiments revealed that ZMYND8 increased the circulating breast cancer cells, to promote their extravasation and colonization, leading to lung metastasis in severe combined immunodeficiency (SCID) mice, whereas in ZMYND8 knockouts, these features were reversed [22].

ZMYND8 may induce angiogenesis in cancer, especially in hypoxic conditions (Figure 4). Under hypoxia, ZMYND8 expression was induced, together with hypoxia-inducible factor-1α (HIF1α) and VEGF, at 72 h post-fertilization in zebrafish [2]. In breast cancer cells, HIF-1 and HIF-2 can induce ZMYND8 expression, and HIFs and ZMYND8 co-activate oncogenes and increase RNA polymerase II phosphorylation, leading to the promotion of cell motility, tumor growth, and lung metastasis [22]. When exposed to hypoxic condition, with 1% O_2 for 12 days, the MDA-MB-231 breast cancer cells with ZMYND8-knockout showed decreased colony formation, migration, and invasion, compared to parental cells [22].

Furthermore, ZMYND8 can induce the expression of VEGFα mRNA and promote angiogenesis in prostate cancer xenografts in zebrafish and tube formation in human umbilical vascular endothelial cell cultures [2]. In zebrafish, ZMYND8 knockdown suppresses tumor angiogenesis in DU145 prostate cancer xenografts, and the re-introduction of ZMYND8 mRNA restores the tumor angiogenesis [2]. However, ZMYND8 overexpression does not increase VEGFα expression in DU145 xenografts, suggesting that ZMYND8 mainly acts on the surrounding zebrafish tissues, to regulate the expression of VEGFα, to induce angiogenesis [2]. ZMYND8 knockout also decreases the microvessel density in the mammary fat pad MDA-MB-231 tumor and subcutaneous MAF-7 tumor in SCID mice, which further supports the induction of angiogenesis by ZMYND8 [22]. In addition, transcriptome analyses reveal an increase in ZMYND8 expression during tumor angiogenesis in prostate cancer xenografts [2]. Furthermore, ZMYND8 is a binding partner of PKC, and PKC isozymes—in particular, PKCβ—are important mediators of VEGF signaling [2,3,39]. Inhibition of PKCβ causes decreased proliferation of endothelial cells and neovascularization of hepatocellular carcinoma, in a syngeneic xenograft model in BALB/c mice [39]. Thus, ZMYND8 can be induced in hypoxic conditions, and it can promote tumor angiogenesis, probably through HIF and VEGF activation, and enhance tumor growth [2,22].

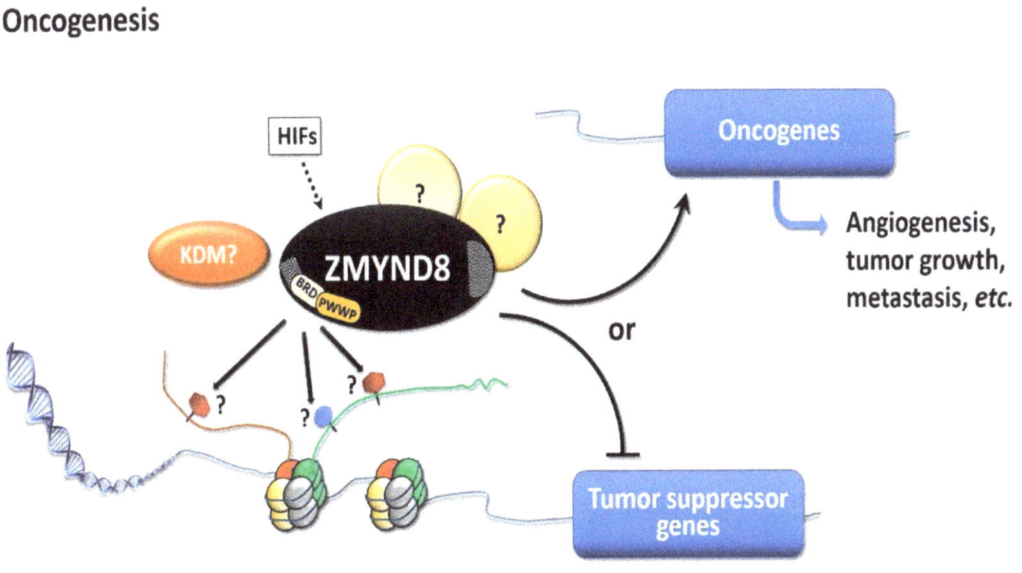

Figure 4. Diagram showing the possible mechanisms of the pro-oncogenic effects of ZMYND8. ZMYND8 can be activated by HIFs and induces angiogenesis, cellular proliferation, and tumor growth. The pro-oncogenic pathways of ZMYND8 are still unclarified. ZMYND8 may cooperate with demethylase, recognize the histone marks, suppress the transcription of tumor suppressor genes, or activate oncogenes, to enhance the tumorigenesis. HIFs: Hypoxia-inducible factors; KDM: Lysine demethylase.

Overall, these results indicate that ZMYND8 may have a crucial role in the tumorigenesis of breast, prostate, colorectal, and cervical cancers [2,21–23]. In addition, ZMYND8 may promote angiogenesis in zebrafish, as well as breast and prostate cancers [2,22]. Therefore, ZMYND8 is important for tumor cell proliferation, angiogenesis, and tumor growth [23]. However, data supporting its oncogenic role are still limited and the pro-oncogenic pathways of ZMYND8 are still unclarified (Figure 4).

6. Conclusions

Aberrant regulation of gene expression and epigenetic mutations play an important role in carcinogenesis. ZMYND8 is a transcription factor, a histone H3-interacting protein, and a putative chromatin reader/effector, important for regulating transcription in normal cells, and its mutation, altered expression, and fusion with other genes, are associated with development and progression of cancer. Increased expression of ZMYND8 is associated with breast, prostate, colorectal, and cervical cancers, and it is pro-oncogenic in breast and prostate cancers [2,21–23]. ZMYND8 is induced during hypoxic conditions, and can promote angiogenesis in zebrafish, as well as in breast and prostate cancers [2,22]. In contrast, lower expression of ZMYND8 is linked to breast, prostate, and nasopharyngeal cancers, and ZMYND8 exerts tumor-suppressive effects on breast and prostate cancers [8,9,24,25]. It suppresses tumor growth by promoting differentiation; inhibiting proliferation, progression of cell cycle, invasiveness, and metastasis; and maintaining the epithelial phenotype in various types of cancer [8,9,24,25]. Although all of these results indicate that ZMYND8 is important in cancer, they are contradictory, and the actual role of ZMYND8 in cancer is still unclear. In addition, the investigations are limited to a few types of cancer, like that of breast and prostate. As ZMYND8 interacts with various transcriptional corepressors, chromatin remodeling complexes, histone demethylase/deacetylase, and acetyl transferase enzymes, the role of ZMYND8 in cancers may be related to not just its direct action, but to multiple factors. Different cell types, fusion with other genes, and the interaction of ZMYND8 with various binding partners may affect the functions of ZMYND8 in cancers. The interaction between ZMYND8 and various binding partners is considered to be crucial in determining whether the function of ZMYND8 is pro-oncogenic or tumor suppressive (Figure 5).

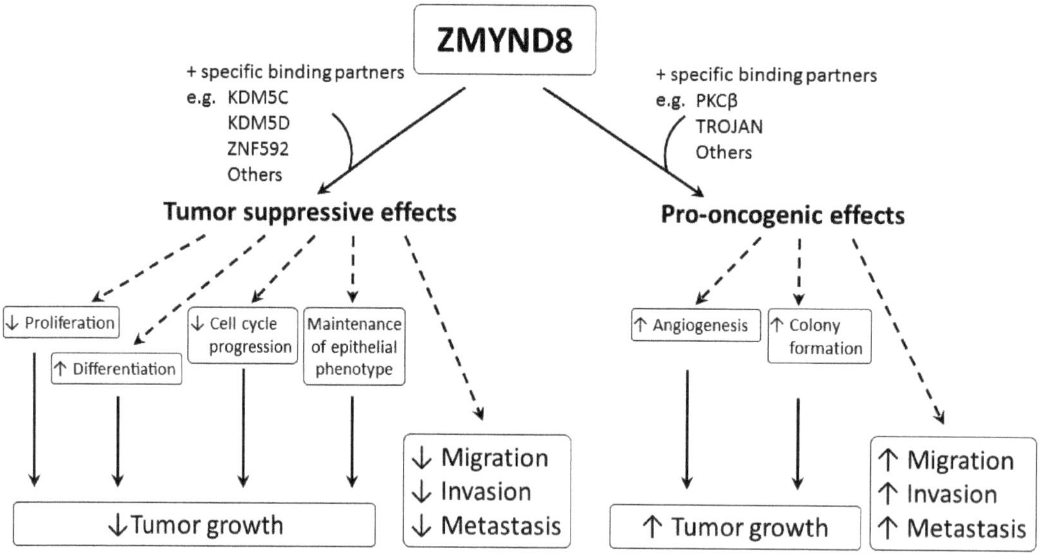

Figure 5. Diagram showing the pro-oncogenic and tumor-suppressive effects of ZMYND8 in cancers. The functions of ZMYND8 were considered through the interaction between ZMYND8 and a specific ZMYND8-binding partner. The ↑ indicates enhancement, and ↓ indicates suppression.

For example, the interaction between ZMYND8 and PKCβ or TROJAN may induce pro-oncogenic effects, while interaction between ZMYND8 and KDM5C, KDM5D, or ZNF592 may cause tumor-suppressive effects. Therefore, more studies are necessary, and they need to be focused not only on ZMYND8, but also on its specific binding partners in different cancer types. Hopefully, in the future, regulation of the expression of ZMYND8 and/or its binding partners may become useful in treating cancer.

Author Contributions: Conceptualization, S.-H.T. and Y.C.; methodology, Y.C., Y.-H.T. and S.-H.T.; investigation, Y.C. and Y.-H.T.; writing—original draft preparation, Y.C. and Y.-H.T.; writing—review and editing, S.-H.T. All authors have read and agreed to the published version of the manuscript.

Funding: This research was funded by the Ministry of Science and Technology, R.O.C., grant numbers MOST 107-2314-B-002-074 and MOST 108-2314-B-002-087.

Conflicts of Interest: The authors declare no conflict of interest.

Sample Availability: Samples are not available.

References

1. Taverna, S.D.; Li, H.; Ruthenburg, A.J.; Allis, C.D.; Patel, D.J. How chromatin-binding modules interpret histone modifications: Lessons from professional pocket pickers. *Nat. Struct. Mol. Biol.* **2007**, *14*, 1025–1040. [CrossRef]
2. Kuroyanagi, J.; Shimada, Y.; Zhang, B.; Ariyoshi, M.; Umemoto, N.; Nishimura, Y.; Tanaka, T. Zinc finger MYND-type containing 8 promotes tumour angiogenesis via induction of vascular endothelial growth factor-A expression. *FEBS Lett.* **2014**, *588*, 3409–3416. [CrossRef] [PubMed]
3. Wada, Y.; Matsuura, M.; Sugawara, M.; Ushijima, M.; Miyata, S.; Nagasaki, K.; Noda, T.; Miki, Y. Development of detection method for novel fusion gene using Gene Chip exon array. *J. Clin. Bioinforma.* **2014**, *4*, 3. [CrossRef] [PubMed]
4. Adhikary, S.; Sanyal, S.; Basu, M.; Sengupta, I.; Sen, S.; Srivastava, D.K.; Roy, S.; Das, C. Selective recognition of H3.1K36 dimethylation/H4K16 acetylation facilitates the regulation of all-trans-retinoic acid (ATRA)-responsive genes by putative chromatin reader ZMYND8. *J. Biol. Chem.* **2016**, *291*, 2664–2681. [CrossRef]
5. Wen, H.; Li, Y.; Xi, Y.; Jiang, S.; Stratton, S.; Peng, D.; Tanaka, K.; Ren, Y.; Xia, Z.; Wu, J.; et al. ZYMND11 links histone H3.3K36me3 to transcription elongation and tumor suppression. *Nature* **2014**, *508*, 263–268. [CrossRef] [PubMed]
6. Gong, F.; Chiu, L.Y.; Cox, B.; Aymard, F.; Clouaire, T.; Leung, J.W.; Cammarata, M.; Perez, M.; Agarwal, P.; Brodbelt, J.S.; et al. Screen identifies bromodomain protein ZMYND8 in chromatin recognition of transcription-associated DNA damage that promotes homologous recombination. *Genes Dev.* **2015**, *29*, 197–211. [CrossRef] [PubMed]
7. Savitsky, P.; Krojer, T.; Fujisawa, T.; Lambert, J.P.; Picaud, S.; Wang, C.Y.; Shanle, E.K.; Krajewski, K.; Friedrichsen, H.; Kanapin, A.; et al. Multivalent histone and DNA engagement by a PHD/BRD/PWWP triple reader cassette recruits ZMYND8 to K14ac-rich chromatin. *Cell Rep.* **2016**, *17*, 2724–2737. [CrossRef]
8. Li, N.; Li, Y.; Lv, J.; Zheng, X.; Wen, H.; Shen, H.; Zhu, G.; Chen, T.Y.; Dhar, S.S.; Kan, P.Y.; et al. ZMYND8 reads the dual histone mark H3K4me1-H3K14ac to antagonize the expression of metastasis-linked genes. *Mol. Cell* **2016**, *63*, 470–484. [CrossRef]
9. Basu, M.; Khan, M.W.; Chakrabarti, P.; Das, C. Chromatin reader ZMYND8 is a key target of all trans retinoic acid-mediated inhibition of cancer cell proliferation. *Biochim. Biophys. Acta* **2017**, *1860*, 450–459. [CrossRef] [PubMed]
10. Basu, M.; Sengupta, I.; Khan, M.W.; Srivastava, D.K.; Chakrabarti, P.; Roy, S.; Das, C. Dual histone reader ZMYND8 inhibits cancer cell invasion by positively regulating epithelial genes. *Biochem. J.* **2017**, *474*, 1919–1934. [CrossRef]
11. Mukherjee, S.; Sen, S.; Adhikary, S.; Sengupta, A.; Mandal, P.; Dasgupta, D.; Chakrabarti, P.; Roy, S.; Das, C. A novel role of tumor suppressor ZMYND8 in inducing differentiation of breast cancer cells through its dual-histone binding function. *J. Biosci.* **2020**, *45*, 2. [CrossRef] [PubMed]
12. Malovannaya, A.; Lanz, R.B.; Jung, S.Y.; Bulynko, Y.; Le, N.T.; Chan, D.W.; Ding, C.; Shi, Y.; Yucer, N.; Krenciute, G.; et al. Analysis of the human endogenous coregulator complexome. *Cell* **2011**, *145*, 787–799. [CrossRef]
13. Ghosh, K.; Tang, M.; Kumari, N.; Nandy, A.; Basu, S.; Mall, D.P.; Rai, K.; Biswas, D. Positive regulation of transcription by human ZMYND8 through its association with P-TEFb complex. *Cell Rep.* **2018**, *24*, 2141–2154. [CrossRef] [PubMed]
14. Spruijt, C.G.; Luijsterburg, M.S.; Menafra, R.; Lindeboom, R.G.; Jansen, P.W.; Edupuganti, R.R.; Baltissen, M.P.; Wiegant, W.W.; Voelker-Albert, M.C.; Matarese, F.; et al. ZMYND8 Co-localizes with NuRD on Target Genes and Regulates Poly(ADP-Ribose)-Dependent Recruitment of GATAD2A/NuRD to Sites of DNA Damage. *Cell Rep.* **2016**, *17*, 783–798. [CrossRef] [PubMed]
15. Gong, F.; Clouaire, T.; Aguirrebengoa, M.; Legube, G.; Miller, K.M. Histone demethylase KDM5A regulates the ZMYND8-NuRD chromatin remodeler to promote DNA repair. *J. Cell Biol.* **2017**, *216*, 1959–1974. [CrossRef] [PubMed]
16. Gong, F.; Miller, K.M. Double duty: ZMYND8 in the DNA damage response and cancer. *Cell Cycle* **2018**, *17*, 414–420. [CrossRef] [PubMed]
17. Gursoy-Yuzugullu, O.; Chelsea Carman, C.; Price, B.D. Spatially restricted loading of BRD2 at DNA double-strand breaks protects H4 acetylation domains and promotes DNA repair. *Sci. Rep.* **2017**, *7*, 12921. [CrossRef] [PubMed]

18. Eberl, H.C.; Spruijt, C.G.; Kelstrup, C.D.; Vermeulen, M.; Mann, M. A map of general and specialized chromatin readers in mouse tissues generated by label-free interaction proteomics. *Mol. Cell* **2013**, *49*, 368–378. [CrossRef]
19. Zeng, W.; Kong, Q.; Li, C.; Mao, B. Xenopus RCOR2 (REST corepressor 2) interacts with ZMYND8, which is involved in neural differentiation. *Biochem. Biophys. Res. Commun.* **2010**, *394*, 1024–1029. [CrossRef] [PubMed]
20. Wang, Y.; Luo, M.; Chen, Y.; Wang, Y.; Zhang, B.; Ren, Z.; Bao, L.; Wang, Y.; Wang, J.E.; Fu, Y.X.; et al. ZMYND8 expression in breast cancer cells blocks T-lymphocyte surveillance to promote tumor growth. *Cancer Res.* **2020**, *81*, 174–186.
21. Bierkens, M.; Krijgsman, O.; Wilting, S.M.; Bosch, L.; Jaspers, A.; Meijer, G.A.; Meijer, C.J.; Snijders, P.J.; Ylstra, B.; Steenbergen, R.D. Focal aberrations indicate EYA2 and hsa-miR-375 as oncogene and tumor suppressor in cervical carcinogenesis. *Genes Chromosomes Cancer* **2013**, *52*, 56–68. [CrossRef] [PubMed]
22. Chen, Y.; Zhang, B.; Bao, L.; Jin, L.; Yang, M.; Peng, Y.; Kumar, A.; Wang, J.E.; Wang, C.; Zou, X.; et al. ZMYND8 acetylation mediates HIF-dependent breast cancer progression and metastasis. *J. Clin. Invest.* **2018**, *128*, 1937–1955. [CrossRef] [PubMed]
23. Chen, J.; He, Q.; Wu, P.; Fu, J.; Xiao, Y.; Chen, K.; Xie, D.; Zhang, X. ZMYND8 expression combined with pN and pM classification as a novel prognostic prediction model for colorectal cancer: Based on TCGA and GEO database analysis. *Cancer Biomark.* **2020**, *28*, 201–211. [CrossRef] [PubMed]
24. Jin, X.; Xu, X.E.; Jiang, Y.Z.; Liu, Y.R.; Sun, W.; Guo, Y.J.; Ren, Y.X.; Zuo, W.J.; Hu, X.; Huang, S.L.; et al. The endogenous retrovirus-derived long noncoding RNA TROJAN promotes triple-negative breast cancer progression via ZMYND8 degradation. *Sci. Adv.* **2019**, *5*, eaat9820. [CrossRef] [PubMed]
25. Shen, H.; Xu, W.; Guo, R.; Rong, B.; Gu, L.; Wang, Z.; He, C.; Zheng, L.; Hu, X.; Hu, Z.; et al. Suppression of enhancer overactivation by a RACK7-histone demethylase complex. *Cell* **2016**, *165*, 331–342. [CrossRef] [PubMed]
26. Lai, A.Y.; Wade, P.A. Cancer biology and NuRD: A multifaceted chromatin remodelling complex. *Nat. Rev. Cancer* **2011**, *11*, 588–596. [CrossRef] [PubMed]
27. Yu, H.; Jiang, Y.; Liu, L.; Shan, W.; Chu, X.; Yang, Z.; Yang, Z.Q. Integrative genomic and transcriptomic analysis for pinpointing recurrent alterations of plant homeodomain genes and their clinical significance in breast cancer. *Oncotarget* **2017**, *8*, 13099–13115. [CrossRef] [PubMed]
28. Eichmuller, S.; Usener, D.; Dummer, R.; Nicorici, D.; Hongisto, V.; Kleivi, K.; Rye, I.H.; Nyberg, S.; Wolf, M.; Borresen-Dale, A.L.; et al. Serological detection of cutaneous T-cell lymphoma-associated antigens. *Proc. Natl. Acad. Sci. USA* **2001**, *98*, 629–634. [CrossRef]
29. Panagopoulos, I.; Micci, F.; Thorsen, J.; Haugom, L.; Buechner, J.; Kerndrup, G.; Tierens, A.; Zeller, B.; Heim, S. Fusion of ZMYND8 and RELA genes in acute erythroid leukemia. *PLoS ONE* **2013**, *8*, e63663. [CrossRef]
30. Edgren, H.; Murumagi, A.; Kangaspeska, S.; Nicorici, D.; Hongisto, V.; Kleivi, K.; Rye, I.H.; Nyberg, S.; Wolf, M.; Borresen-Dale, A.L.; et al. Identification of fusion genes in breast cancer by paired-end RNA-sequencing. *Genome Biol.* **2011**, *12*, R6. [CrossRef]
31. Park, J.; Betel, D.; Gryfe, R.; Michalickova, K.; Di Nicola, N.; Gallinger, S.; Hogue, C.W.; Redston, M. Mutation profiling of mismatch repair-deficient colorectal cncers using an in silico genome scan to identify coding microsatellites. *Cancer Res.* **2002**, *62*, 1284–1288. [PubMed]
32. The Cancer Genome Atlas Research Network: Integrated genomic analyses of ovarian carcinoma. *Nature* **2011**, *474*, 609–615. [CrossRef]
33. Ricketts, C.J.; Linehan, W.M. Gender specific mutation incidence and survival associations in clear cell renal cell carcinoma (CCRCC). *PLoS ONE* **2015**, *10*, e0140257. [CrossRef]
34. Rondinelli, B.; Rosano, D.; Antonini, E.; Frenquelli, M.; Montanini, L.; Huang, D.; Segalla, S.; Yoshihara, K.; Amin, S.B.; Lazarevic, D.; et al. Histone demethylase JARID1C inactivation triggers genomic instability in sporadic renal cancer. *J. Clin. Invest.* **2016**, *126*, 4387. [CrossRef] [PubMed]
35. Stein, J.; Majores, M.; Rhode, M.; Lim, S.; Schneider, S.; Krappe, E.; Ellinger, J.; Dietel, M.; Stephan, C.; Jung, K.; et al. KDM5C is overexpressed in prostate cancer ans is a prognostic marker for prostate-specific antigen-relapse following radical prostatectomy. *Am. J. Pathol.* **2014**, *184*, 2430–2437. [CrossRef] [PubMed]
36. Chen, J.; Liu, J.; Chen, X.; Li, Y.; Li, Z.; Shen, C.; Chen, K.; Zhang, X. Low expression of ZMYND8 correlates with aggressive features and poor prognosis in nasopharyngeal carcinoma. *Cancer Manag. Res.* **2019**, *11*, 7835–7843. [CrossRef] [PubMed]
37. Li, N.; Dhar, S.S.; Chen, T.Y.; Kan, P.Y.; Wei, Y.; Kim, J.H.; Chan, C.H.; Lin, H.K.; Hung, M.C.; Lee, M.G. JARID1D is a suppressor and prognostic marker of prostate cancer invasion and metastasis. *Cancer Res.* **2016**, *76*, 831–843. [CrossRef] [PubMed]
38. Kalluri, R.; Weinberg, R.A. The basics of epithelial-mesenchymal transition. *J. Clin. Invest.* **2009**, *119*, 1420–1428. [CrossRef]
39. Yoshiji, H.; Kuriyama, S.; Ways, D.K.; Yoshii, J.; Miyamoto, Y.; Kawata, M.; Ikenaka, Y.; Tsujinoue, H.; Nakatani, T.; Shibuya, M.; et al. Protein kinase C lies on the signaling pathway for vascular endothelial growth factor-mediated tumor development and angiogenesis. *Cancer Res.* **1999**, *59*, 4413–4418.

molecules

MDPI

Article

Comparison of Transcriptomic Profiles of MiaPaCa-2 Pancreatic Cancer Cells Treated with Different Statins

Silvie Rimpelová [1,*], Michal Kolář [2], Hynek Strnad [2], Tomáš Ruml [1], Libor Vítek [3] and Helena Gbelcová [4,*]

1 Department of Biochemistry and Microbiology, University of Chemistry and Technology Prague, Technická 3, 166 28 Prague, Czech Republic; tomas.ruml@vscht.cz
2 Laboratory of Genomics and Bioinformatics, Institute of Molecular Genetics, Czech Academy of Sciences, Vídeňská 1083, 142 20 Prague, Czech Republic; michal.kolar@img.cas.cz (M.K.); hynek.strnad@img.cas.cz (H.S.)
3 Institute of Medical Biochemistry and Laboratory Diagnostics, and 4th Department of Internal Medicine, 1st Faculty of Medicine, Charles University, 128 08 Prague, Czech Republic; vitek@cesnet.cz
4 Institute of Medical Biology, Genetics and Clinical Genetics, Faculty of Medicine, Comenius University, Špitálska 24, 813 72 Bratislava, Slovakia
* Correspondence: silvie.rimpelova@vscht.cz (S.R.); helena.gbelcova@fmed.uniba.sk (H.G.)

Abstract: Statins have been widely used for the treatment of hypercholesterolemia due to their ability to inhibit HMG-CoA reductase, the rate-limiting enzyme of de novo cholesterol synthesis, via the so-called mevalonate pathway. However, their inhibitory action also causes depletion of downstream intermediates of the pathway, resulting in the pleiotropic effects of statins, including the beneficial impact in the treatment of cancer. In our study, we compared the effect of all eight existing statins on the expression of genes, the products of which are implicated in cancer inhibition and suggested the molecular mechanisms of their action in epigenetic and posttranslational regulation, and in cell-cycle arrest, death, migration, or invasion of the cancer cells.

Keywords: statins; pancreatic cancer; DNA microarray; pitavastatin; cerivastatin; simvastatin; fluvastatin; atorvastatin; pravastatin; HMG-CoA reductase inhibitors

Citation: Rimpelová, S.; Kolář, M.; Strnad, H.; Ruml, T.; Vítek, L.; Gbelcová, H. Comparison of Transcriptomic Profiles of MiaPaCa-2 Pancreatic Cancer Cells Treated with Different Statins. *Molecules* **2021**, *26*, 3528. https://doi.org/10.3390/molecules26123528

Academic Editors: Marialuigia Fantacuzzi and Alessandra Ammazzalorso

Received: 16 March 2021
Accepted: 26 May 2021
Published: 9 June 2021

1. Introduction

Statins (Figure 1) are the inhibitors of *de novo* cholesterol synthesis in the cell due to their ability to competitively inhibit the β-hydroxy-β-methylglutaryl coenzyme A (HMG-CoA) reductase. They represent the most prescribed drugs in the treatment of cardiovascular diseases [1]. Currently, there are eight existing statins, namely atorvastatin, cerivastatin, fluvastatin, lovastatin, pitavastatin, pravastatin, rosuvastatin, and simvastatin [2]. Although all statins have the same mechanism of hypolipidemic action, they differ in their chemical structure, physico-chemical properties, pharmacokinetic effects, and effects on lipid profile [3]. The inhibition of HMG-CoA conversion to mevalonate caused by HMG-CoA reductase inhibition results in the depletion of downstream intermediates of the mevalonate pathway.

Mevalonate is the precursor of, i.e., farnesyl pyrophosphate (FPP), geranylgeranyl pyrophosphate (GGPP), isopentenyl adenine, dolichol, and the polyisoprenoid side chains of heme A and ubiquinone, which are essential molecules that play a vital role in almost any cell process [3]. From these, FPP and GGPP play an important role in the posttranslational modification of cellular proteins involved in cell division and differentiation, gene expression, cytoskeleton formation, intracellular protein and lipid transport, and defense against pathogens [4]. Another intermediate in the mevalonate pathway, isopentenyl adenine, is essential for proper tRNA function and protein synthesis. Dolichol acts as an important scavenger of free radicals in cell membranes, and ubiquinone is involved in mitochondrial respiration and inhibition of lipid peroxidation. A decrease in the intracellular level of ubiquinone leads to mitochondrial damage, oxidative stress, and cell damage. The involvement of the aforementioned mevalonate pathway intermediates in various cell processes explains the pleiotropic activity exhibited by statins, in addition to their hypolipidemic effect.

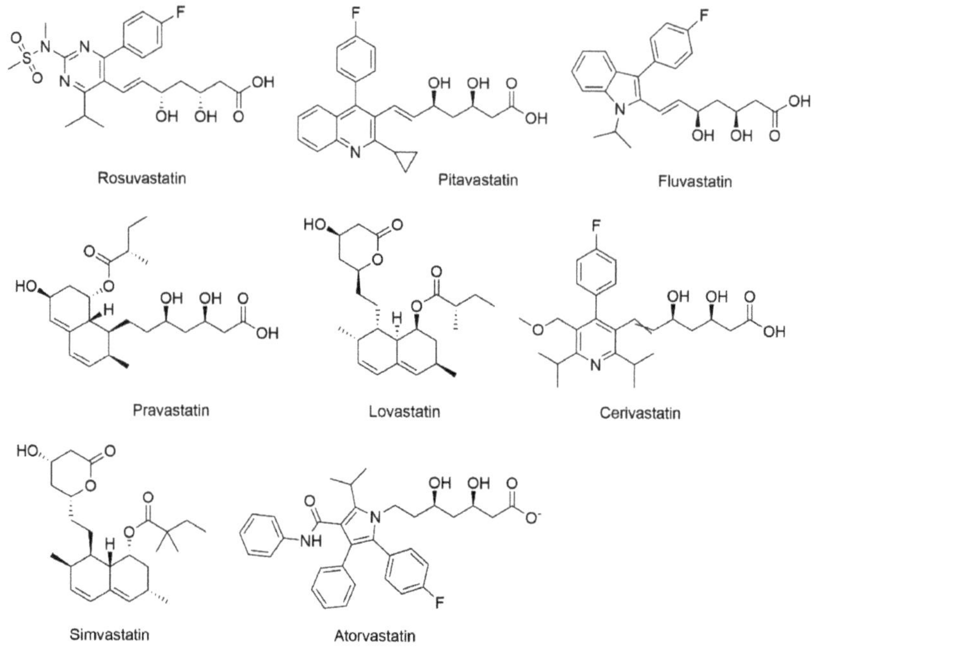

Figure 1. Chemical structures of statins.

Based on this, it is clear that statins significantly affect basic physiological processes of cells and organs that also are connected with oncogenesis [5]. The results of lipid-lowering therapy in animals initially indicated an increased risk of carcinogenesis [6]. However, the dose of statins administered in that study was very high and not applicable for humans [7]. The results of studies on tissue-specific cancer development in individuals on statins therapy (as hypolipidemic drugs) have been controversial. An increased incidence of breast cancer after statin administration was observed in one study [8], but another study did not confirm these findings [9]. Contrary to that, a reduced incidence of melanomas has been reported after statin administration [9]. A similar beneficial effect of statins was observed in connection with reduced incidence of colon carcinomas [10]. However, most of these studies were not originally designed to investigate the relationship between statin intake and cancer development, but rather between statins and cardiovascular diseases. Indeed, some reports have shown a statistically significantly lower incidence of cancer in patients receiving statin therapy, despite relatively short follow-up times and inappropriate patient selection [11–16]. Moreover, extensive studies conducted on 500,000 U.S. war veterans have shown that statin use is associated with a two- to fivefold lower incidence of lung [17], breast [18], and prostate cancers [19]. Based on other meta-analyses, statins appear to be particularly effective in the chemoprevention of colorectal cancer [10,20]. While there have been several in vitro and in vivo studies directly targeting and confirming the marked effect of statins on the growth of a wide variety of tumor types, such as hepatocellular [21], lung [22], and colorectal carcinoma [23], clinical trials targeting statin efficacy in cancer treatment have been very rare, so far. One of them showed that patients suffering from hepatocellular carcinoma exhibited statistically significantly longer survival rates for pravastatin therapy [24] than untreated. On the other hand, beneficial effects of lovastatin therapy on the survival rate of patients suffering from glioblastoma multiforme or advanced gastric adenocarcinoma have not been observed [25,26]. The findings of the meta-analyses suggested an association between pravastatin treatment and cancer in elderly patients [27] but did not support the potential role of statins in the prevention of hematological malignancies [28] or the hypothesis that statins reduce the risk of pancreatic cancer development [29].

The setting of the experimental conditions of the present study was based on the results of our previous published studies [30,31], in which we reported on the differences in the individual anticancer potential of individual statins in cells derived from pancreatic carcinoma. Moreover, we were inspired by the aforementioned findings, as well as recent reviews shedding light on statins as cancer inhibitors with several possible mechanisms of action [32–35]. Therefore, using DNA microarray analysis, we sought after statin-induced changes in the expression of genes, the products of which are connected with tumorigenesis, inhibition of tumor growth, or metastasis. We focused on the pancreatic cancer cells because, in the very recent meta-analysis of 26 studies containing more than 3 million participants and 170,000 pancreatic cancer patients, statin therapy was shown to significantly reduce the risk of pancreatic cancer [36].

2. Results

From eight existing statins, only six (cerivastatin, pitavastatin, simvastatin, lovastatin, fluvastatin, and atorvastatin) significantly affected the gene expression in the MiaPaCa-2 pancreatic cancer cell line after 24 h of treatment with 12 μM statin concentration. The concentration was selected based on our previous studies [30,31], in which we determined the IC_{50} of individual statins in cells from pancreatic carcinoma after 24, 48, and 72 h. The value 12 μM corresponds to the IC_{50} of simvastatin in MiaPaCa-2 cells after 24 h of treatment. Other statins were compared at the same concentration since simvastatin was at the time of analysis one of the most potent clinically used statins (cerivastatin had been withdrawn from the market at the time of analysis).

2.1. Effect of Statins on Lipid Metabolism and Synthesis of Steroids

Lipids, particularly cholesterol, and their derivatives play several roles in tumorigenesis and cancer cell metabolism [37,38]. In contrast to noncancerous cells, malignant cells exhibit enhanced *de novo* synthesis of fatty acids, which serve as substrates for β-oxidation, or conversion to triglycerides for storage of phospholipids for membrane formation.

DNA microarray analysis showed that out of the eight statins evaluated, six effective ones significantly affected steroid biosynthesis in MiaPaCa-2 cells. They upregulated the gene encoding HMG-CoA reductase, representing the key target of statins. In addition, they even more markedly triggered upregulation of the gene encoding HMG-CoA synthase, catalyzing the synthesis of HMG-CoA, the substrate for the aforementioned enzyme covalently inhibited by statins. The inhibition of the mevalonate pathway resulted in a switch from cholesterol synthesis to the triacylglyceroles and phospholipid synthesis via the Kennedy pathway. Genes encoding enzymes of the Kennedy pathway were directly upregulated by the action of only the most effective statins; i.e., cerivastatin, pitavastatin, and simvastatin (Table 1). However, in terms of knowledge of the lipid metabolism of tumors, this observation indicated a procarcinogenic effect rather than an antitumor effect of statins. The changes in the expression of the genes involved in the mevalonate pathway are shown in Figure 2.

Table 1. Genes involved in the metabolism of lipids and steroids that were affected by statin treatment of MiaPaCa-2 cells. Numeric columns display fold changes of the gene expression between cells treated by individual statins at 12 μM concentration for 24 h and untreated cells. Cer.—cerivastatin; Pit.—pitavastatin; Sim.—simvastatin; Flu.—fluvastatin; Ato.—atorvastatin; Lov.—lovastatin. Pravastatin and rosuvastatin did not induce any significant change in MiaPaCa-2 cell gene expression.

Gene Symbol	Ref. ID	Product Name	Cer.	Pit.	Sim.	Flu.	Ato.	Lov.
			Fold Change					
HMGCS1	NM_002130	HMG-CoA synthase (EC 2.3.3.10)	5.67	2.99	4.13	2.96	2.90	2.80
HMGCR	NM_000859	HMG-CoA reductase (EC 1.1.1.34)	3.91	3.16	3.04	2.66	2.35	2.08
MVD	NM_002461	Mevalonate pyrophosphate decarboxylase (EC 4.1.1.33)	3.66	2.11	2.32	2.01	-	-
PPAP2A	NM_003711	Phosphatidic acid phosphatase 2a (EC 3.1.3.4)	3.41	2.78	2.15	-	-	-
AGPAT2	NM_006412	1-acyl-glycerol-phosphate acyltransferase 2 (EC 2.3.1.51)	2.63	2.28	-	-	-	-

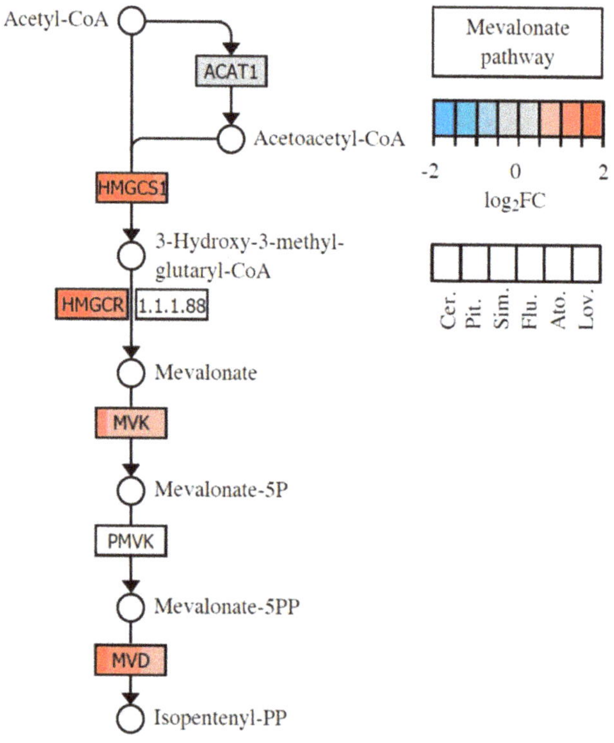

Figure 2. Mevalonate pathway and the changes induced by statin treatment in the expression of the genes that code for enzymes of the pathway. The color fill of the nodes indicates the base-2 logarithm of the fold change in gene expression upon treatment by a statin. Different statins are shown in the distinct position of the node as indicated in the bottom key.

On the other hand, statins are responsible for a decrease in the cholesterol content in lipid rafts by inhibiting the mevalonate pathway and, thus, induce apoptosis via inhibition of the Akt signaling pathway [39]. Interestingly, in our study, the Akt signaling pathway was not affected by the evaluated statins at 12 μM after 24 h treatment of MiaPaCa-2 cells.

In tumors with deregulated Hedgehog signaling, the depletion of cholesterol results in impairment of Hedgehog signal transduction and inhibition of cancer cell growth [40]. Cholesterol itself serves as a substrate for the post-translational modification of Hedgehog ligands, which is required for their proper trafficking [41]. This means that all statins should indirectly inhibit the Hedgehog signaling by inhibiting the cholesterol synthesis. Moreover, we found that pitavastatin and cerivastatin significantly upregulated the *GAS1* (growth arrest-specific gene 1) (data not shown), the product of which positively regulates the Hedgehog signaling [42,43]. The possible explanation for *GAS1* gene upregulation after statin treatment was the effort of affected cells to reactivate the statins-suppressed Hedgehog signaling.

Finally, to maintain cancer cell proliferation, the increased activation of SREBPs (sterol regulatory element-binding proteins) is required [44]; therefore, SREBP inhibitors are used in molecular-targeted cancer therapies [45,46]. SREBPs are transcription factors that regulate the expression of genes required for the synthesis of fatty acids, triglycerides, and cholesterol. Intracellular cholesterol level is controlled by SREBP-1 and SREBP-2. These transcription factors upregulate the synthesis of enzymes involved in the sterol biosynthesis upon binding to specific sterol regulatory element DNA sequences. Sterols in turn inhibit the cleavage of SREBPs, and therefore, synthesis of additional sterols is reduced via a negative feedback loop. Statin-mediated inhibition of sterol synthesis was reported to activate the SREBPs in many tumor types [45]. In our experiment, statins at a concentration (12 μM) sufficient to induce a more or less intensive antiproliferative effect on MiaPaCa-2 pancreatic cancer cells (IC_{50}: cerivastatin 10 μM, simvastatin 12 μM, lovastatin 13 μM, pitavastatin 20 μM, fluvastatin 26 μM, atorvastatin 27 μM, pravastatin 29 μM, rosuvastatin 36 μM) did not significantly affect the expression of genes encoding SREBPs (data not shown).

2.2. Statins in the Role of Epigenetic Regulators

Recently, it was described that acetyl-CoA metabolism supports multistep pancreatic tumorigenesis. In pancreatic adenocarcinoma, both upregulated gene expression of the mevalonate pathway and histone acetylation was detected [47]. Dysregulation between activities of histone acetyltransferases (HATs) and histone deacetylases (HDACs) is frequent in human tumors [48]. The expression of genes encoding HATs or HDACs was not altered by statins in our experiments (data not shown); however, genes encoding histone H4 were downregulated, in contrast to genes for histone H2B that were upregulated by cerivastatin, pitavastatin, and simvastatin (Table 2). STRING enrichment analysis of epigenetic regulators significantly affected by statin treatment is shown in Figure 3.

Table 2. Epigenetic regulator genes that were affected by statin treatment of MiaPaCa-2 cells. Numeric columns display fold changes of the gene expression between cells treated by individual statins at 12 μM concentration for 24 h and untreated cells. Cer.—cerivastatin; Pit.—pitavastatin; Sim.—simvastatin; Flu.—fluvastatin. Atorvastatin, lovastatin, pravastatin, and rosuvastatin did not induce any significant change in MiaPaCa-2 cells' gene expression.

Gene Symbol	Ref. ID	Product Name	Cer.	Pit.	Sim.	Flu.
				Fold Change		
HIST1H4C	NM_003542.3	Histone H4	0.41	0.34	0.49	-
HIST1H2BF	NM_003522.3	Histone H2B type 1-K	0.33	0.41	0.43	0.49
HIST2H3C	NM_021059.2	Histone H3C type 2	-	0.50	-	-
H2AFX	NM_002105.2	Histone H2A family member X	-	0.43	-	-
HIST2H2BE	NM_003528.2	Histone H2B type 2-E	4.32	4.33	2.05	-
HIST1H2BD	NM_138720.1	Histone H2B type 1-D	4.15	4.55	2.01	-
HIST1H2BK	NM_080593.1	Histone H2B type 1-K	2.10	2.67	-	-
HIST3H2A	NM_033445.2	Histone H2A type 3	-	2.02	-	-

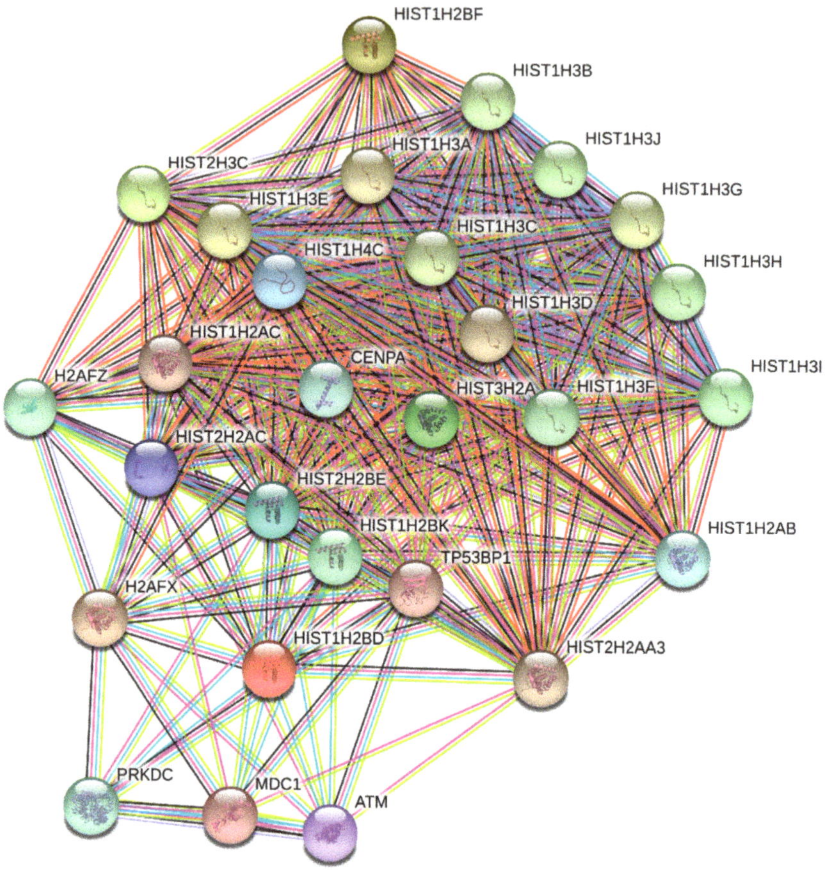

Figure 3. STRING enrichment analysis of epigenetic regulators significantly affected by statin treatment (mainly by cerivastatin and pitavastatin) of MiaPaCa-2 cells at 12 µM concentration for 24 h. Individual nodes represent affected gene products and their interactions. Input nodes represent the genes listed in Table 2 (*HIST1H4C, HIST1H2BF, HIST2H3C, H2AFX, HIST2H2BE, HIST1H2BD, HIST1H2BK*, and *HIST3H2A*). The evidence view of the association network was generated according to the known and predicted interactions in *Homo sapiens*. Known interactions: turquoise—from curated databases; violet—experimentally determined. Predicted interactions: green—gene neighborhood; red—gene fusions; blue—gene co-occurrence. Others: grass green—text-mining; black—co-expression; light blue—protein homology. A complete description of the nodes is given in Supplementary Table S1.

2.3. Statins and Their Potential Role as Posttranslational Regulators

Statins deplete the cellular pool of isoprene precursors, thereby having an impact on protein prenylation; i.e., farnesylation and geranylgeranylation. Among prenylated proteins, the low-molecular-weight guanosine triphosphate-binding proteins Ras and Ras-related growth modulators were monitored (Table 3). The overall effect on the RAS signaling pathway is shown in Figure 4.

Table 3. Genes involved in posttranslational regulation affected by statin treatment of MiaPaCa-2 cells. Numeric columns display fold changes of the gene expression between cells treated by individual statins at 12 µM concentration for 24 h and untreated cells. Cer.—cerivastatin; Pit.—pitavastatin; Sim.—simvastatin; Flu.—fluvastatin; Ato.—atorvastatin; Lov.—lovastatin. Pravastatin and rosuvastatin did not induce any significant change in MiaPaCa-2 cell gene expression.

Gene Symbol	Ref. ID	Product Name	Cer.	Pit.	Sim.	Flu.	Ato.	Lov.
			Fold Change					
RHOB	NM_004040.2	Ras homolog gene family, member B	12.48	11.90	10.81	7.11	5.59	4.92
RASL10A	NM_001007279.1	RAS-like, family 10, member A	4.14	3.58	2.65	2.17	2.01	-
KRAS	NM_033360.2	Kirsten rat sarcoma viral oncogene homolog	3.23	2.64	2.58	2.00	-	-
RAB40B	NM_006822.1	Member RAS oncogene family	3.14	2.89	2.16	-	-	-
RRAS	NM_006270.3	Related RAS viral (r-ras) oncogene homolog	2.58	2.53	2.04	-	-	-
RAB5B	NM_002868.2	RAS oncogene family member	2.46	2.04	-	-	-	-
RAB6B	NM_016577.3	RAS oncogene family member	2.32	2.31	-	-	-	-
RHOA	NM_001664.2	Ras homolog gene family, member A	2.21	2.40	2.03	-	-	-
ARHGEF3	NM_019555.1	Rho guanine nucleotide exchange factor (GEF) 3	2.21	2.09	-	-	-	-
RHOQ	NM_012249.3	Ras homolog gene family, member Q	2.17	-	-	-	-	-
RRAGC	NM_022157.2	Ras-related GTP binding C	2.06	-	-	-	-	-
RAB38	NM_022337.1	Member RAS oncogene family	0.41	-	-	-	-	-
ARHGAP19	NM_032900.4	Rho GTPase activating protein 19	0.47	0.38	-	-	-	-

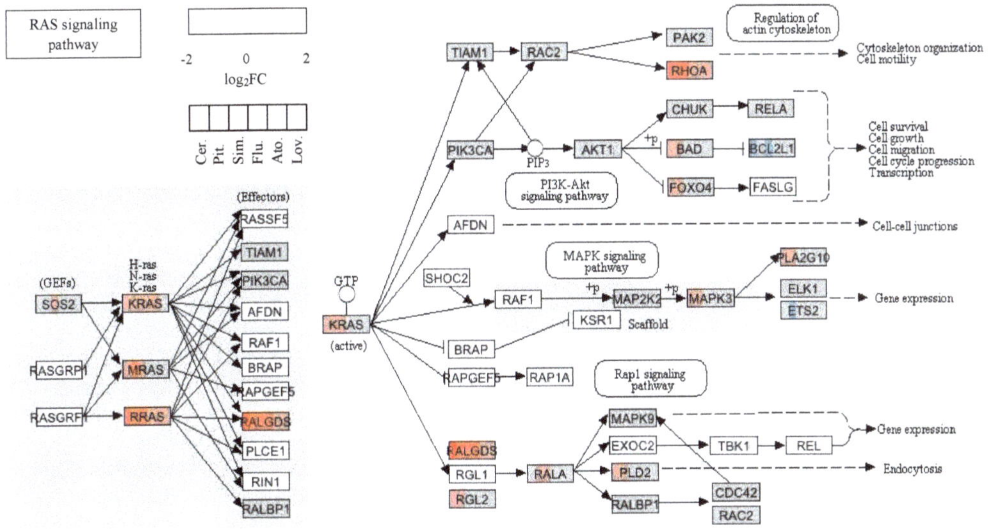

Figure 4. RAS signaling pathway and the changes induced by statin treatment in the expression of the genes that code for members of the pathway. The color fill of the nodes indicates the base-2 logarithm of the fold change in gene expression upon treatment by a statin. Different statins are shown in the distinct position of the node as indicated in the key.

RHOB, the most dramatically upregulated gene by statins (Table 3), belongs to the Rho protein family of proteins regulating diverse cellular processes, including cytoskeletal organization, gene transcription, cell cycle progression, and cytokinesis [49,50]. While most Rho proteins have been shown to have positive roles in proliferation and malignant transformation, RhoB rather appears to act as a negative regulator of these processes [51,52]. R-Ras promotes the formation of focal adhesions, cell spreading, and activation of integrins [53]. Cerivastatin, pitavastatin, simvastatin, and fluvastatin also increased the expression of the *KRAS* gene, the most frequently mutated gene in pancreatic cancer, and frequently mutated in cancer in general. As the K-Ras is the protein related to many functional pathways, such as the mitogen-activated protein kinase (MAPK) signaling pathway, the receptor tyrosine-protein kinase (ErbB) signaling pathway, dorso-ventral axis formation, axon guidance, the vascular endothelial growth factor (VEGF) signaling pathway, tight junctions, gap junctions, natural killer cell-mediated cytotoxicity, the T-cell receptor signaling pathway, the B-cell receptor signaling pathway, the Fc epsilon RI signaling pathway, long-term potentiation, long-term depression, regulation of actin cytoskeleton, the insulin signaling pathway, and the gonadotropin-releasing hormone (GnRH) signaling pathway, the pleiotropic effect of statins is comprehensible. Moreover, the *KRAS* gene upregulation after statin treatment adverts to the unavailability of K-Ras protein for the cell signaling without its correct posttranslational modification due to the mevalonate pathway inhibition. Similarly, this mechanism could also explain the upregulation of other Ras and Ras-related proteins induced by treatment with simvastatin. Genes encoding guanine nucleotide exchange factor (GEF), GTPase-activating proteins (GAP), or guanosine nucleotide dissociation inhibitor (GDI) of Ras and Ras-related proteins were not significantly up- or downregulated by statins.

2.4. *Statins' Effect on Cell Cycle and Cell Death*

The effect of statins on the expression of genes related to the cell cycle and cell death is of special interest concerning their cancerostatic capability. The expression levels of genes associated with DNA replication were significantly affected only by pitavastatin, cerivastatin, and simvastatin, and they were mostly downregulated (Table 4). The changes in the cell-cycle circuit are shown in Figure 5.

The origin recognition complex (ORC) is a highly conserved six-subunit protein complex essential for the initiation of DNA replication in eukaryotic cells. The ORC binds specifically to origins of replication and serves as a platform for the assembly of additional initiation factors such as minichromosome maintenance (MCM) proteins. ORC1L is the largest subunit of the ORC complex. While the levels of other ORC subunits are stable throughout the whole cell cycle, the level of ORC1L changes in various phases of the cell cycle. These changes are controlled by ubiquitin-mediated proteolysis after the initiation of DNA replication [54]. From this, it seems that statins blocked the progression of the cell cycle through the S phase. From the quantum of genes encoding proteins involved in the cell-cycle regulation, such as cyclins, cyclin-dependent kinases (CDK), and cell-cycle negative regulators, only the expression of those denoted in Table 4 were affected by statins. CDC2 (CDK1) is the catalytic subunit of a highly conserved protein kinase complex known as the M-phase promoting factor (MPF), which is essential for the G1/S and G2/M phase transitions in the cell cycle of eukaryotic cells. Mitotic cyclins stably associate with this protein and function as regulatory subunits. The kinase activity of this protein is controlled by cyclin accumulation and degradation through the cell cycle [55].

M-phase inducer phosphatase 2 (CDC25B), a member of the cell division control protein 25 (CDC25) family of phosphatases, activates the cyclin-dependent kinase (CDC2) and is required for entry into the mitosis [56]. Whereas the *CDC2* gene was downregulated by simvastatin treatment of MiaPaCa-2 cells, the *CDC25B* gene was upregulated (Table 4). Some other genes encoding proteins related to the S phase (SKP2, E2F2) were downregulated by cerivastatin and pitavastatin. The SKP2 (S-phase kinase-associated protein 2) is an essential element of the cyclin A/CDK2 S-phase kinase [57]. E2F2 is a member of the E2F family of transcription factors and plays a crucial role in the control of the cell cycle. Expression of the S-phase genes is not activated when E2F is repressed [58].

Table 4. Genes involved in the cell cycle and DNA replication affected by statin treatment of MiaPaCa-2 cells. Numeric columns display fold changes of the gene expression between cells treated by individual statins at 12 μM concentration for 24 h and untreated cells. Cer.—cerivastatin; Pit.—pitavastatin; Sim.—simvastatin; Flu.—fluvastatin; Ato.—atorvastatin; Lov.—lovastatin. Pravastatin and rosuvastatin did not induce any significant change in MiaPaCa-2 cell gene expression.

Gene Symbol	Ref. ID	Product Name	Cer.	Pit.	Sim.	Flu.	Ato.	Lov.
					Fold Change			
CDKN1A	NM_000389.2	Cyclin-dependent kinase inhibitor 1A (p21, Cip1)	3.64	4.21	2.74	2.59	2.33	2.40
SFN	NM_006142.3	Stratifin	2.40	2.57	-	-	-	-
CDKN1C	NM_057735.1	Cyclin-dependent kinase inhibitor 1C (p57, Kip2)	-	2.37	-	-	-	-
CCNE2	NM_057735.1	Cyclin E2	0.30	0.29	-	-	-	-
CDC25A	NM_001789.2	Cell division cycle 25 homolog A	0.30	0.33	-	-	-	-
ORC1L	NM_004153.2	Origin recognition complex, subunit 1-like	0.30	0.22	-	-	-	-
ORC6L	NM_014321.2	Origin recognition complex, subunit 6 like	0.31	0.30	-	-	-	-
SKP2	NM_005983.2	S-phase kinase-associated protein 2 (p45)	0.34	0.37	-	-	-	-
MCM7	NM_005916.3	Minichromosome maintenance complex component 7	0.38	0.45	-	-	-	-
E2F2	NM_004091.2	E2F transcription factor 2	0.39	0.40	-	-	-	-
CDC45L	NM_003504.3	CDC45 cell division cycle 45-like	0.39	0.27	-	-	-	-
MCM2	NM_004526.2	Minichromosome maintenance complex component 2	0.40	0.30	-	-	-	-
MCM3	NM_002388.3	Minichromosome maintenance complex component 3	0.41	0.33	-	-	-	-
CDC6	NM_001254.3	Cell division cycle 6 homolog	0.41	0.47	-	-	-	-
CDC2	NM_001786.2	Cell division cycle 2, G1 to S and G2 to M	0.41	0.32	-	-	-	-
CCND1	NM_053056.2	Cyclin D1	0.43	-	-	-	-	-
MCM4	NM_005914.2	Minichromosome maintenance complex component 4	0.43	0.36	-	-	-	-
MCM5	NM_006739.3	Minichromosome maintenance complex component 5	0.45	0.35	-	-	-	-
PCNA	NM_182649.1	Proliferating cell nuclear antigen (PCNA), transcript variant 2	0.46	0.45	-	-	-	-
CDK2	NM_001798.2	Cyclin-dependent kinase 2	0.48	0.44	-	-	-	-
PKMYT1	NM_182687.1	Protein kinase, membrane associated tyrosine/threonine 1	0.49	0.30	-	-	-	-
MAD2L1	NM_002358.2	MAD2 mitotic arrest deficient-like 1	0.49	0.36	-	-	-	-
CCNA2	NM_001237.2	Cyclin A2	-	0.31	-	-	-	-
TTK	NM_003318.3	TTK protein kinase	-	0.41	-	-	-	-
CDC20	NM_001255.2	Cell division cycle 20 homolog	-	0.46	-	-	-	-
CDC25C	NM_001790.3	Cell division cycle 25 homolog C	-	0.46	-	-	-	-
PLK1	NM_005030.3	Polo-like kinase 1	-	0.47	-	-	-	-
BUB1	NM_004336.2	BUB1 budding uninhibited by benzimidazoles 1 homolog	-	0.48	-	-	-	-

In our experimental setup, one of the genes most affected by statin treatment was *TNFRSF10D* (Table 5). Its product, the tumor necrosis factor receptor superfamily member 10D precursor (known also as TNF-related apoptosis-inducing ligand receptor 4, or TRAIL receptor 4) is a member of the TNF-receptor superfamily, which is closely connected with apoptosis. TNFRSF10D has been shown to play an inhibitory role in TRAIL-induced cell apoptosis [59]. Upregulation of another gene, *GABARAPL* (also known as early estrogen-regulated protein; Table 5) suggests that statin treatment may induce cell death by autophagy [53]. STRING enrichment analysis of products of genes involved in cell death significantly affected by statin treatment is shown in Figure 6.

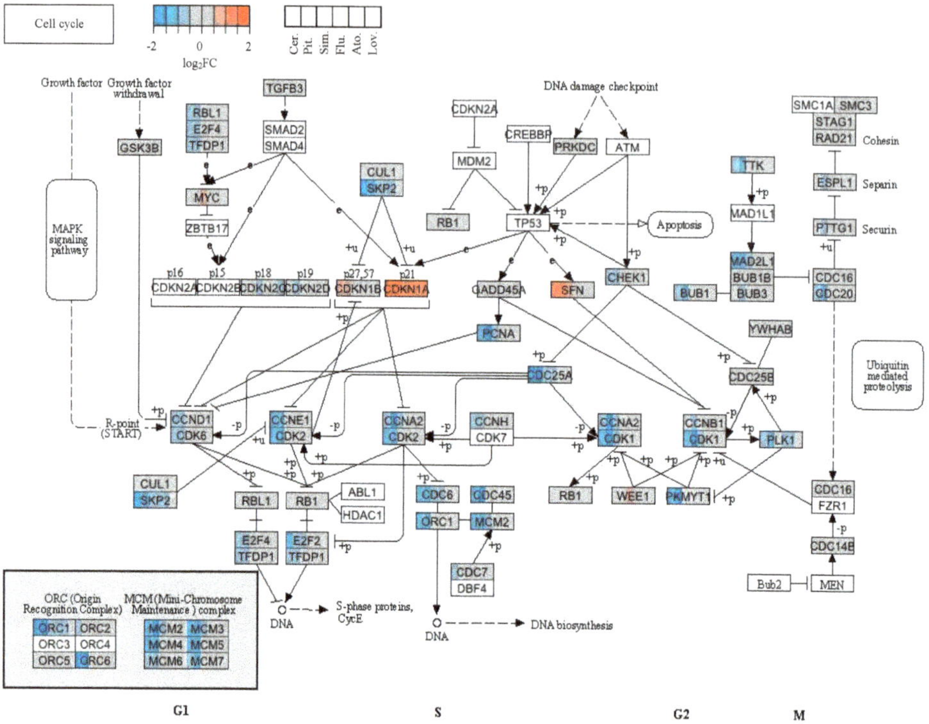

Figure 5. Cell-cycle signalization and the changes induced by statin treatment in the expression of the genes that code for members of the circuit. The color fill of the nodes indicates the base-2 logarithm of the fold change in gene expression upon treatment by a statin. Different statins are shown in the distinct position of the node as indicated in the key.

Table 5. Genes involved in cell death affected by statin treatment of MiaPaCa-2 cells. Numeric columns display fold changes of the gene expression between cells treated by individual statins at 12 μM concentration for 24 h and untreated cells. Cer.—cerivastatin; Pit.—pitavastatin; Sim.—simvastatin; Flu.—fluvastatin; Ato.—atorvastatin; Lov.—lovastatin. Pravastatin and rosuvastatin did not induce any significant change in MiaPaCa-2 cell gene expression.

Gene Symbol	Ref. ID	Product Name	Cer.	Pit.	Sim.	Flu.	Ato.	Lov.
					Fold Change			
TNFRSF10D	NM_003840.3	Tumor necrosis factor receptor superfamily, member 10d	3.71	3.17	4.68	3.06	2.76	2.60
SLC6A12	NM_003044.2	Solute carrier family 6 (betaine/GABA), member 12	2.45	2.16	2.84	2.45	-	-
DRAM	NM_018370.2	Damage-regulated autophagy modulator	2.18	2.41	-	-	-	-
CASP9	NM_032996.1	Caspase 9, apoptosis-related cysteine peptidase	2.16	-	-	-	-	-
GABARAPL1	NM_031412.2	GABA(A) receptor-associated protein like 1	2.13	3.76	2.49	2.13	-	-
ATG2A	NM_015104.1	ATG2 autophagy related 2 homolog A	2.08	-	-	-	-	-
TNFAIP1	NM_021137.3	Tumor necrosis factor, alpha-induced protein 1	2.01	-	-	-	-	-
CARD10	NM_014550.3	Caspase recruitment domain family, member 10	0.43	0.49	-	-	-	-
TNFRSF6B	NM_032945.2	Tumor necrosis factor receptor superfamily, member 6b	0.48	-	-	-	-	-

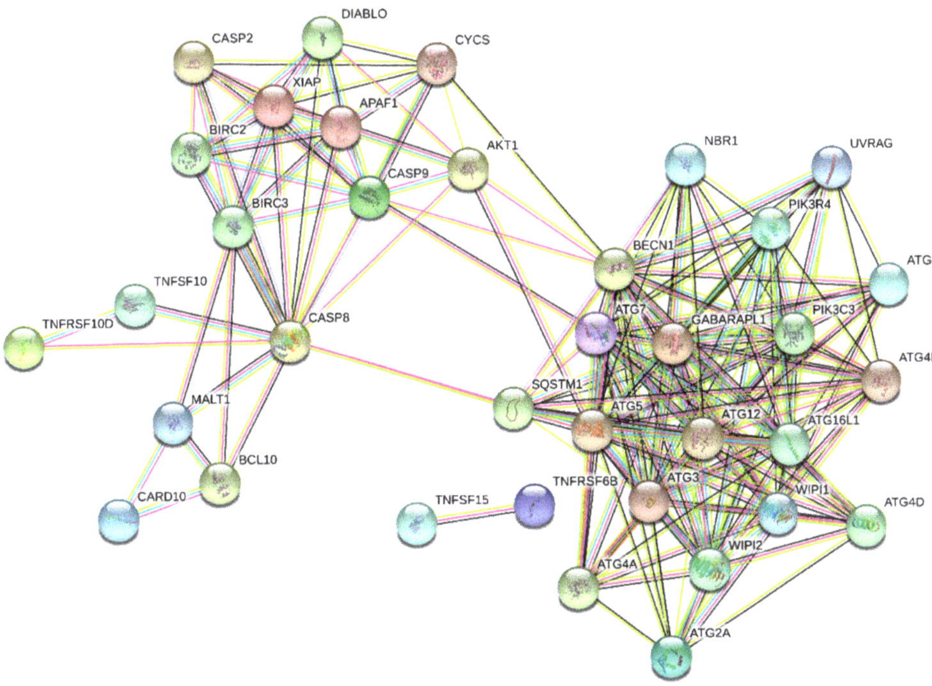

Figure 6. STRING enrichment analysis of products of genes involved in cell death significantly affected by statin treatment (mainly by cerivastatin and pitavastatin) of MiaPaCa-2 cells at 12 μM concentration for 24 h. Individual nodes represent affected gene products and their interactions. Input nodes were based on the genes listed in Table 5 (*TNFRSF10D, SLC6A12, DRAM, CASP9, GABARAPL1, ATG2A, TNFAIP1, CARD10,* and *TNFRSF6B*). A complete description of the nodes is given in Supplementary Table S1. See Figure 3's caption for color coding of the edges.

2.5. Statins' Effect on Migration and Invasion of Cancer Cells

Since statins are known to affect migration and invasion of various cancer cells [60–64], which is also in accordance with our preliminary unpublished data, we also concentrated on the analyses of changes in the transcription of genes involved in cell migration and cytoskeleton architecture. The pancreatic cancer cells used in our study were firmly attached to the cultivation surface. However, the statin treatment induced a change in the cell shape and facilitated their detachment (data not shown). This is consistent with the effect of statins on the expression of the genes encoding the cytoskeletal proteins (Table 6). STRING enrichment analysis of products of genes involved in cytoskeleton maintenance significantly affected by statin treatment is shown in Figure 7.

Intermediate filaments (IF) of the cytoplasmic cytoskeleton are composed of keratins that are the major structural proteins of epithelial cells. They interact with desmosomes and hemidesmosomes, by which they assist in cell–cell adhesion [65].

TNNT1 is a subunit of troponin, which is a regulatory complex located on the thin filament of the sarcomere. This complex regulates striated muscle contraction in response to fluctuations in intracellular calcium concentration [66]. Gelsolin is an actin-binding protein that is a key regulator of actin filament assembly and disassembly. Among the lipid-binding actin regulatory proteins, gelsolin is one of the few that exhibit preferential binding toward polyphosphoinositide. The activity of gelsolin is stimulated by calcium ions (Ca^{2+}) [67]. Kinesins belong to a class of motor proteins found in eukaryotic cells. Kinesins move along microtubule cables powered by the dephosphorylation of adenosine triphosphate (ATP). The active movement of kinesins supports several cellular functions, including mitosis, meiosis, and transport of cargo [68]. Catenins are proteins found in complexes with cadherin cell adhesion molecules of animal cells. Junction plakoglobin (catenin gamma) was originally identified as a component of desmosomes (a cell structure specialized for cell-to-cell adhesion) [69]. Ezrin is the cytoplasmic peripheral membrane protein that serves as an intermediate between the plasma membrane and the actin cytoskeleton. This protein plays a key role in cell-surface structure adhesion, migration, and organization, and it has been implicated in various human cancers [70]. CDH10 is an integral membrane protein that mediates calcium-dependent cell–cell adhesion [71].

Table 6. Genes involved in cytoskeleton maintenance affected by statin treatment of MiaPaCa-2 cells. Numeric columns display fold changes of the gene expression between cells treated by individual statins at 12 μM concentration for 24 h and untreated cells. Cer.—cerivastatin; Pit.—pitavastatin; Sim.—simvastatin; Flu.—fluvastatin; Ato.—atorvastatin; Lov.—lovastatin. Pravastatin and rosuvastatin did not induce any significant change in MiaPaCa-2 cell gene expression.

Gene Symbol	Ref. ID	Product Name	Cer.	Pit.	Sim.	Flu.	Ato.	Lov.
			Fold Change					
LOC400578	XR_017543.1	Similar to keratin, type I cytoskeletal 14 (Cytokeratin-14)	15.80	12.21	5.44	3.62	3.32	2.59
KRT16	NM_005557.2	Keratin 16	13.85	12.21	4.60	3.52	3.28	2.23
MGC102966	XR_015970.1	Similar to keratin, type I cytoskeletal 16 (Cytokeratin-16)	13.54	11.95	4.84	3.53	3.18	2.31
KRT15	NM_002275.2	Homo sapiens keratin 15	5.97	5.86	3.85	3.43	3.02	3.25
KLHL24	NM_017644.3	Kelch-like 24	5.78	4.56	2.89	2.21	2.21	-
JUP	NM_002230.1	Junction plakoglobin	5.33	4.09	2.78	2.51	2.00	-
TUBB1	NM_030773.2	Tubulin, beta 1	4.02	-	-	2.23	-	-
KRT13	NM_002274.3	Keratin 13	3.16	4.35	3.38	2.84	2.68	3.05
KRT19	NM_002276.3	Keratin 19	3.13	2.88	2.50	2.20	2.11	-
GSN	NM_198252.2	Gelsolin (amyloidosis, Finnish type)	2.97	2.32	2.45	2.00	-	-
KIF1A	NM_004321.4	Kinesin family member 1A	2.73	3.05	2.26	-	-	-
TNNT1	NM_003283.3	Troponin T, slow skeletal muscle	2.70	3.57	2.10	-	-	-
ITGB4	NM_001005619.1	Homo sapiens integrin, beta 4	2.45	2.49	2.18	2.03	-	2.20
VIL2	NM_003379.3	Villin 2 (ezrin)	2.16	2.18	2.01	-	-	-
NAV1	NM_020443.2	Neuron navigator 1	2.14	2.38	2.13	-	-	-
GSN	NM_198252.2	Gelsolin (amyloidosis, Finnish type)	-	-	-	-	-	-
CDH10	NM_006727.2	Cadherin 10, type 2 (T2-cadherin)	0.31	0.28	0.33	0.48	0.45	-
SYNM	NM_015286.5	Synemin, intermediate filament protein	0.48	0.50	-	-	-	-

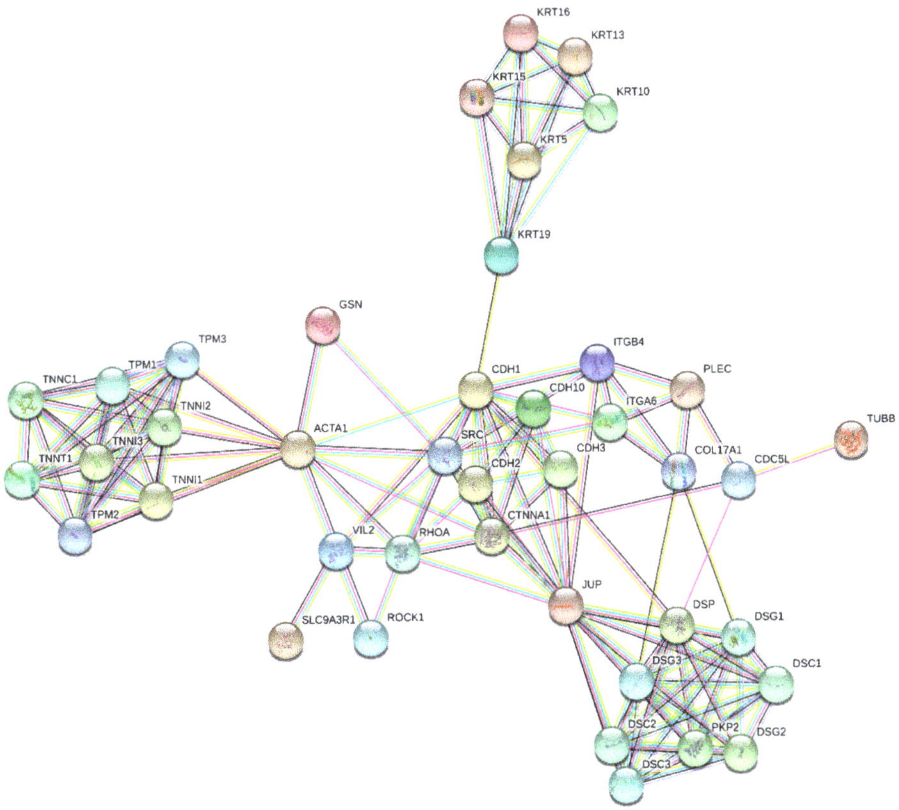

Figure 7. STRING enrichment analysis of products of genes involved in cytoskeleton maintenance significantly affected by statin treatment (mainly by cerivastatin, pitavastatin, and simvastatin) of MiaPaCa-2 cells at 12 μM concentration for 24 h. Individual nodes represent affected gene products and their interactions. Input nodes were based on the genes listed in Table 6 (*LOC400578, KRT16, MGC102966, KRT15, KLHL24, JUP, TUBB1, KRT13, KRT19, GSN, KIF1A, TNNT1, ITGB4, VIL2, NAV1, GSN, CDH10,* and *SYNM*). A complete description of the nodes is given in Supplementary Table S1. See Figure 3's caption for color coding of the edges.

3. Materials and Methods

3.1. DNA Microarray Analysis

Description of an experimental method for the studying of the effects of individual statins on the gene-expression profile of MiaPaCa-2 cells was reported by Gbelcová et al. [30]. We compared the effect of statins to simvastatin because it was chosen as the most effective clinically used statin tested *in vitro* in our previous study. Briefly, pure forms (≥98 %) of all commercially available statins were used: atorvastatin, lovastatin, simvastatin, fluvastatin, cerivastatin, pravastatin, rosuvastatin, and pitavastatin (LKT Laboratories, USA). Statins were dissolved in methanol and tested in 12 μM concentrations, representing the IC_{50} value for simvastatin after 24 h of treatment of MiaPaCa-2 cancer cells. Human pancreatic cancer cells MiaPaCa-2 (ATCC, Manassas, VA) were cultured in DMEM medium (Sigma Aldrich, Germany) supplemented with 10 % fetal bovine serum. Illumina HumanWG-6_V3 chips (Illumina, USA) were used for the microarray analysis following the standard protocol. Annotation of differentially expressed transcripts was done with R/BioConductor packages [72] against the Ensembl database (version 47) [73]. The transcripts with a false discovery rate smaller than 0.05 and fold change smaller than 0.5 or greater than 2 were reported and used in the downstream analysis. Changes in the gene expression were visualized using the Pathview package [74] on the pathways provided by the KEGG database [75].

3.2. *RT-qPCR Analysis*

Validation of the selected gene expression changes was performed using quantitative RT-PCR. The amount of 1×10^8 cells was washed with phosphate-buffered saline and lysed using the RLT buffer (Qiagen, Hilden, Germany) supplemented with β-mercaptoethanol. The total RNA was extracted by the RNeasy Micro kit (Qiagen) according to the manufacturer's protocol. All extracts were treated with DNase I (Qiagen) to remove contaminating genomic DNA. The quality and quantity of the RNA were evaluated with an Agilent 2100 Bioanalyzer instrument using the RNA 6000 Nano kit (both Agilent Technologies, Santa Clara, CA, USA). Expression levels of the mRNA were determined using a two-step RT-qPCR method. First, cDNA was reverse-transcribed from 1 μg of total RNA in a final reaction volume of 20 μL using a QuantiTect reverse transcription kit (Qiagen) according to the manufacturer's instructions. Then, the cDNA concentration was quantified using a LightCycler 480 instrument in LightCycler 480 SYBR Green I master mix (both Roche Applied Sciences, Penzberg, Germany) with a custom primer mix (see Supplementary Table S1 for primer sequences). For each condition, two biological replicates were analyzed (three for the control group).

Data analysis was performed using the delta–delta Cq method [76] within the R statistical environment [77]. Cq values were truncated at the value of 40. Three housekeeping genes (RPS9, TBP, and GAPDH) were used as reference genes for RNA quantity normalization using the geNorm algorithm [78]. Relative expression levels were computed assuming the perfect efficiency of the PCR.

3.3. *STRING Analysis*

A functional association network of known and predicted functional partners or selected genes identified as significantly changed in the microarray analysis in MiaPaCa-2 cells treated with 12 μM concentration of statins for 24 h was created using STRING database 11.0 [79]. STRING is an interaction network database for functional enrichment analysis of protein–protein interaction networks. Input nodes were chosen based on the most important hits identified by the microarray analysis and depicted in Figure 3, Figure 6, and Figure 7. The evidence view diagrams were generated by STRING to illustrate the known protein–protein interactions of all connected nodes. The view of the association network was done for *Homo sapiens* according to the known and predicted from curated databases, experimentally determined, gene neighborhood, gene fusions, gene co-occurrence, text-mining, co-expression, and protein homology. The confidence score was set to high, equal to 0.700, with a maximum of 30 interactions. Disconnected nodes in the networks were hidden.

4. Discussion and Conclusions

Statins have been intensively studied drugs based on their deep impact on the human organism caused, in particular by their cholesterol-lowering activity. However, their effects also include remarkable and potentially clinically relevant antitumor effects.

Although lipids are not genetically encoded, the genome changes can reflect cholesterol homeostasis indirectly. The changes in gene expression following statin treatment studied by microarray technology have been reported since the year 2000. The interpretation of our microarray analysis indicates a significant correlation between our and previously reported results. On the other hand, many differences are resulting from distinct experimental conditions due to the type of statin used, its concentration and duration of its activity, the experimental model (the type of a cell line or organism), etc.

Previously, we have demonstrated substantial differences in cancer cell antiproliferative effects of all commercially available statins in an experimental model of human pancreatic cancer [31]. Various statins exhibited significantly different inhibitory efficacy, and we have also observed notable differences in statin sensitivity between pancreatic cancer cell lines, concerning the level of differentiation and harboring of G12C-activating mutation in the *KRAS* gene. Cerivastatin, pitavastatin, and simvastatin were the most effective, whereas rosuvastatin and pravastatin were the least effective, and their effectiveness correlated with the properties of the cell lines tested (the level of differentiation, and presence of G12C *KRAS* mutation) [31]. In the present study, we observed that depletion of farnesylated K-Ras protein caused by the three most effective statins led to significant upregulation of gene-encoding K-Ras.

The pleiotropic effect of statins is comprehensible, since K-Ras is related to many functional pathways, such as the MAPK signaling pathway, the ErbB signaling pathway, dorso-ventral axis formation, axon guidance, the VEGF signaling pathway, tight junction, gap junction, natural killer cell-mediated cytotoxicity, the T-cell receptor signaling pathway, the B-cell receptor signaling pathway, the Fc epsilon RI signaling pathway, long-term potentiation, long-term depression, regulation of actin cytoskeleton, the insulin signaling pathway, and the GnRH signaling pathway. Moreover, the upregulation of KRAS after the statin treatment seemed to be a result of the unavailability of farnesylated K-Ras protein for cell signaling due to the mevalonate pathway inhibition. Similarly, this mechanism could also explain the upregulation of other Ras and Ras-related proteins induced by statin treatment (Table 3). However, the products of the mevalonate pathway are required not only for post-translational modifications of many proteins, but also for regulation of the transcription of many proteins, including proteins of the cytoskeleton. For example, expression of keratin 13 is known to be regulated by nuclear receptor ligands such as retinoids, 1α, 25-dihydroxy vitamin D3, or estrogen [65]. Except for the metabolism of lipids (biosynthesis of steroids and sphingolipid metabolism), the inhibition of the mevalonate pathway by statins directly affected the energy metabolism due to ubiquinone depletion, as ubiquinone is involved in mitochondrial respiration [80].

Genetic heterogeneity is an important factor that affects the sensitivity of particular cancer cells to the antiproliferative/proapoptotic effects of statins. Despite the level of cancer cell differentiation, pancreatic cancer cell lines harboring activating K-Ras mutation were more sensitive to the antiproliferative effect of statins than cells harboring wild-type K-Ras [31]. Similarly, Wong et al. demonstrated that only 8 of 17 multiple myeloma cell lines evaluated were sensitive to lovastatin-induced apoptosis, while resistant cell lines had different genetic profiles [81].

The first effect of statins, specifically simvastatin, studied by microarray analysis was focused on actomyosin contraction, gap formation, and barrier dysfunction produced by thrombin. The experiment was performed in human pulmonary artery endothelial cells (EC) treated with 5 μM simvastatin for 24 h. Several genes related to thrombin-mediated cytoskeletal dynamics and barrier regulation, including caldesmon and the thrombin receptor PAR-1, were dramatically downregulated. In addition, ITGB4, a protein known to be involved in cell–cell adhesion, was dramatically upregulated. *RhoA* and *RhoC* genes were also upregulated similarly to Rac1 and specific GEFs, potential regulators of preferential Rho GTPase activity. In contrast, the RhoGDP dissociation inhibitor was downregulated, which was interpreted as a compensatory response [82]. Consistent with these data, our results also indicated that statins directly affected the expression of specific genes related to the Rho GTPase signaling and cytoskeletal regulation. However, from all the Rho family members, only *RhoB* was significantly upregulated by all effective statins (pravastatin and rosuvastatin were not effective in our microarray study), and *RhoA* was significantly upregulated only by the most effective statins (cerivastatin, pitavastatin, and simvastatin). No changes were observed in the expression of genes encoding specific GEFs. Also, downregulation of caldesmon or the thrombin receptor PAR-1 was not observed in our study. This could vary in different types of cell lines evaluated.

Interestingly, a gene encoding the integrin beta 4 subunit of a receptor for the laminins; i.e., *Itgb4*, was the most significantly upregulated gene (fold change—7.57) of all the tested genes [83]. The reason for the enhanced transcription of a gene involved in the biology of invasive carcinoma is unclear. Another notable finding is that no changes were observed in the expression of the *RhoB* gene after treatment of EC with 5 μM simvastatin [84], whereas in our study, the *RhoB* gene was the more affected gene compared to the Itgb4 gene after treatment with all effective statins.

In the other study, the DNA microarrays were used to identify gene expression patterns in the cerebral cortex of mice treated with simvastatin (50 mg/kg b.wt.) by daily oral doses for 21 days. The maximum average concentration of simvastatin was determined as 600 pmol/g in brains. This study revealed the influence of simvastatin on the expression of several genes involved in cell growth and signaling. *C-fos*, *c–myc*, and *Bcl-2* were of particular interest due to the linkage of simvastatin with cell growth and apoptosis. Simvastatin significantly reduced the expression of the proto-oncogene *c-fos*. On the other hand, it significantly increased the expression of the oncogene *c-myc* and antiapoptotic gene *Bcl-2* [84,85]. In contrast to these data, neither the expression of previously mentioned genes nor of other genes attributed to apoptotic cell death (e.g., genes encoding death receptors or caspases, the only exception to which was caspase 9, which was upregulated by cerivastatin) were affected by statins in our microarray analysis. However, as demonstrated by the analysis of the most affected functional pathways, statins affected some processes related to DNA repair, such as base excision repair or mismatch repair [30]. It is known that failure of these processes could be followed by programmed necrosis [86]. Finally, the upregulation of the *GABARAPL* gene related to autophagy was observed (Table 5). Autophagy does not always result in programmed cell death, but it represents the important mechanism for catabolic production of ATP during nutrient stress, and also plays an important role in the turnover of proteins and organelles under nutrient-replete conditions [87]. The statin-treated cells were in nutrient stress due to inhibition of the mevalonate pathway. From many end products of this pathway, ubiquinone is required in a process of ATP formation during oxidative phosphorylation. Moreover, oxidative phosphorylation is also reported as one of the significantly affected functional pathways by statins [30]. Interestingly, it was published that ubiquitinated hydrophobic proteins that are prone to aggregation are kept on the surface of lipid droplets and subjected to autophagy, as well as proteasomal degradation [88].

The cell-cycle arrest represents another frequently discussed event associated with statins. Many reports describe the effect of individual statins on the expression of cell-cycle-related genes. For example, changes in the expression of genes related to the cell cycle in chronic myelogenous leukemia cells K562 were described. Fifteen downregulated and 9 upregulated cell-cycle-related genes were observed in the presence of 20 μM simvastatin for 48 h. The results of flow cytometry showed that the cell cycle was arrested in the G1 phase [89]. Assmus et al. performed a microarray analysis of about 12,000 genes in endothelial progenitor cells (a primary cell line) treated with 0.1 μM atorvastatin for 10 h. The expression of cyclins and proliferating cell nuclear antigen (PCNA) was increased after atorvastatin treatment. Moreover, the expression of the cell-cycle inhibitory protein p27 was reduced [90]. In the next study, downregulation of cyclin D1, PCNA, and c-myc, and upregulation of p21 and p19, were provided by the treatment of human breast cancer cells with cerivastatin [91].

In our microarray analysis, the expression of genes encoding cyclin D1 was affected only by cerivastatin, cyclin A2 by pitavastatin, and cyclin E2 by both mentioned statins, similar to the *PCNA* gene. Other statins did not affect the expression of genes encoding cyclins or PCNA. The expression of the *p21* gene was increased by all effective statins. Moreover, the genes associated with DNA replication, such as *ORC1L*, *MCM2*, or *MCM3*, were downregulated by cerivastatin and pitavastatin (Table 4). This suggests that statins blocked the progress of the cell cycle through the S phase of MiaPaCa-2 cells. The downregulation of the genes encoding histone H4 and upregulation of the gene encoding histone H2B by the three most effective statins (cerivastatin, pitavastatin, and simvastatin) also was very interesting. The effect of simvastatin on expression of the gene encoding histone was also observed in a report by Johnson-Anuna et al., in which the expression level of the gene encoding the linker histone H1.2 was increased after simvastatin therapy [84]. Likewise, other proteins related to the S phase (SKP2, E2F2) or M phase (CDC2, CDC25B) were downregulated by cerivastatin and pitavastatin treatment of MiaPaCa-2 cells in our study, indicating that except for the G1 phase, the most effective statins blocked the cell-cycle entry into the M phase. This was not surprising, as lovastatin is used in the cell-cycle synchronization protocols [92] and as a pharmacological tool for controlling the growth of neoplastic cells both in vitro and in vivo [23,93,94]. Furthermore, lovastatin is commercially available as an inhibitor of the cell cycle in the G1 and G2/M phases (Sigma, USA). The G1 block has been attributed to the inhibition of either cytokinesis or cell spreading following cytokinesis [95]. Several authors have also noted the retardation or arrest of the cell cycle at the G2/M transition [93,94,96]. However, the mechanism of the cell-cycle arrest by statins is not exactly clear. Despite a piece of evidence that lovastatin suppresses cell proliferation through inhibition of proteasome-mediated degradation of p21 and p27 [97], it was concluded that lovastatin neither synchronizes cells nor arrests the cells in the G1 phase of the division cycle [98].

To explain the reported results, the distinct impact of statins on gene expression profiles in MiaPaCa-2 cells should be related to their inhibitory activity interfering with the mevalonate pathway. Quantum biochemistry computations indicated some variations among the attractive forces of four tested statins (atorvastatin, rosuvastatin, simvastatin, and fluvastatin) and the HMG-CoA reductase binding site. The highest binding energies was determined for atorvastatin followed by rosuvastatin, while the lowest were found for simvastatin and fluvastatin; i.e., binding energies of 320, 310, 290, and 290 $kcal \cdot mol^{-1}$, respectively [99]. However, in this study, cerivastatin, lovastatin, and pitavastatin were not included in the calculations. In another study, the crystal structures of the catalytic moiety of HMG-CoA reductase in a complex with six statins documented van der Waals interactions of the rigid hydrophobic moieties of the statins through a shallow nonpolar binding pocket and a part of the binding surface for CoA [100]. These interactions prevented the binding of the substrate HMG-CoA to the active site of the enzyme. No dramatic differences were found among the numbers of binding interactions among the statins evaluated, namely: compactin, simvastatin, fluvastatin, cerivastatin, atorvastatin, and rosuvastatin. Atorvastatin, simvastatin, lovastatin, fluvastatin, and cerivastatin are relatively lipophilic and are metabolized by the cytochrome P450 system. The other lipophilic compound pitavastatin is metabolized poorly via this pathway. Very limited P450-mediated metabolization was reported also for hydrophilic pravastatin and rosuvastatin, which were only nonsignificantly metabolized. Interestingly, high systemic bioavailability was reported for both cerivastatin and pitavastatin (60% [101] and 80% [102], respectively), which could explain their large impact on changes in gene expression. Except for pravastatin, all the other statins were efficiently bound to plasma proteins. However, the unbound pravastatin was poorly distributed in tissues due to its high hydrophilic nature [103].

Further, the distinct efficacy of individual statins on both antiproliferative activity and changes in gene expression could be also correlated with the statin levels inside cells. This correlation was the strongest for the least efficient statins (rosuvastatin and pravastatin); whereas for the most bioavailable statins (in particular lovastatin), this correlation was not so strong [30]. Thus, the statin effects on whole gene expression correlated with their bioavailability, as well as the impact on cell viability, only to a limited extent. This hypothesis held for cerivastatin; however, not so for pitavastatin and lovastatin, which led us to the conclusion that other crucial factors played an important role in the differences of statin effects on pancreatic cancer cell proliferation.

In summary, differences in the efficacy of individual statins are known depending on their structure, concentration, duration of action, or microenvironment. Although tumor cells exhibit many identical properties, the effect of statins depends also on the cell type [104]. The antitumor effect of statins is not only a function of the mechanism of their action, but also of how they are metabolized. In general, healthy cells are generally more resistant to statins than tumor cells [105]. The use of statins in the treatment of cancer as monotherapeutics is not effective enough, but their use in combination with other therapeutic approaches would significantly increase the effectiveness of cancer treatments and patient survival [106,107].

Supplementary Materials: The following are available online: Table S1: Legend for figures from STRING database.

Author Contributions: Conceptualization, L.V., H.G., S.R.; methodology, L.V., H.S., H.G. software, M.K., S.R.; validation, H.S.; formal analysis, M.K., H.G.; investigation, L.V., H.S., H.G.; resources, S.R., M.K., H.G.; data curation, M.K., H.G., S.R.; writing—original draft preparation, H.G., S.R.; writing—review and editing, M.K., T.R., L.V.; visualization S.R., M.K.; supervision, L.V., T.R; project administration, L.V.; funding acquisition, L.V., T.R. All authors have read and agreed to the published version of the manuscript.

Funding: This research was funded by grant no. APVV-15-0217 given by the Slovak Research and Devel-opment Agency; by the Operational Programme Research, Development, and Education (Reg. No. CZ.02.1.01/0.0/0.0/16_019/0000785); and by grant no. RVO-VFN64165/2021 given by the Czech Ministry of Health.

Institutional Review Board Statement: Not applicable.

Informed Consent Statement: Not applicable.

Data Availability Statement: The gene microarray data have been deposited in the ArrayExpress database (accession number E-MTAB-3263).

Acknowledgments: We gratefully acknowledge Martina Krausová, Jana Šáchová, and Miluše Hradilová for excellent technical support.

Conflicts of Interest: The authors declare no conflict of interest.

References

1. Goldstein, J.L.; Brown, M.S. A century of cholesterol and coronaries: From plaques to genes to statins. *Cell* **2015**, *161*, 161–172. [CrossRef] [PubMed]
2. Alexandrova, R.; Dinev, D.; Glavcheva, M.; Danova, J.; Yetik-Anacak, G.; Krasilnikova, J.; Podlipnik, C. Briefly about anticancer properties of statins. *Biomed. J. Sci. Tech. Res.* **2019**, *7*, 12655–12659. [CrossRef]
3. Mohammadkhani, N.; Gharbib, S.; Rajani, H.F.; Farzaneh, A.; Mahjoobe, G.; Hoseinsalari, A.; Korsching, E. Statins: Complex outcomes but increasingly helpful treatment options for patients. *European J. Pharmacol.* **2019**, *863*, 1–8. [CrossRef] [PubMed]
4. Tavintharan, S.; Ong, C.N.; Jeyaseelan, K.; Sivakumar, M.; Lim, S.C.; Sum, C.F. Reduced mitochondrial coenzyme Q10 levels in HepG2 cells treated with high-dose simvastatin: A possible role in statin-induced hepatotoxicity? *Toxicol. Appl. Pharmacol.* **2007**, *223*, 173–179. [CrossRef] [PubMed]
5. Svoboda, M.; Vyskočil, J.; Nováková, J. Statiny v onkologii. *Klin. Farmakol. Farm.* **2005**, *19*, 155–159.
6. Newman, T.B.; Hulley, S.B. Carcinogenicity of lipid-lowering drugs. *JAMA* **1996**, *275*, 55–60. [CrossRef] [PubMed]
7. Dalen, J.E.; Dalton, W.S. Does lowering cholesterol cause cancer? *JAMA* **1996**, *275*, 67–69. [CrossRef]
8. Sacks, F.M.; Pfeffer, M.A.; Moye, L.A.; Rouleau, J.L.; Rutherford, J.D.; Cole, T.G.; Brown, L.; Warnica, J.W.; Arnold, J.M.; Wun, C.C.; et al. The effect of pravastatin on coronary events after myocardial infarction in patients with average cholesterol levels. Cholesterol and recurrent events trial investigators. *N. Engl. J. Med.* **1996**, *335*, 1001–1009. [CrossRef]
9. Downs, J.R.; Clearfield, M.; Weis, S.; Whitney, E.; Shapiro, D.R.; Beere, P.A.; Langendorfer, A.; Stein, E.A.; Kruyer, W.; Gotto, A.M., Jr. Primary prevention of acute coronary events with lovastatin in men and women with average cholesterol levels: Results of AFCAPS/TexCAPS. Air Force/Texas Coronary Atherosclerosis Prevention Study. *JAMA* **1998**, *279*, 1615–1622. [CrossRef]
10. Graaf, M.R.; Beiderbeck, A.B.; Egberts, A.C.; Richel, D.J.; Guchelaar, H.J. The risk of cancer in users of statins. *Am. J. Clin. Oncol.* **2004**, *22*, 2388–2394. [CrossRef]
11. Scandinavian Simvastatin Survival Study Group. Randomised trial of cholesterol lowering in 4444 patients with coronary heart disease: The Scandinavian Simvastatin Survival Study (4S). *Lancet* **1994**, *344*, 1383–1389. [CrossRef]
12. Shepherd, J.; Cobbe, S.M.; Ford, I.; Isles, C.G.; Lorimer, A.R.; MacFarlane, P.W.; McKillop, J.H.; Packard, C.J. West of Scotland Coronary Prevention Study Group. Prevention of coronary heart disease with pravastatin in men with hypercholesterolemia. *N. Engl. J. Med.* **1995**, *333*, 1301–1307. [CrossRef]
13. Lewis, S.J.; Sacks, F.M.; Mitchell, J.S.; East, C.; Glasser, S.; Kell, S.; Letterer, R.; Limacher, M.; Moye, L.A.; Rouleau, J.L.; et al. Effect of pravastatin on cardiovascular events in women after myocardial infarction: The cholesterol and recurrent events (CARE) trial. *J. Am. Coll. Cardiol.* **1998**, *32*, 40–46. [CrossRef]

14. Ridker, P.M.; Rifai, N.; Pfeffer, M.A.; Sacks, F.M.; Moye, L.A.; Goldman, S.; Flaker, G.C.; Braunwald, E. Inflammation, pravastatin, and the risk of coronary events after myocardial infarction in patients with average cholesterol levels. Cholesterol and recurrent events (CARE) investigators. *Circulation* **1998**, *98*, 839–844. [CrossRef]
15. Long-Term Intervention with Pravastatin in Ischaemic Disease (LIPID) Study Group. Prevention of cardiovascular events and death with pravastatin in patients with coronary heart disease and a broad range of initial cholesterol levels. *N. Engl. J. Med.* **1998**, *339*, 1349–1357. [CrossRef]
16. Athyros, V.G.; Papageorgiou, A.A.; Mercouris, B.R.; Athyrou, V.V.; Symeonidis, A.N.; Basayannis, E.O.; Demitriadis, D.S.; Kontopoulos, A.G. Treatment with atorvastatin to the National Cholesterol Educational Program goal versus 'usual' care in secondary coronary heart disease prevention. The GREek Atorvastatin and Coronary-heart-disease Evaluation (GREACE) study. *Curr. Med. Res. Opin.* **2002**, *18*, 220–228. [CrossRef]
17. Khurana, V.; Bejjanki, H.R.; Caldito, G.; Owens, M.W. Statins reduce the risk of lung cancer in humans: A large case-control study of US Veterans. *Chest* **2007**, *131*, 1282–1288. [CrossRef]
18. Kochhar, R.; Khurana, V.; Bejjanki, H.; Caldito, G.; Fort, C. Statins reduce breast cancer risk: A case control study in US female veterans. *J. Clin. Oncol.* **2005**, *23*, 514. [CrossRef]
19. Singal, R.; Khurana, V.; Caldito, G.; Fort, C. Statins and prostate cancer risk. *J. Clin. Oncol.* **2005**, *23*, 1004. [CrossRef]
20. Poynter, J.N.; Gruber, S.B.; Higgins, P.D.; Almog, R.; Bonner, J.D.; Rennert, H.S.; Low, M.; Greenson, J.K.; Rennert, G. Statins and the risk of colorectal cancer. *N. Engl. J. Med.* **2005**, *352*, 2184–2192. [CrossRef]
21. Kawata, S.; Nagase, T.; Yamasaki, E.; Ishiguro, H.; Matsuzawa, Y. Modulation of the mevalonate pathway and cell growth by pravastatin and dlimonene in a human hepatoma cell line (Hep G2). *Br. J. Cancer* **1994**, *69*, 1015–1020. [CrossRef]
22. Hawk, M.A.; Cesen, K.T.; Siglin, J.C.; Stoner, G.D.; Ruch, R.J. Inhibition of lung tumor cell growth *in vitro* and mouse lung tumor formation by lovastatin. *Cancer Lett.* **1996**, *109*, 217–222. [CrossRef]
23. Feleszko, W.; Jakobisiak, M. Lovastatin augments apoptosis induced by chemotherapeutic agents in colon cancer cells. *Clin. Cancer Res.* **2000**, *6*, 1198–1199.
24. Kawata, S.; Yamasaki, E.; Nagase, T.; Inui, Y.; Ito, N.; Matsuda, Y.; Inada, M.; Tamura, S.; Noda, S.; Imai, Y.; et al. Effect of pravastatin on survival in patients with advanced hepatocellular carcinoma. A randomized controlled trial. *Br. J. Cancer* **2001**, *84*, 886–891. [CrossRef]
25. Kim, W.S.; Kim, M.M.; Choi, H.J.; Yoon, S.S.; Lee, M.H.; Park, K.; Park, C.H.; Kang, W.K. Phase II study of high-dose lovastatin in patients with advanced Bystric adenocarcinoma. *Incest. New Drugs* **2001**, *19*, 81–83. [CrossRef]
26. Larner, J.; Jane, J.; Laws, E.; Packer, R.; Myers, C.; Shaffrey, M. A phase I-II trial of lovastatin for anaplastic astrocytoma and glioblastoma multiforme. *Am. J. Clin. Oncol.* **1998**, *21*, 579–583. [CrossRef]
27. Bonovas, S.; Filioussi, K.; Sitaras, N.M. Statins are not associated with a reduced risk of pancreatic cancer at the population level, when taken at low doses for managing hypercholesterolemia: Evidence from a meta-analysis of 12 studies. *Am. J. Gastroenterol.* **2008**, *103*, 2646–3651. [CrossRef]
28. Bonovas, S.; Filioussi, K.; Tsantes, A.; Sitaras, N.M. Use of statins and risk of haematological malignancies: A meta-analysis of six randomized clinical trials and eight observational studies. *Br. J. Clin. Pharmacol.* **2007**, *64*, 255–262. [CrossRef]
29. Bonovas, S.; Sitaras, N.M. Does pravastatin promote cancer in elderly patients? A metaanalysis. *CMAJ* **2007**, *176*, 649–654. [CrossRef]
30. Gbelcová, H.; Rimpelová, S.; Ruml, T.; Fenclová, M.; Kosek, V.; Hajšlová, J.; Strnad, H.; Kolář, M.; Vítek, L. Variability in statin-induced changes in gene expression profiles of pancreatic cancer. *Sci. Rep.* **2017**, *7*, 44219. [CrossRef]
31. Gbelcová, H.; Leníček, M.; Zelenka, J.; Knejzlík, Z.; Dvořáková, G.; Zadinová, M.; Poučková, P.; Kudla, M.; Balaž, P.; Ruml, T.; et al. Differences in antitumor effects of various statins on human pancreatic cancer. *Int. J. Cancer* **2008**, *122*, 1214–1221. [CrossRef] [PubMed]
32. Longo, J.; van Leeuwen, J.E.; Elbaz, M.; Branchard, E.; Penn, L.Z. Statins as anticancer agents in the era of precision medicine. *Clin. Cancer Res.* **2020**, *26*, 5791–5800. [CrossRef] [PubMed]
33. Mullen, P.J.; Yu, R.; Longo, J.; Archer, M.C.; Penn, L.Z. The interplay between cell signalling and the mevalonate pathway in cancer. *Nat. Rev. Cancer* **2016**, *16*, 718–731. [CrossRef] [PubMed]
34. Di Bello, E.; Zwergel, C.; Mai, A.; Valente, S. The innovative potential of statins in cancer: New targets for new therapies. *Front. Chem.* **2020**, *8*, 516. [CrossRef] [PubMed]
35. Ahmadi, M.; Amiri, S.; Pecic, S.; Machaj, F.; Rosik, J.; Łos, M.J.; Alizadeh, J.; Mahdian, R.; da Silva Rosa, S.C.; Schaafsma, D.; et al. Pleiotropic effects of statins: A focus on cancer. *Biochim. Biophys. Acta Mol. Basis Dis.* **2020**, *1866*, 165968. [CrossRef] [PubMed]
36. Zhang, Y.; Liang, M.; Sun, C.; Qu, G.; Shi, T.; Min, M.; Wu, Y.; Sun, Y. Statin use and risk of pancreatic cancer an updated meta-analysis of 26 studies. *Pancreas* **2019**, *48*, 142–150. [CrossRef] [PubMed]
37. Riscal, R.; Skuli, N.; Simon, M.C. Even cancer cells watch their cholesterol! *Mol. Cell* **2019**, *76*, 220–231. [CrossRef]
38. Zhuang, L.; Kim, J.; Adam, R.M.; Solomon, K.R.; Freeman, M.R. Cholesterol targeting alters lipid raft composition and cell survival in prostate cancer cells and xenografts. *J. Clin. Investig.* **2005**, *115*, 959–968. [CrossRef]
39. Gordon, R.E.; Zhang, L.; Peri, S.; Kuo, Y.M.; Du, F.; Egleston, B.L.; Ng, J.M.Y.; Andrews, A.J.; Astsaturov, I.; Curran, T.; et al. Statins synergize with hedgehog pathway inhibitors for treatment of medulloblastoma. *Clin. Cancer Res.* **2018**, *24*, 1375–1388. [CrossRef]
40. Eaton, S. Multiple roles for lipids in the Hedgehog signalling pathway. *Nat. Rev. Mol. Cell. Biol.* **2008**, *9*, 437–445. [CrossRef]

41. Allen, B.L.; Tenzen, T.; McMahon, A.P. The hedgehog-binding proteins GAS1 and CDO cooperate to positively regulate SHH signalling during mouse development. *Genes Dev.* **2007**, *21*, 1244–1257. [CrossRef]
42. Martinelli, D.C.; Fan, C.M. Gas1 extends the range of hedgehog action by facilitating its signalling. *Genes Dev.* **2007**, *21*, 1231–1243. [CrossRef]
43. Shao, W.; Espenshade, P.J. Expanding roles for SREBP in metabolism. *Cell Metab.* **2012**, *16*, 414–419. [CrossRef]
44. Li, X.; Chen, Y.T.; Hu, P.; Huang, W.C. Fatostatin displays high antitumor activity in prostate cancer by blocking SREBP-regulated metabolic pathways and androgen receptor signaling. *Mol. Cancer Ther.* **2014**, *13*, 855–866. [CrossRef]
45. Wen, Y.A.; Xiong, X.; Zaytseva, Y.Y.; Napier, D.L.; Vallee, E.; Li, A.T.; Wang, C.; Weiss, H.L.; Evers, B.M.; Gao, T. Downregulation of SREBP inhibits tumor growth and initiation by altering cellular metabolism in colon cancer. *Cell Death Dis.* **2018**, *9*, 265. [CrossRef]
46. Carrer, A.; Trefely, S.; Zhao, S.; Campbell, S.L.; Norgard, R.J.; Schultz, K.C.; Sidoli, S.; Parris, J.L.D.; Affronti, H.C.; Sivanand, S.; et al. AcetylCoA metabolism supports multistep pancreatic tumorigenesis. *Cancer Discov.* **2019**, *9*, 416–435. [CrossRef]
47. Fraga, M.F.; Ballestar, E.; Villar-Garea, A.; Boix-Chornet, M.; Espada, J.; Schotta, G.; Bonaldi, T.; Haydon, C.; Ropero, S.; Petrie, K.; et al. Loss of acetylation at Lys16 and trimethylation at Lys20 of histone H4 is a common hallmark of human cancer. *Nat. Genet.* **2005**, *37*, 391–400. [CrossRef]
48. Sahai, E.; Marshall, C.J. Rho-GTPases and cancer. *Nat. Rev. Cancer* **2002**, *21*, 133–142. [CrossRef]
49. Ridley, A.J. Rho proteins and cancer. *Breast Cancer Res. Treat.* **2004**, *84*, 13–19. [CrossRef]
50. Mazieres, J.; Tillement, V.; Allal, C.; Clanet, C.; Bobin, L.; Chen, Z.; Sebti, S.M.; Favre, G.; Pradines, A. Geranylgeranylated, but not farnesylated, RhoB suppresses Ras transformation of NIH-3T3 cells. *Exp. Cell Res.* **2005**, *304*, 354–364. [CrossRef]
51. Prendergast, G.C. Actin' up: RhoB in cancer and apoptosis. *Nat. Rev. Cancer* **2001**, *1*, 162–168. [CrossRef]
52. Furuhjelm, J.; Peränen, J. The C-terminal end of R-Ras contains a focal adhesion targeting signal. *J. Cell Sci.* **2003**, *116*, 3729–3738. [CrossRef]
53. Nowak, J.; Archange, C.; Tardivel-Lacombe, J.; Pontarotti, P.; Pébusque, M.J.; Vaccaro, M.I.; Velasco, G.; Dagorn, J.C.; Iovanna, J.L. The TP53INP2 protein is required for autophagy in mammalian cells. *Mol. Biol. Cell* **2008**, *20*, 870–881. [CrossRef]
54. NCBI. Available online: https://www.ncbi.nlm.nih.gov/sites/entrez?db=gene&cmd=Retrieve&dopt=Graphics&list_uids=4998 (accessed on 9 February 2021).
55. NCBI. Available online: http://www.ncbi.nlm.nih.gov/sites/entrez?db=gene&cmd=Retrieve&dopt=Graphics&list_uids=983 (accessed on 9 February 2021).
56. NCBI. Available online: http://www.ncbi.nlm.nih.gov/sites/entrez?db=gene&cmd=Retrieve&dopt=Graphics&list_uids=994 (accessed on 9 February 2021).
57. NCBI. Available online: http://www.ncbi.nlm.nih.gov/sites/entrez?db=gene&cmd=Retrieve&dopt=Graphics&list_uids=6502 (accessed on 9 February 2021).
58. NCBI. Available online: http://www.ncbi.nlm.nih.gov/sites/entrez?db=gene&cmd=Retrieve&dopt=Graphics&list_uids=1870 (accessed on 9 February 2021).
59. NCBI. Available online: http://www.ncbi.nlm.nih.gov/sites/entrez?db=gene&cmd=Retrieve&dopt=Graphics&list_uids=8793 (accessed on 9 February 2021).
60. Corpataux, J.M.; Naik, J.; Porter, K.E.; London, N.J. The effect of six different statins on the proliferation, migration, and invasion of human smooth muscle cells. *J. Surg. Res.* **2005**, *129*, 52–56. [CrossRef]
61. Fromigue, O.; Hamidouche, Z.; Vaudin, P.; Lecanda, F.; Patino, A.; Barbry, P.; Mari, B.; Marie, P.J. CYR61 downregulation reduces osteosarcoma cell invasion, migration, and metastasis. *J. Bone Miner. Res.* **2011**, *26*, 1533–1542. [CrossRef]
62. Kidera, Y.; Tsubaki, M.; Yamazoe, Y.; Shoji, K.; Nakamura, H.; Ogaki, M.; Satou, T.; Itoh, T.; Isozaki, M.; Kaneko, J.; et al. Reduction of lung metastasis, cell invasion, and adhesion in mouse melanoma by statin-induced blockade of the Rho/Rho-associated coiled-coil-containing protein kinase pathway. *J. Exp. Clin. Cancer Res.* **2010**, *29*, 127. [CrossRef]
63. Brown, M.; Hart, C.; Tawadros, T.; Ramani, V.; Sangar, V.; Lau, M.; Clarke, N. The differential effects of statins on the metastatic behaviour of prostate cancer. *Br. J. Cancer* **2012**, *106*, 1689–1696. [CrossRef]
64. Wang, G.; Cao, R.; Wang, Y.; Qian, G.; Dan, H.C.; Jiang, W.; Ju, J.; Wu, M.; Xiao, Y.; Wang, X. Simvastatin induces cell cycle arrest and inhibits proliferation of bladder cancer cells via PPARγ signalling pathway. *Sci. Rep.* **2016**, *6*, 35783. [CrossRef]
65. Sheng, S.; Barnett, D.H.; Katzenellenbogen, B.S. Differential estradiol and selective estrogen receptor modulator (SERM) regulation of Keratin 13 gene expression and its underlying mechanism in breast cancer cells. *Mol. Cell Endocrinol.* **2008**, *296*, 1–9. [CrossRef]
66. NCBI. Available online: http://www.ncbi.nlm.nih.gov/sites/entrez?db=gene&cmd=Retrieve&dopt=Graphics&list_uids=7138 (accessed on 9 February 2021).
67. Sun, H.Q.; Yamamoto, M.; Mejillano, M.; Yin, H.L. Gelsolin, a multifunctional actin regulatory protein. *J. Biol. Chem.* **1999**, *274*, 33179–33182. [CrossRef]
68. Schnitzer, M.J.; Block, S.M. Kinesin hydrolyses one ATP per 8-nm step. *Nature* **1997**, *388*, 386–390. [CrossRef] [PubMed]
69. NCBI. Available online: http://www.ncbi.nlm.nih.gov/sites/entrez?db=gene&cmd=Retrieve&dopt=Graphics&list_uids=3728 (accessed on 9 February 2021).
70. NCBI. Available online: http://www.ncbi.nlm.nih.gov/sites/entrez?db=gene&cmd=Retrieve&dopt=Graphics&list_uids=7430 (accessed on 9 February 2021).

71. NCBI. Available online: http://www.ncbi.nlm.nih.gov/sites/entrez?db=gene&cmd=Retrieve&dopt=Graphics&list_uids=1008 (accessed on 9 February 2021).
72. Durinck, S.; Moreau, Y.; Kasprzyk, A.; Davis, S.; De Moor, B.; Brazma, A.; Huber, W. BioMart and Bioconductor: A powerful link between biological databases and microarray data analysis. *Bioinformatics* **2005**, *21*, 3439–3440. [CrossRef] [PubMed]
73. Hubbard, J.P.; Aken, B.L.; Beal, K.; Ballester, B.; Caccamo, M.; Chen, Y.; Clarke, L.; Coates, G.; Cunningham, F.; Cutts, T.; et al. Ensembl 2007. *Nuc. Acids Res.* **2007**, *35*, D610–D617. [CrossRef] [PubMed]
74. Luo, W.; Brouwer, C. Pathview: An R/Bioconductor package for pathway-based data integration and visualization. *Bioinformatics* **2013**, *29*, 1830–1831. [CrossRef]
75. Kanehisa, M.; Goto, S. KEGG: Kyoto encyclopedia of genes and genomes. *Nucl. Acids Res.* **2000**, *28*, 27–30. [CrossRef]
76. Livak, K.J.; Schmittgen, T.D. Analysis of relative gene expression data using real-time quantitative PCR and the 2(-Delta Delta C(T)) Method. *Methods* **2001**, *25*, 402–408. [CrossRef]
77. R Core Team. R: A Language and Environment for Statistical Computing; R Foundation for Statistical Computing; Vienna, Austria. Available online: https://www.R-project.org/ (accessed on 20 February 2021).
78. Vandesompele, J.; De Preter, K.; Pattyn, F.; Poppe, B.; Van Roy, N.; De Paepe, A.; Speleman, F. Accurate normalization of real-time quantitative RT-PCR data by geometric averaging of multiple internal control genes. *Genome Biol.* **2002**, *3*, research0034.1. [CrossRef]
79. STRING. Available online: https://string-db.org/ (accessed on 9 February 2021).
80. Stocker, R.; Bowry, V.W.; Frei, B. Ubiquinol-10 protects human low density lipoprotein more efficiently against lipid peroxidation than doe's α-tocopherol. *Med. Sci.* **1991**, *88*, 1646–1650. [CrossRef]
81. Wong, W.W.; Clendening, J.W.; Martirosyan, A.; Boutros, P.C.; Bros, C.; Khosravi, F.; Jurisica, I.; Stewart, A.K.; Bergsagel, P.L.; Penn, L.Z. Determinants of sensitivity to lovastatin-induced apoptosis in multiple myeloma. *Mol. Cancer Ther.* **2007**, *6*, 1886–1897. [CrossRef]
82. Jacobson, J.R.; Wong, W.W.; Dimitroulakos, J.; Minden, M.D.; Penn, L.Z. HMG-CoA reductase inhibitors and the malignant cell: The statin family of drugs as triggers of tumor-specific apoptosis. *Leukemia* **2002**, *16*, 508–519. [CrossRef]
83. Jacobson, J.R.; Dudek, S.M.; Birukov, K.G.; Ye, S.Q.; Grigoryev, D.N.; Girgis, R.E.; Garcia, J.G. Cytoskeletal activation and altered gene expression in endothelial barrier regulation by simvastatin. *Am. J. Respir. Cell Mol. Biol.* **2004**, *30*, 662–670. [CrossRef]
84. Johnson-Anuna, L.N.; Eckert, G.P.; Keller, J.H.; Igbavboa, U.; Franke, C.; Fechner, T.; Schubert-Zsilavecz, M.; Karas, M.; Müller, W.E.; Wood, W.G. Chronic administration of statins alters multiple gene expression patterns in mouse cerebral cortex. *J. Pharmacol. Exp. Ther.* **2005**, *312*, 786–793. [CrossRef]
85. Adamkov, M.; Halasova, E.; Rajcani, J.; Bencat, M.; Vybohova, D.; Rybarova, S.; Galbavy, S. Relation between expression pattern of p53 and survivin in cutaneous basal cell carcinomas. *Med. Sci. Monit.* **2011**, *17*, BR74–BR80. [CrossRef]
86. Zong, W.X.; Ditsworth, D.; Bauer, D.E.; Wang, Z.Q.; Thompson, C.B. Alkylating DNA damage stimulates a regulated form of necrotic cell death. *Genes Dev.* **2004**, *18*, 1272–1282. [CrossRef]
87. Klionsky, D.J.; Emr, S.D. Autophagy as a regulated pathway of cellular degradation. *Science* **2000**, *290*, 1717–1721. [CrossRef]
88. Fujimoto, T.; Ohsaki, Y. Proteasomal and autophagic pathways converge on lipid droplets. *Autophagy* **2006**, *2*, 299–301. [CrossRef]
89. Yang, Y.C.; Huang, W.F.; Chuan, L.M.; Xiao, D.W.; Zeng, Y.L.; Zhou, D.A.; Xu, G.Q.; Liu, W.; Huang, B.; Hu, Q. *In vitro* and *in vivo* study of cell growth inhibition of simvastatin on chronic myelogenous leukemia cells. *Chemotherapy* **2008**, *54*, 438–446. [CrossRef]
90. Assmus, B.; Urbich, C.; Aicher, A.; Hofmann, W.K.; Haendeler, J.; Rössig, L.; Spyridopoulos, I.; Zeiher, A.M.; Dimmeler, S. HMG-CoA reductase inhibitors reduce senescence and increase proliferation of endothelial progenitor cells via regulation of cell cycle regulatory genes. *Circ. Res.* **2003**, *92*, 1049–1055. [CrossRef]
91. Denoyelle, C.; Albanese, P.; Uzan, G.; Hong, L.; Vannier, J.P.; Soria, J.; Soria, C. Molecular mechanism of the anti-cancer activity of cerivastatin, an inhibitor of HMG-CoA reductase, on aggressive human breast cancer cells. *Cell Signal.* **2003**, *15*, 327–338. [CrossRef]
92. Keyomarsi, K.; Sandoval, L.; Band, V.; Pardee, A.B. Synchronization of tumor and normal cells from G1 to multiple cell cycles by lovastatin. *Cancer Res.* **1991**, *51*, 3602–3609.
93. Maltese, W.A.; Sheridan, K.M. Differentiation of neuroblastoma cells induced by an inhibitor of mevalonate synthesis: Relation of neurite outgrowth and acetylcholinesterase activity to changes in cell proliferation and blocked isoprenoid synthesis. *J. Cell Physiol.* **1985**, *125*, 540–558. [CrossRef]
94. Jakóbisiak, M.; Bruno, S.; Skierski, J.S.; Darzynkiewicz, Z. Cell cycle-specific effects of lovastatin. *Proc. Natl. Acad. Sci. USA* **1991**, *88*, 3628–3632. [CrossRef]
95. Ghosh, P.M.; Mott, G.E.; Ghosh-Choudhury, N.; Radnik, R.A.; Stapleton, M.L.; Ghidoni, J.J.; Kreisberg, J.I. Lovastatin induces apoptosis by inhibiting mitotic and post-mitotic events in cultured mesangial cells. *Biochim. Biophys. Acta.* **1997**, *1359*, 13–24. [CrossRef]
96. Engelke, K.J.; Hacker, M.P. A non-characteristic response of L1210 cells to lovastatin. *Biochem. Biophys. Res. Commun.* **1994**, *203*, 400–407. [CrossRef]
97. Rao, S.; Porter, D.C.; Chen, X.; Herliczek, T.; Lowe, M.; Keyomarsi, K. Lovastatin-mediated G1 arrest is through inhibition of the proteasome, independent of hydroxymethyl glutaryl-CoA reductase. *Proc. Natl. Acad. Sci. USA* **1999**, *96*, 7797–7802. [CrossRef]
98. Cooper, S. Reappraisal of G1-phase arrest and synchronization by lovastatin. *Cell Biol. Int.* **2002**, *26*, 715–727. [CrossRef]

99. da Costa, R.F.; Freire, V.N.; Bezerra, E.M.; Cavada, B.S.; Caetano, E.W.; de Lima Filho, J.L.; Albuquerque, E.L. Explaining statin inhibition effectiveness of HMG-CoA reductase by quantum biochemistry computations. *Phys. Chem. Chem. Phys.* **2012**, *14*, 1389–1398. [CrossRef]
100. Istvan, E.S.; Deisenhofer, J. Structural mechanism for statin inhibition of HMG-CoA reductase. *Science* **2001**, *292*, 1160–1164. [CrossRef]
101. Mück, W.; Ritter, W.; Ochmann, K.; Unger, S.; Ahr, G.; Wingender, W.; Kuhlmann, J. Absolute and relative bioavailability of the HMG-CoA reductase inhibitor cerivastatin. *Int. J. Clin. Pharmacol. Ther.* **1997**, *35*, 255–260. [PubMed]
102. Kajinami, K.; Mabuchi, H.; Saito, Y. NK-104: A novel synthetic HMG-CoA reductase inhibitor. *Expert Opin. Investig. Drugs.* **2000**, *9*, 2653–2661. [CrossRef]
103. Hamelin, B.A.; Turgeon, J. Hydrophilicity/lipophilicity: Relevance for the pharmacology and clinical effects of HMG-CoA reductase inhibitors. *Trends Pharmacol. Sci.* **1998**, *19*, 26–37. [CrossRef]
104. Menter, D.G.; Ramsauer, V.P.; Harirforoosh, S.; Chakraborty, K.; Yang, P.; Hsi, L.; Newman, R.A.; Krishnan, K. Differential effects of pravastatin and simvastatin on the growth of tumor cells from different organ sites. *PLoS ONE* **2011**, *6*, e28813. [CrossRef] [PubMed]
105. Hindler, K.; Cleeland, C.S.; Rivera, E.; Collard, C.D. The role of statins in cancer therapy. *Oncologist* **2006**, *11*, 306–315. [CrossRef] [PubMed]
106. Chimento, A.; Casaburi, I.; Avena, P.; Trotta, F.; De Luca, A.; Rago, V.; Pezzi, V.; Sirianni, R. Cholesterol and its metabolites in tumor growth: Therapeutic potential of statins in cancer treatment. *Front Endocrinol. (Lausanne)* **2019**, *9*, 807. [CrossRef]
107. Sopková, J.; Vidomanová, E.; Strnádel, J.; Škovierová, H.; Halašová, E. The role of statins as therapeutic agents in cancer. *Gen. Phys. Biophys.* **2017**, *36*, 501–511. [CrossRef]

molecules

MDPI

Article

Saponins Extracted from Tea (*Camellia Sinensis*) Flowers Induces Autophagy in Ovarian Cancer Cells

Yaomin Wang [1,2,3,†], Chen Xia [1,†], Lianfu Chen [1], Yi Charlie Chen [4,*] and Youying Tu [1,*]

1 Department of Tea Science, Zhejiang University, Hangzhou 310058, Zhejiang, China; wangym@mail.hzau.edu.cn (Y.W.); lukexia@tealab.cn (C.X.); c.lianfu@foxmail.com (L.C.)
2 Key Laboratory of Horticulture Plant Biology, Ministry of Education, College of Horticulture & Forestry Sciences, Huazhong Agricultural University, Wuhan 430070, Hubei, China
3 Key Laboratory of Urban Agriculture in Central China, Ministry of Agriculture, Wuhan 430070, Hubei, China
4 College of Health, Science, Technology and Mathematics, Alderson Broaddus University, Philippi, WV 26416, USA
* Correspondence: chenyc@ab.edu (Y.C.C.); youytu@zju.edu.cn (Y.T.)
† These authors contributed equally to this work.

Academic Editors: Marialuigia Fantacuzzi and Alessandra Ammazzalorso
Received: 19 October 2020; Accepted: 9 November 2020; Published: 11 November 2020

Abstract: Tea flower saponins (TFS) possess effective anticancer properties. The diversity and complexity of TFS increases the difficulty of their extraction and purification from tea flowers. Here, multiple methods including solvent extraction, microporous resin separation and preparative HPLC separation were used to obtain TFS with a yield of 0.34%. Furthermore, we revealed that TFS induced autophagy—as evidenced by an increase in MDC-positive cell populations and mCherry-LC3B-labeled autolysosomes and an upregulation of LC3II protein levels. 3-MA reversed the decrease in cell viability induced by TFS, showing that TFS induced autophagic cell death. TFS-induced autophagy was not dependent on the Akt/mTOR/p70S6K signaling pathway. TFS-induced autophagy in OVCAR-3 cells was accompanied by ERK pathway activation and reactive oxygen species (ROS) generation. This paper is the first report of TFS-mediated autophagy of ovarian cancer cells. These results provide new insights for future studies of the anti-cancer effects of TFS.

Keywords: saponins; phytochemicals; tea (*Camellia sinensis*) flower; ovarian cancer; autophagy

---

1. Introduction

Epithelial ovarian cancer continues to be a deadly disease due to its high mortality rate and poor long-term prognosis [1–4]. In recent years, much attention has been focused on studying natural products and searching for compounds which possess anti-cancer effects [5–7]. The effectiveness of tea (*Camellia sinensis*) against different types of cancer has been extensively studied owing to the numerous bioactive constituents contained in the tea plant [8–11]. Tea flowers are the reproductive organs of tea, and recent studies have demonstrated the effective anti-cancer effects of tea flowers and compounds extracted from tea flowers [12]. Tea flowers contain a number of bioactive constituents including polyphenols, polysaccharides, amino acids and saponins [13–16]. Tea flower saponins in particular have attracted attention for their anticancer effects [17]. However, the diversity and complexity of tea flower saponins increases the difficulty of their extraction and separation from tea flowers, which limits the research of tea flower saponins.

Apoptosis and autophagy are two major modalities of programed cell death (PCD). Targeting PCD pathways is becoming an important strategy for drug discovery from natural compounds [18]. Apoptosis and autophagy may share common upstream signals; thus, apoptosis and autophagy may occur simultaneously [19–21]. Natural saponins have been reported to induce combined apoptosis and autophagy in various cancer cell lines in vitro [22–24]. Our previous study revealed that tea flower saponins (TFS) induced apoptosis in A2780/CP70 human ovarian cancer cells and OVCAR-3 cells, as well as S-phase arrest [17]. Nonetheless, an autophagic effect caused by TFS has never been reported.

In this study, we extracted and isolated TFS from tea flowers, then demonstrated for the first time that TFS induced autophagy, and evaluated the molecular mechanisms in OVCAR-3 human ovarian cancer cells.

2. Results

2.1. Extraction of TFS from Tea Flowers

Multiple processes were used to extract highly purified TFS from tea flowers. As shown in Figure 1, 210 g dried tea flowers were used for the extraction of TFS, which involved 70% methanol extraction followed by solvent extraction and then microporous resin separation. TFS was mainly present in the 75% and 90% ethanol fractions. The 45% and 60% ethanol fractions also contained smaller amounts of TFS (Figure S3). We thus collected the 75% and 90% ethanol fractions for subsequent HPLC separation, resulting in three TFS fractions. We previously characterized the high purity TFS fraction 2 (Figure S2) and found it contains 14 triterpenoid saponins [17]. TFS fractions 1 and 3 also have high purities (Figure S4). The total yield was 0.34%.

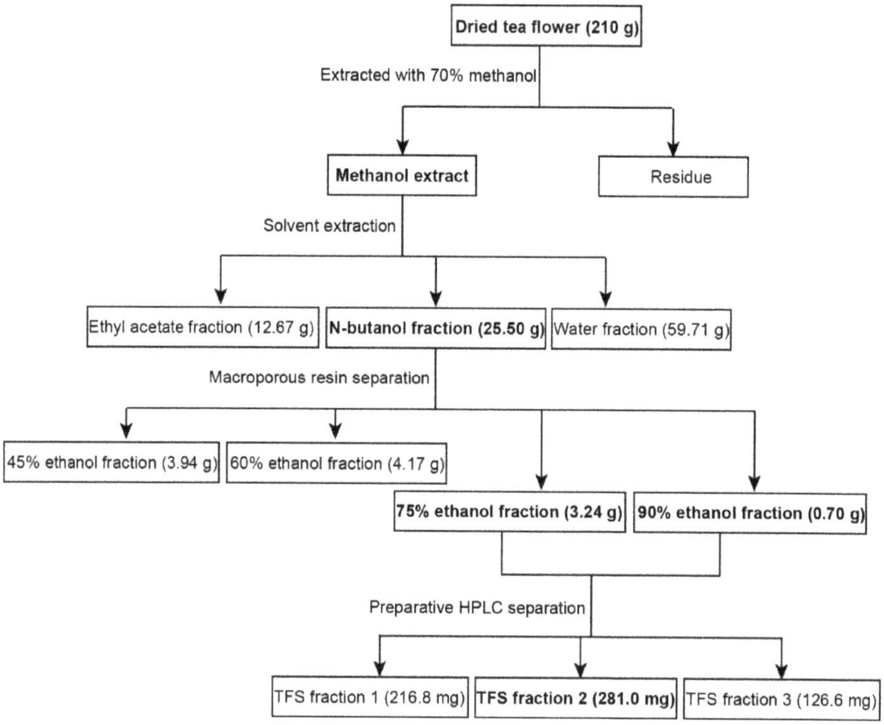

Figure 1. Extraction and isolation scheme of tea flower saponins (TFS) from tea flowers.

2.2. TFS Decreased Cell Viability and Induced Morphological Changes in OVCAR-3 Cells

To test whether TFS possesses an anti-cancer effect, we determined cell viability using an MTS assay after OVCAR-3 cells were treated with TFS for 24 h. As shown in Figure 2, TFS decreased cell viability in a dose-dependent manner. We additionally observed the morphology of OVCAR-3 cells by microscopy after treatment with TFS for 24 h. As shown in Figure 2, TFS induced morphological changes in OVCAR-3 cells, as the cells exhibited round bodies and clustered in groups.

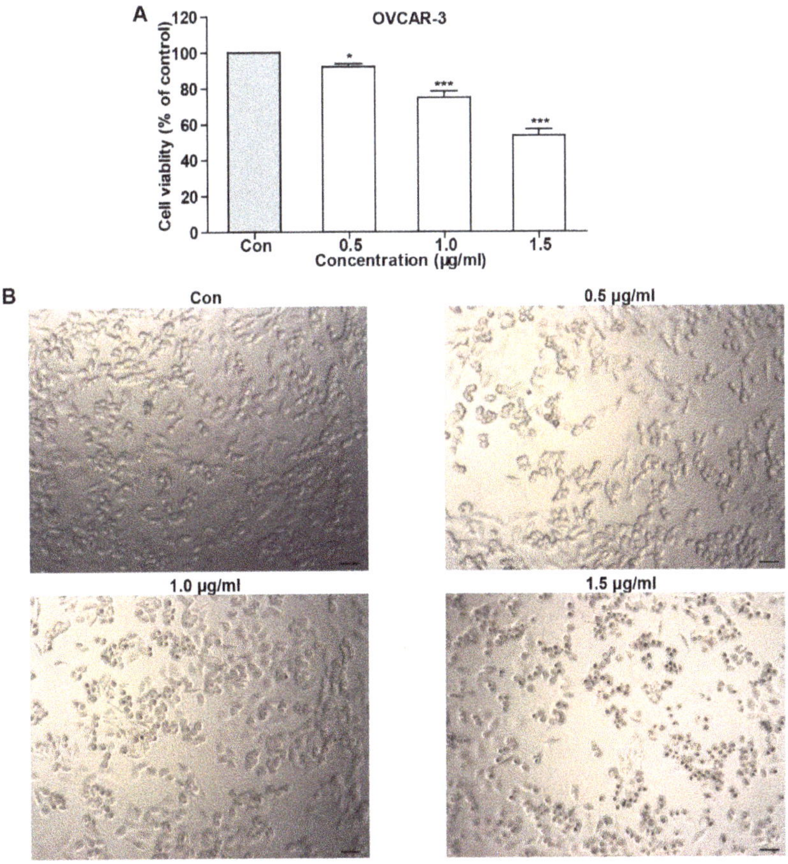

Figure 2. TFS decreased cell viability and induced morphology changes in OVCAR-3 cells. (**A**) The effect of TFS on cell viability was conducted using an MTS assay. Results were obtained from three independent experiments and expressed as mean ± SEM. Significant difference verse control (* $p < 0.05$ and *** $p < 0.001$. (**B**) OVCAR-3 cells were treated with the indicated concentrations of TFS for 24 h. Cell morphology was observed using microscopy (magnification 10×), scale bar = 50 µm.

2.3. *TFS Triggers Autophagy in OVCAR-3 Cells*

MDC staining was conducted to determine whether TFS induces autophagy and decreased viability of OVCAR-3 cells. MDC is an eosinophilic fluorescent dye that binds to the ubiquitin-like binding system Apg8, which requires the formation of autophagic vacuoles. Under excitation by ultraviolet light, the autophagic vacuoles demonstrated bright green fluorescence [25]. As shown in Figure 3, the presence of MDC-positive cells increased dose-dependently following treatment with TFS for 24 h. As indicated by the white arrows, bright green fluorescence appeared within the cells. The number of autophagic cells in the group treated with 1.5 µg/mL TFS for 24 h was significantly greater than the number of autophagic cells in the control group.

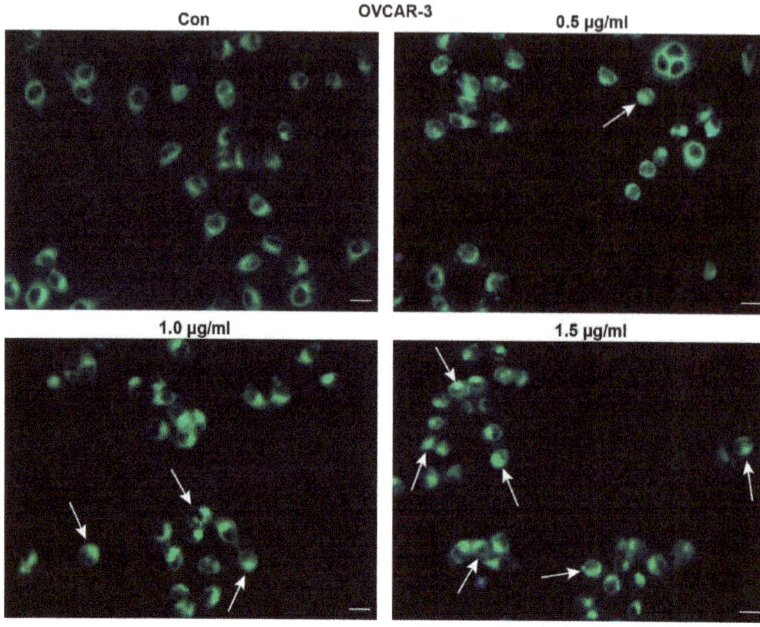

Figure 3. TFS induced autophagic vacuoles in OVCAR-3 cells. OVCAR-3 cells were treated with TFS (0, 0.5, 1.0 and 1.5 μg/mL) for 24 h then stained with MDC dye and visualized by fluorescence microscopy. White arrows indicate autophagic cells (magnification 20×), scale bar = 20 μm.

To further confirm the induction of autophagy by TFS, autophagic lysosomes were detected by mCherry-LC3B plasmid transfection. The mCherry-LC3B fusion fluorescent protein aggregates on autophagic lysosomes during autophagy, and specific spots of bright red fluorescence can be visualized under confocal microscopy. In this study, mCherry-LC3B plasmids were transfected into OVCAR-3 cells, and then the cells were treated with TFS for 24 h. Confocal microscopy images were captured with an inverted laser scanning confocal microscope. As shown in Figure 4A, the number of autophagic lysosomes marked by red fluorescence in the OVCAR-3 cells increased with higher concentrations of TFS.

We quantified the effect of TFS treatment on the expression of LC3 protein in OVCAR-3 cells by western blotting. Under normal conditions, LC3 protein is cleaved by Atg4 at the carboxyl end to form LC3-I (16 kD) and localizes to the cytoplasm. When autophagy occurs, ubiquitin-like systems such as Atg7 and Atg3 modify LC3-I, causing it to bind with phosphatidylethanolamine found on the surface of the autophagosome membrane to produce LC3II (14 kD) where it remains localized on the autophagic membrane. LC3-II expression is directly proportional to the activity of autophagic vesicles. Therefore, the change of expression between LC3-I and LC3-II could indicate whether autophagy is occurring. As shown in Figure 4B,C, the expression of LC3-II protein in OVCAR-3 cells increased significantly after treatment with TFS in a dose-dependent manner after 24 h. Taken together, the results from MDC staining, mCherry-LC3B plasmid transfection, and Western blotting for LC3 protein clearly indicated that TFS induced autophagy in OVCAR-3 cells.

Next, we added the autophagy inhibitor 3-MA to determine whether TFS-induced autophagy in OVCAR-3 cells promoted cancer cell survival or caused cancer cell death. As shown in Figure 4D, cell viability increased from 47% to 79% following treatment with 1.5 μg/mL of 3-MA for 24 h, indicating that TFS-induced autophagy promoted cell death of OVCAR-3 cells. Thus, these results revealed that TFS treatment led to the autophagic death of OVCAR-3 cells.

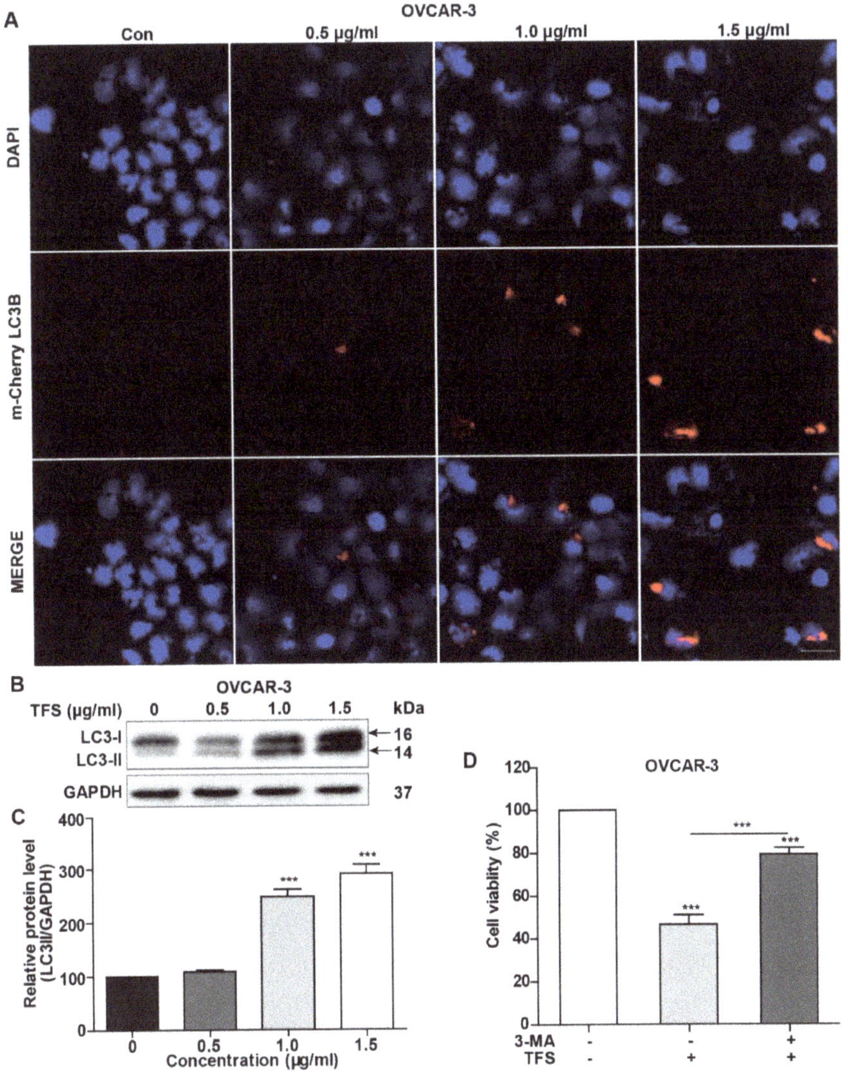

Figure 4. TFS treatment induced autophagic cell death in OVCAR-3 cells. (**A**) OVCAR-3 cells were transfected with mCherry-LC3B plasmid and treated with TFS (0, 0.5, 1.0, 1.5 μg/mL) for 24 h. Cells were imaged with an inverted laser scanning confocal microscope (magnification 40×), scale bar = 50 μm. (**B**,**C**) OVCAR-3 Cells were treated with different concentrations of TFS (0, 0.5, 1.0, 1.5 μg/mL) for 24 h. Western blotting was conducted to evaluate the levels of LC3I and LC3II protein with GAPDH used as an internal control. (**D**) OVCAR-3 cells were treated with 3-MA and TFS (1.5 μg/mL) for 24 h and then detected for cell viability. Each data point represents three independent experiments, significant difference versus control (*** $p < 0.001$).

2.4. TFS-Induced Autophagy in OVCAR-3 Cells Independently from the Akt/mTOR/p70S6K Pathway and Was Accompanied by ERK Activation

We further evaluated the possible molecular mechanisms of TFS-induced autophagy by Western blot analysis, first by measuring Akt/mTOR/p70S6K pathway-related proteins. The Akt/mTOR/p70S6K pathway is a major autophagy regulatory pathway which negatively regulates autophagy [24,26,27].

As shown in Figure 5A, protein levels of p-Akt and Akt remained unchanged following treatment with TFS (0, 0.5, 1.0, 1.5 μg/mL) for 24 h. Phosphorylation of p70S6K was upregulated dose-dependently by TFS in OVCAR-3 cancer cell lines. Taken together, these results demonstrated that TFS-induced autophagy in OVCAR-3 cells was independent of the Akt/mTOR/p70S6K pathway. It has been reported that MAPK signaling pathways, which include ERK1/2, p38, and JNK, play a pivotal role in autophagy induction [22,27,28]. Accordingly, we evaluated the levels of MAPK signaling pathway proteins following treatment with TFS for 24 h. As shown in Figure 5B, TFS treatment significantly upregulated protein levels of p-ERK while total ERK expression remained unchanged. No obvious changes to p-p38, p38, and JNK expression were observed. These results indicated that the ERK pathway was activated in OVCAR-3 cancer cells.

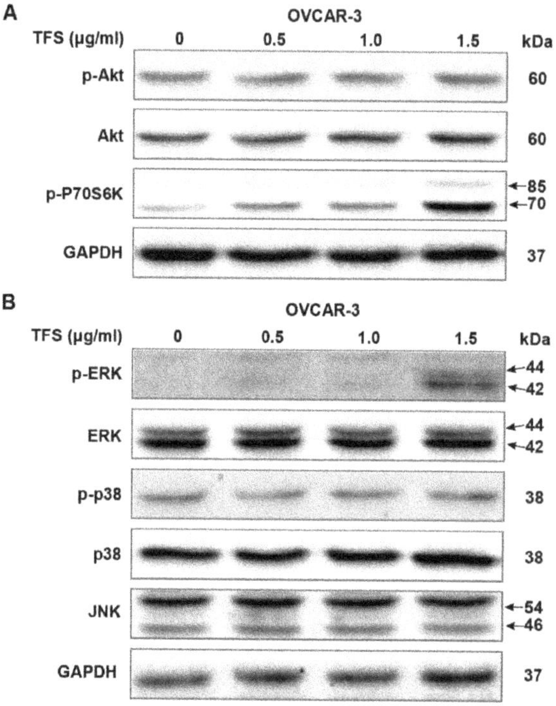

Figure 5. Effects of TFS on Akt pathways and MAPK pathways in OVCAR-3 cells. Protein expression of (**A**) Akt pathways related proteins p-Akt, Akt, p-P70S6K and (**B**) MAPK pathways related proteins p-ERK, ERK, p-p38, p38, JNK were analyzed by Western blot after being treated with different concentrations of TFS (0, 0.5, 1.0, 1.5 μg/mL) for 24 h, GAPDH was used as internal control.

2.5. TFS-Induced Autophagy in OVCAR-3 Cells Is Accompanied by ROS Generation

Reactive oxygen species (ROS) generation is considered to be associated with the autophagy initiation and contributes to autophagy-mediated cell death [5,29]. We measured ROS generation using DCFH-DA following treatment with TFS. As shown in Figure 6, DCFH-DA positive cells increased after treatment with TFS, indicating that TFS treatment significantly enhanced ROS generation in OVCAR-3 cells. The results suggested that ROS generation is possibly involved in TFS-induced autophagy and this finding will need to be further elucidated.

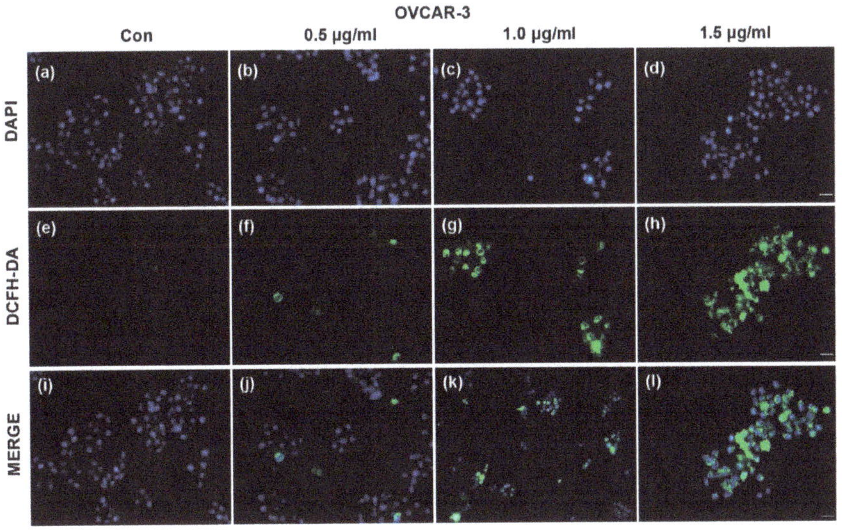

Figure 6. Effects of TFS on reactive oxygen species (ROS) generation in OVCAR-3 cells. ROS generation in OVCAR-3 cells was evaluated by DAPI and DCFH-DA double staining. Representative images are shown. After treatment with TFS (0, 0.5, 1.0 and 1.5 μg/mL) for 24 h, cells were stained with DCFH-DA and DAPI and visualized by fluorescence microscopy (magnification 20×), scale bar = 50 μm. The top line of images (**a**–**d**) shows cells stained with DAPI. The middle line of images (**e**–**h**) shows cells which generated ROS as represented by staining with DCFH-DA. The bottom line of images (**i**–**l**) shows merged fluorescence images of cells stained by DAPI and DCFH-DA.

3. Discussion

Natural saponins from tea (*Camellia sinensis*) flowers possess remarkable structural diversity and have become increasingly important compounds for the prevention and treatment of cancer and other diseases [29–31]. Several triterpenoid saponins have demonstrated the ability to induce autophagy of cancer cells in various cancer cells lines [32,33]. To better understand the mechanisms underlying this observed anticancer effect, we performed a chemical extraction of triterpenoid saponins from tea flowers. We first extracted dried tea flowers with 70% methanol, which was the most efficient extraction solution according to our previous studies. We then performed solvent extraction, microporous resin separation, and preparative HPLC separation to obtain three TFS fractions with a total yield of 0.34%. Our previous study showed that TFS induced apoptosis and S phase arrest in A2780/CP70 and OVCAR-3 cells [17]. In our present study, we have shown for the first time that TFS can induce autophagic cell death in OVCAR-3 cells.

To confirm that TFS induced autophagy in OVCAR-3 cells, MDC staining was conducted following treatment with TFS for 24 h, showing a dramatic increase of MDC-positive cells. Autophagic lysosomes in OVCAR-3 cells increased significantly after transfection with mCherry-LC3B plasmids and TFS treatment. Western blot analysis was conducted to evaluate expression changes of LC3 in OVCAR-3 cells. LC3-II is considered to be the most reliable autophagic biomarker as LC3-II expression levels are proportional to the formation of autophagosomes [18,33]. In our study, we found that TFS dose-dependently upregulated protein levels of LC3-II in OVCAR-3 cells. These results indicated that TFS induced autophagy in ovarian cancer cells. Moreover, the autophagy inhibitor 3-MA reversed the decrease of cell viability caused by TFS, which further indicated that TFS induced autophagic cell death in OVCAR-3 cells.

Inhibition of the Akt/mTOR/p70S6K pathway is crucial for the induction of autophagy. p70S6K is the downstream target of Akt, and expression levels of p-p70S6K can be used as a marker for mTOR activity [22]. The natural compound delicaflavone can induce autophagy via the Akt/mTOR/p70S6K pathway in human lung cancer cells [26]. However, in our study, proteins levels of p-Akt and Akt remained unchanged while p-P70S6K was upregulated in OVCAR-3 cells. These results suggest that TFS-induced autophagy in ovarian cancer cells does not involve the Akt/mTOR/p70S6K pathway, which is consistent with previous reports that Platycodin D triggered autophagy in HepG2 cells [34].

We further evaluated the effects of TFS on MAPK signaling pathways and ROS generation. ERK, p38, and JNK are important regulatory proteins of MAPK signaling pathways which could also regulate autophagy processes [35,36]. In our present study, TFS significantly upregulated protein levels of p-ERK in OVCAR-3 cells. Protein levels of p-p38, p38, and JNK were not affected after treatment with TFS. These results indicated that the ERK pathway was activated by TFS-induced autophagy in ovarian cancer cells. Our findings were also consistent with several reports that ERK activation occurs in autophagy induced by different compounds in various cancer cell lines [22,37,38]. To better elucidate the role of ERK pathway in TFS-induced autophagy, ERK inhibitor such as U0126 should be applied to future experiment and clarify whether ERK inhibition attenuates TFS-induced autophagy in ovarian cancer cells. Additionally, TFS treatment significantly enhanced ROS generation in OVCAR-3 cells. As ROS generation is considered to be an essential aspect of apoptosis and autophagy [29], we previously reported that TFS induces apoptosis in A2780/CP70 and OVCAR-3 cells [17]. The specific role of ROS generation in TFS-induced cell death however, needs to be further elucidated by pretreatment with ROS inhibitor N-acetyl-L-cysteine (NAC), then to detect the expression levels of autophagy related proteins to clarify the role of ROS in TFS-induced autophagy in OVCAR-3 cells. Taken together, we conclude that TFS-induced autophagy in OVCAR-3 cells is accompanied by ERK activation and ROS generation, the mechanisms of which will merit further study.

4. Materials and Methods

4.1. Materials and Reagents

Dried tea flowers (Figure S1) were purchased from Zhejiang Yilongfang Co., Ltd. (Hangzhou, China). Analytical grades of methanol, ethanol, N-butanol, Ethyl acetate and other extraction chemical regents used in this study were obtained from Sinopharm Chemical Reagent Co., Ltd. (Shanghai, China). Monodansylcadaverine (MDC) was purchased from Nanjing KeyGen Biotech Co., Ltd. (Nanjing, China). 3-Methyladenine (3-MA) was purchased from Dalian Meilun Biotech Co., Ltd. m-Cherry LC3B plasmid was purchased from Hanheng Biotech Co., Ltd. (Shanghai, China). Lipofectamine 2000 Reagent was purchased from Invitrogen (Grand Island, NY, USA). Primary rabbit polyclonal antibodies against LC3B, p-Akt, Akt, p-P70S6K, p-p38, p38 and JNK were obtained from Cell Signaling Inc. (Danvers, MA, USA). Secondary antibodies, p-ERK, ERK, and GAPDH were obtained from Santa Cruz Biotechnology (Santa Cruz, CA, USA). 2′,7′-dichlorodihydrofluorescein diacetate (DCFH-DA) and CellTiter 96 Aqueous One Solution Cell Proliferation were purchased from Sigma-Aldrich (St. Louis, MO, USA) and Promega (Madison, WI, USA), respectively.

4.2. Extraction and Isolation of TFS

Dried tea flowers (210 g) were pulverized and extracted with 70% methanol two separate times for 2 h under reflux at 60 °C. Seventy per cent methanol extracts were concentrated by a rotary evaporator to obtain a 70% methanol concentrate. The methanol extract was suspended in H_2O and extracted with equal volumes of ethyl acetate and *N*-butanol three times, successively. The solvents were then evaporated to obtain the ethyl acetate fraction (12.67 g), *N*-butanol fraction (25.50 g) and water fraction (59.71 g). The 25.50 g *N*-butanol fraction was resolved in 10% ethanol and loaded in a D101 macroporous adsorption resin column and successively eluted with 0%, 15%, 30%, 45%, 60%, 75%, and 90% ethanol. The 45%, 60%, 75%, and 90% ethanol eluents were collected, then evaporated and freeze-dried to obtain the 45% ethanol fraction (3.94 g), 60% ethanol fraction (4.17 g), 75% ethanol fraction (3.24 g), and 90% ethanol fraction (0.70 g). The 75% and 90% ethanol fractions were mixed and separated using preparative HPLC to obtain three fractions, TFS fraction 1 (216.8 mg), TFS fraction 2 (281.0 mg), and TFS fraction 3 (126.6 mg). TFS fraction 2 was identified previously and marked as "TFS" in later experiments [17].

4.3. Cell Lines and Cell Culture

The human ovarian cancer cell line OVCAR-3 was provided by Dr. Jiang from West Virginia University. The cells were cultured in RPMI-1640 medium supplemented with 10% fetal bovine serum (FBS) at 37 °C with 5% CO_2 in a humidified incubator.

4.4. MTS Assay

OVCAR-3 cells were seeded in a 96-well plate at a density of 1.0×10^4 cells per well and incubated overnight for attachment. The cells were then treated with different concentrations of TFS with or without 3-MA for 24 h. MTS reagents were added to each well and absorbance was measured at 490 nm using a microplate reader.

4.5. Morphology Observation

OVCAR-3 cells were exposed to different concentrations of TFS (0, 0.5, 1.0, 1.5 μg/mL) for 24 h. Cell morphology was then observed by microscopy (ZEISS, Heidelberg, Germany). Images were captured using a digital camera attached to the microscope at magnification × 10.

4.6. Labeling of Autophagic Vacuoles with MDC Staining

OVCAR-3 cells were seeded in a 24-well plate at a density of 1.0×10^5 cells per well after a growth period of 24 h. The cells were then treated with different concentrations of TFS (0, 0.5, 1.0, 1.5 μg/mL) for another 24 h. After media change and wash with PBS, 50 μM MDC was added to each well and the plate was incubated for 30 min, after which fluorescence images were captured using an Olympus DP70 fluorescence microscope.

4.7. Transfection of mCherry-LC3B Plasmid

OVCAR-3 cells were grown with medium (without antibiotics) in a 24-well plate (1.0×10^5 cells per well) for 24 h. The cells were ready for transfection once cell confluence reached 90%. The transfection mixture was prepared as follows: 0.5 μg mCherry-LC3B plasmid and 2 μL Lipofectamine 2000 were diluted with 50 μL OPTI-MEMI medium, respectively, and incubated at room temperature for 5 min. The diluted mCherry-LC3B plasmid was mixed with diluted Lipofectamine 2000 to prepare the transfection mixture and incubated at room temperature for 20 min. The culture medium was discarded and washed with PBS twice. Next, 400 μL of serum-free culture medium (without antibiotics) was added to each well and 100 μL of transfection mixture was then added. After a transfection period of 6 h in the incubator, the cells were then incubated with different concentrations of TFS for 24 h. Imaging slides were mounted with DAPI and images were captured using an FV1000 Laser Scanning Confocal Microscope (Olympus, Tokyo, Japan).

4.8. Reactive Oxygen Species (ROS) Detection

ROS generation was measured by DCFH-DA staining. Briefly, OVCAR-3 cells were grown in a 96-well plate (1.0×10^4 cells per well) for 24 h and different concentrations of TFS (0, 0.5, 1.0, 1.5 μg/mL) were added to the indicated wells. After a 24 h incubation period, the cells were then incubated with DCFH-DA (10 μM) at 37 °C for 30 min. Imaging slides were mounted with DAPI and images were captured with an Olympus DP70 fluorescence microscope.

4.9. Western Blotting

Cells were treated with different concentrations of TFS for 24 h, washed with PBS twice, harvested, and total protein was extracted using protein extraction reagent supplemented with 1% protease inhibitor. Protein content was detected by a BCA protein assay kit. Equal amounts of protein were loaded into 10% SDS-PAGE gels for separation and transferred onto nitrocellulose membranes. The membranes were blocked with 5% non-fat milk for 1 h, then incubated with indicated primary antibody overnight followed by secondary antibody for 2 h at room temperature. Protein bands were visualized using the ChemiDoc MP System (Bio Rad, Hercules, CA, USA). GAPDH was used to normalize relative values of each protein.

4.10. Statistical Analysis

Data represents the mean of three independent experiments. Statistical significance was analyzed by Graphpad Prism software using the Newman–Keuls test. * $p < 0.05$, ** $p < 0.01$ and *** $p < 0.001$ were considered as significant p-values.

5. Conclusions

In the present study, we demonstrated an efficient extraction and purification method for TFS with a yield of 0.34%. We showed for the first time that TFS induced autophagic cell death in ovarian cancer cells. The specific autophagic effect mediated by TFS occurred independently from Akt/mTOR/p70S6K pathway signaling and the TFS-induced autophagy in ovarian cancer cells was found to be accompanied by ERK activation and ROS generation. Thus, our research provides an important basis for future study on the autophagic effects of TFS in ovarian cancer cells.

Supplementary Materials: The following are available online, Figure S1: Dried tea (*Camellia sinensis*) flowers, Figure S2: Saponins isolated from dried tea (*Camellia sinensis*) flowers, Figure S3: HPLC chromatograms of eluted fractions of 45%, 60%, 75%, 90% ethanol, Figure S4: Chromatograms of TFS 1, TFS 2and TFS 3 detected by LC/MS.

Author Contributions: Conceptualization, Y.W., Y.T. and Y.C.C.; methodology, Y.W. and C.X.; formal analysis, Y.W., C.X., and L.C.; resources, Y.T. and Y.C.; writing—original draft preparation, Y.W., C.X., and L.C.; writing—review and editing, Y.W., Y.T., and Y.C.C.; funding acquisition, Y.T. and Y.W. All authors have read and agreed to the published version of the manuscript.

Funding: This work was funded by the Key research and development projects in Zhejiang Province "Industrialization model projects on exploring functional components and related products from tea flowers and fruits" (Grant No: 2018C02012), the National key research and development plan "Processing of tea products, key technology of quality control during storage and equipment development" (Grant No: 2017YFD0400803), and the Natural Science Foundation of Hubei Province (Grant No: 2019CFB187). The authors are very grateful to Yul Huh for language editing.

Conflicts of Interest: The authors declare no conflict of interest.

Abbreviations

TFS	Tea flower saponins
ERK	Extracellular signal-regulated kinase
LC3	Microtubule-associated protein light chain 3
ROS	Reactive oxygen species
MDC	Dansylcadaverine
MAPK	Mitogen-activated protein kinase
p70S6K	p70 ribosomal protein S6 kinase

References

1. Piver, M.S.; Frank, T.S. Epidemiology of Ovarian Cancer. In *Diagnosis and Management of Ovarian Disorders*; Altchek, A., Deligdisch, L., Kase, N.G., Eds.; Academic Press: San Diego, CA, USA, 2003; pp. 209–218.
2. Bast, R.C., Jr.; Hennessy, B.; Mills, G.B. The biology of ovarian cancer: New opportunities for translation. *Nat. Rev. Cancer* **2009**, *9*, 415–428. [CrossRef] [PubMed]

3. Jayson, G.C.; Kohn, E.C.; Kitchener, H.C.; Ledermann, J.A. Ovarian cancer. *Lancet* **2014**, *384*, 1376–1388. [CrossRef]
4. Yeung, T.-L.; Leung, C.S.; Li, F.; Wong, S.S.T.; Mok, S.C. Targeting Stromal-Cancer Cell Crosstalk Networks in Ovarian Cancer Treatment. *Biomolecules* **2016**, *6*, 3. [CrossRef] [PubMed]
5. Kim, A.D.; Kang, K.A.; Kim, H.S.; Kim, D.H.; Choi, Y.H.; Lee, S.J.; Kim, H.S.; Hyun, J.W. A ginseng metabolite, compound K, induces autophagy and apoptosis via generation of reactive oxygen species and activation of JNK in human colon cancer cells. *Cell Death Dis.* **2013**, *4*, e750. [CrossRef] [PubMed]
6. Huang, H.; Chen, A.Y.; Rojanasakul, Y.; Ye, X.; Rankin, G.O.; Chen, Y.C. Dietary compounds galangin and myricetin suppress ovarian cancer cell angiogenesis. *J. Funct. Foods* **2015**, *15*, 464–475. [CrossRef]
7. Gao, Y.; Rankin, G.O.; Tu, Y.Y.; Chen, Y.C. Theaflavin-3, 3′-digallate decreases human ovarian carcinoma OVCAR-3 cell-induced angiogenesis via Akt and Notch-1 pathways, not via MAPK pathways. *Int. J. Oncol.* **2016**, *48*, 281–292. [CrossRef]
8. Lee, A.H.; Su, D.; Pasalich, M.; Binns, C.W. Tea consumption reduces ovarian cancer risk. *Cancer Epidemiol.* **2013**, *37*, 54–59. [CrossRef]
9. Trudel, D.; Labbe, D.P.; Bairati, I.; Fradet, V.; Bazinet, L.; Tetu, B. Green tea for ovarian cancer prevention and treatment: A systematic review of the in vitro, in vivo and epidemiological studies. *Gynecol. Oncol.* **2012**, *126*, 491–498. [CrossRef]
10. Rha, C.S.; Jeong, H.W.; Park, S.; Lee, S.; Jung, Y.S.; Kim, D.O. Antioxidative, Anti-Inflammatory, and Anticancer Effects of Purified Flavonol Glycosides and Aglycones in Green Tea. *Antioxidants* **2019**, *8*, 278. [CrossRef]
11. Naponelli, V.; Ramazzina, I.; Lenzi, C.; Bettuzzi, S.; Rizzi, F. Green Tea Catechins for Prostate Cancer Prevention: Present Achievements and Future Challenges. *Antioxidants* **2017**, *6*, 26. [CrossRef]
12. Way, T.-D.; Lin, H.-Y.; Hua, K.-T.; Lee, J.-C.; Li, W.-H.; Lee, M.-R.; Shuang, C.-H.; Lin, J.-K. Beneficial effects of different tea flowers against human breast cancer MCF-7 cells. *Food Chem.* **2009**, *114*, 1231–1236. [CrossRef]
13. Wang, L.; Xu, R.J.; Hu, B.; Li, W.; Sun, Y.; Tu, Y.Y.; Zeng, X.X. Analysis of free amino acids in Chinese teas and flower of tea plant by high performance liquid chromatography combined with solid-phase extraction. *Food Chem.* **2010**, *123*, 1259–1266. [CrossRef]
14. Han, Q.A.; Yu, Q.Y.; Shi, J.A.; Xiong, C.Y.; Ling, Z.J.; He, P.M. Structural Characterization and Antioxidant Activities of 2 Water-Soluble Polysaccharide Fractions Purified from Tea (*Camellia sinensis*) Flower. *J. Food Sci.* **2011**, *76*, C462–C471. [CrossRef]
15. Matsuda, H.; Hamao, M.; Nakamura, S.; Kon'i, H.; Murata, M.; Yoshikawa, M. Medicinal Flowers. XXXIII. Anti-hyperlipidemic and Anti-hyperglycemic Effects of Chakasaponins I–III and Structure of Chakasaponin IV from Flower Buds of Chinese Tea Plant (*Camellia sinensis*). *Chem. Pharm. Bull.* **2012**, *60*, 674–680. [CrossRef] [PubMed]
16. Lin, Y.S.; Wu, S.S.; Lin, J.K. Determination of tea polyphenols and caffeine in tea flowers (*Camellia sinensis*) and their hydroxyl radical scavenging and nitric oxide suppressing effects. *J. Agr. Food Chem.* **2003**, *51*, 975–980. [CrossRef]
17. Wang, Y.M.; Ren, N.; Rankin, G.O.; Li, B.; Rojanasakul, Y.; Tu, Y.Y.; Chen, Y.C. Anti-proliferative effect and cell cycle arrest induced by saponins extracted from tea (*Camellia sinensis*) flower in human ovarian cancer cells. *J. Funct. Foods* **2017**, *37*, 310–321. [CrossRef]
18. Ouyang, L.; Shi, Z.; Zhao, S.; Wang, F.T.; Zhou, T.T.; Liu, B.; Bao, J.K. Programmed cell death pathways in cancer: A review of apoptosis, autophagy and programmed necrosis. *Cell Prolif.* **2012**, *45*, 487–498. [CrossRef]
19. Marino, G.; Niso-Santano, M.; Baehrecke, E.H.; Kroemer, G. Self-consumption: The interplay of autophagy and apoptosis. *Nat. Rev. Mol. Cell Biol.* **2014**, *15*, 81–94. [CrossRef]
20. Maiuri, M.C.; Zalckvar, E.; Kimchi, A.; Kroemer, G. Self-eating and self-killing: Crosstalk between autophagy and apoptosis. *Nat. Rev. Mol. Cell Biol.* **2007**, *8*, 741–752. [CrossRef]
21. Mrakovcic, M.; Frohlich, L.F. p53-Mediated Molecular Control of Autophagy in Tumor Cells. *Biomolecules* **2018**, *8*, 14. [CrossRef]
22. Li, T.; Xu, X.H.; Tang, Z.H.; Wang, Y.F.; Leung, C.H.; Ma, D.L.; Chen, X.P.; Wang, Y.T.; Chen, Y.; Lu, J.J. Platycodin D induces apoptosis and triggers ERK- and JNK-mediated autophagy in human hepatocellular carcinoma BEL-7402 cells. *Acta Pharmacol. Sin.* **2015**, *36*, 1503–1513. [CrossRef] [PubMed]
23. Sy, L.K.; Yan, S.C.; Lok, C.N.; Man, R.Y.K.; Che, C.M. Timosaponin A-III Induces Autophagy Preceding Mitochondria-Mediated Apoptosis in HeLa Cancer Cells. *Cancer Res.* **2008**, *68*, 10229–10237. [CrossRef] [PubMed]

24. Chun, J.; Kang, M.; Kim, Y.S. A triterpenoid saponin from Adenophora triphylla var. japonica suppresses the growth of human gastric cancer cells via regulation of apoptosis and autophagy. *Tumor Biol.* **2014**, *35*, 12021–12030. [CrossRef] [PubMed]
25. Shen, Z.Y.; Xu, L.Y.; Li, E.M.; Zhuang, B.R.; Lu, X.F.; Shen, J.; Wu, X.Y.; Li, Q.S.; Lin, Y.J.; Chen, Y.W.; et al. Autophagy and endocytosis in the amnion. *J. Struct. Biol.* **2008**, *162*, 197–204. [CrossRef] [PubMed]
26. Sui, Y.X.; Yao, H.; Li, S.G.; Jin, L.; Shi, P.Y.; Li, Z.J.; Wang, G.; Lin, S.L.; Wu, Y.J.; Li, Y.X.; et al. Delicaflavone induces autophagic cell death in lung cancer via Akt/mTOR/p70S6K signaling pathway. *J. Mol. Med.* **2017**, *95*, 311–322. [CrossRef] [PubMed]
27. Chang, C.H.; Lee, C.Y.; Lu, C.C.; Tsai, F.J.; Hsu, Y.M.; Tsao, J.W.; Juan, Y.N.; Chiu, H.Y.; Yang, J.S.; Wang, C.C. Resveratrol-induced autophagy and apoptosis in cisplatin-resistant human oral cancer CAR cells: A key role of AMPK and Akt/mTOR signaling. *Int. J. Oncol.* **2017**, *50*, 873–882. [CrossRef]
28. Cagnol, S.; Chambard, J.C. ERK and cell death: Mechanisms of ERK-induced cell death—apoptosis, autophagy and senescence. *FEBS J.* **2010**, *277*, 2–21. [CrossRef]
29. Scherz-Shouval, R.; Shvets, E.; Fass, E.; Shorer, H.; Gil, L.; Elazar, Z. Reactive oxygen species are essential for autophagy and specifically regulate the activity of Atg4. *EMBO J.* **2007**, *26*, 1749–1760. [CrossRef]
30. Xu, X.H.; Li, T.; Fong, C.M.V.; Chen, X.P.; Chen, X.J.; Wang, Y.T.; Huang, M.Q.; Lu, J.J. Saponins from Chinese Medicines as Anticancer Agents. *Molecules* **2016**, *21*, 1326. [CrossRef]
31. Xing, J.J.; Hou, J.G.; Liu, Y.; Zhang, R.B.; Jiang, S.; Ren, S.; Wang, Y.P.; Shen, Q.; Li, W.; Li, X.D.; et al. Supplementation of Saponins from Leaves of Panax quinquefolius Mitigates Cisplatin-Evoked Cardiotoxicity via Inhibiting Oxidative Stress-Associated Inflammation and Apoptosis in Mice. *Antioxidants* **2019**, *8*, 347. [CrossRef]
32. Shi, J.M.; Bai, L.L.; Zhang, D.M.; Yiu, A.; Yin, Z.Q.; Han, W.L.; Liu, J.S.; Li, Y.; Fu, D.Y.; Ye, W.C. Saxifragifolin D induces the interplay between apoptosis and autophagy in breast cancer cells through ROS-dependent endoplasmic reticulum stress. *Biochem. Pharmacol.* **2013**, *85*, 913–926. [CrossRef] [PubMed]
33. Sanchez-Sanchez, L.; Escobar, M.L.; Sandoval-Ramirez, J.; Lopez-Munoz, H.; Fernandez-Herrera, M.A.; Hernandez-Vazquez, J.M.V.; Hilario-Martinez, C.; Zenteno, E. Apoptotic and autophagic cell death induced by glucolaxogenin in cervical cancer cells. *Apoptosis* **2015**, *20*, 1623–1635. [CrossRef] [PubMed]
34. Li, T.; Tang, Z.H.; Xu, W.S.; Wu, G.S.; Wang, Y.F.; Chang, L.L.; Zhu, H.; Chen, X.P.; Wang, Y.T.; Chen, Y.; et al. Platycodin D triggers autophagy through activation of extracellular signal-regulated kinase in hepatocellular carcinoma HepG2 cells. *Eur. J. Pharmacol.* **2015**, *749*, 81–88. [CrossRef]
35. Zhou, Y.Y.; Li, Y.; Jiang, W.Q.; Zhou, L.F. MAPK/JNK signalling: A potential autophagy regulation pathway. *Biosci. Rep.* **2015**, *35*, e00199. [CrossRef] [PubMed]
36. Martinez-Lopez, N.; Singh, R. ATGs Scaffolds for MAPK/ERK signaling. *Autophagy* **2014**, *10*, 535–537. [CrossRef]
37. Ellington, A.A.; Berhow, M.A.; Singletary, K.W. Inhibition of Akt signaling and enhanced ERK1/2 activity are involved in induction of macroautophagy by triterpenoid B-group soyasaponins in colon cancer cells. *Carcinogenesis* **2006**, *27*, 298–306. [CrossRef]
38. Ye, Y.C.; Wang, H.J.; Xu, L.; Liu, W.W.; Liu, B.B.; Tashiro, S.I.; Onodera, S.; Ikejima, T. Oridonin induces apoptosis and autophagy in murine fibrosarcoma L929 cells partly via NO-ERK-p53 positive-feedback loop signaling pathway. *Acta Pharmacol. Sin.* **2012**, *33*, 1055–1061. [CrossRef]

Sample Availability: Samples of the compounds TFS are not available from the authors.

molecules

MDPI

Article

Standardized Saponin Extract from Baiye No.1 Tea (*Camellia sinensis*) Flowers Induced S Phase Cell Cycle Arrest and Apoptosis via AKT-MDM2-p53 Signaling Pathway in Ovarian Cancer Cells

Youying Tu [1], Lianfu Chen [1,2], Ning Ren [1,2], Bo Li [1], Yuanyuan Wu [1], Gary O. Rankin [3], Yon Rojanasakul [4], Yaomin Wang [5,*] and Yi Charlie Chen [2,*]

1 Department of Tea Science, Zhejiang University, Hangzhou 310058, China; youytu@zju.edu.cn (Y.T.); c.lianfu@foxmail.com (L.C.); ningren@zju.edu.cn (N.R.); drlib@zju.edu.cn (B.L.); yywu@zju.edu.cn (Y.W.)

2 College of Health, Science, Technology and Mathematics, Alderson Broaddus University, Philippi, WV 26416, USA

3 Department of Biomedical Sciences, Joan C. Edwards School of Medicine, Marshall University, Huntington, WV 25755, USA; rankin@marshall.edu

4 Department of Pharmaceutical Sciences and WVU Cancer Institute, West Virginia University, Morgantown, WV 26506, USA; yrojan@hsc.wvu.edu

5 Key Laboratory of Horticulture Plant Biology, Ministry of Education, College of Horticulture & Forestry Sciences, Huazhong Agricultural University, Wuhan 430070, China

* Correspondence: wangym@mail.hzau.edu.cn (Y.W.); chenyc@ab.edu (Y.C.C.)

Academic Editors: Marialuigia Fantacuzzi and Alessandra Ammazzalorso
Received: 22 June 2020; Accepted: 29 July 2020; Published: 31 July 2020

Abstract: Ovarian cancer is considered to be one of the most serious malignant tumors in women. Natural compounds have been considered as important sources in the search for new anti-cancer agents. Saponins are characteristic components of tea (*Camellia sinensis*) flower and have various biological activities, including anti-tumor effects. In this study, a high purity standardized saponin extract, namely Baiye No.1 tea flower saponin (BTFS), which contained Floratheasaponin A and Floratheasaponin D, were isolated from tea (*Camellia sinensis* cv. Baiye 1) flowers by macroporous resin and preparative liquid chromatography. Then, the component and purity were detected by UPLC-Q-TOF/MS/MS. This high purity BTFS inhibited the proliferation of A2780/CP70 cancer cells dose-dependently, which is evidenced by the inhibition of cell viability, reduction of colony formation ability, and suppression of PCNA protein expression. Further research found BTFS induced S phase cell cycle arrest by up-regulating p21 proteins expression and down-regulating Cyclin A2, CDK2, and Cdc25A protein expression. Furthermore, BTFS caused DNA damage and activated the ATM-Chk2 signaling pathway to block cell cycle progression. Moreover, BTFS trigged both extrinsic and intrinsic apoptosis—BTFS up-regulated the expression of death receptor pathway-related proteins DR5, Fas, and FADD and increased the ratio of pro-apoptotic/anti-apoptotic proteins of the Bcl-2 family. BTFS-induced apoptosis seems to be related to the AKT-MDM2-p53 signaling pathway. In summary, our results demonstrate that BTFS has the potential to be used as a nutraceutical for the prevention and treatment of ovarian cancer.

Keywords: tea (*Camellia sinensis*) flowers; BTFS; A2780/CP70 ovarian cancer cells; apoptosis; S phase cell cycle arrest

1. Introduction

Ovarian cancer is a malignant tumor of the female reproductive system that causes high mortality in women. Worldwide, 4.4% of cancer-related deaths are due to ovarian cancer [1]. Recent statistics have shown that there were 52,100 new cases of ovarian cancer and about 22,500 deaths in China [2]. In the US, there were 22,240 new cases of ovarian cancer with a death toll of 14,070; the survival rate is only 37% [3]. Currently, the standard treatment for ovarian cancer is radical surgery combined with adjuvant chemotherapy drugs, which has certain effects on early patients. In clinic, most ovarian cancer patients are diagnosed in the middle and late stages due to the vague early symptoms and the lack of detection methods. Accordingly, ovarian cancer is easily prone to relapse and drug resistance, and ultimately leads to high mortality [4]. Thus, it is particularly necessary to find new compounds from natural products, which could effectively prevent and treat ovarian cancer.

Infinite proliferation is the main feature of cancer cells and drugs that inhibit cell division are often used in cancer treatment. Disorders of the cell cycle can cause cells to proliferate indefinitely and induce cancer. Cyclin dependent kinases (CDKs), Cyclin, and CKI are highly correlated with the occurrence, development, and prognosis of ovarian cancer [5]. CDK2, CDK4, Cyclin A, Cyclin D, and the expression of Cyclin E are upregulated significantly in ovarian cancer tissues [6], while the protein expression of p21 and p27 are significantly lower than that of non-cancerous ovarian tissue. Many studies have improved the therapeutic effect through the action of drugs on cell cycle checkpoints. Apoptosis is a kind of programmed cell under physiological conditions. The abnormal regulation of apoptosis is closely related to the occurrence and development of cancer. Targeting extrinsic (death receptor-mediated) and intrinsic (mitochondrial-mediated) apoptosis is an important strategy in cancer treatment [7].

Saponins are a class of glycoside compounds with polycyclic compounds as ligands that are widely present in ginseng [8], Chonglou [9], Camellia [10], and other plants. Recent studies demonstrate that saponins show a strong inhibitory effect against ovarian cancer. Chonglou Saponin II induced G2 phase cell cycle arrest in SKOV3 ovarian cancer cells [11]. Baiying steroidal saponin aescin up-regulates the activity of Caspase-3 and promotes the apoptosis of SKOV3 cells [12]. Moreover, several other studies have demonstrated the potency of saponins by inhibiting cell proliferation, inducing apoptosis and cell cycle arrest, as well as inhibiting angiogenesis and weakening the invasion and metastasis, which has made saponins important natural sources in the search for new chemopreventive agents [13–15].

Tea is a popular beverage globally, and many functional ingredients have multiple health functions for the human body. Tea saponins are widely distributed in the roots, stems, leaves, and flowers [13]. However, compared to tea leaves, tea flowers contain a much higher amount of saponins. Moreover, tea flowers have become important food resources and it is an urgent need to explore the health benefits of tea flowers saponins. In recent years, tea flower saponins have demonstrated strong anticancer activity, as confirmed by several research. Kitagawa et al. showed that Chakasaponin I, II, and Floratheasaponin A have inhibitory effects on human gastrointestinal cancer cells HSC-2, HSC-4, MKN-45, and Caco-2, and the effect is stronger than catechin, flavonoids, and caffeine. The inhibition of HSC-2 cell proliferation may be due to the induction of cell cycle arrest in the G2/M phase and activation of apoptosis [16]. Previously, we also reported the effects of tea flower saponins containing Chakasaponin II and other 13 monomers on ovarian cancer cells; the results demonstrated that tea flower saponins shows strong anticancer activity by inducing apoptosis and S phase cell cycle arrest in human OVCAR-3 and A2780/CP70 cancer cells [17]. Now, further-purified tea flower saponins is needed to better elucidate anticancer properties and mechanisms. Thus, the aim of this paper is to obtain high-purity tea flower saponins and further elucidate its antiproliferative effect and mechanisms on human ovarian cancer cell. Our results show that high-purity BTFS extracted from Baiye No.1 tea flowers induced cell cycle arrest in the S phase and induced apoptosis in A2780/CP70 cells by targeting both extrinsic and intrinsic apoptotic pathways.

2. Results

2.1. Analysis and Identification of BTFS

We found, through UPLC-Q-TOF/MS/MS analysis, that BTFS extracted from tea flowers contained 3 triterpenoid saponins (Figure 1A,B). Based on the published literature [18–20] and combined with the retention time, molecular weight, molecular formula, and secondary ion fragment information of the corresponding peak, we inferred that the saponins in BTFS are Floratheasaponin D (58.5%), Floratheasaponin A (36.7%), and an unnamed saponin (4.9%) (Table 1) [20]. Our previous study showed that Floratheasaponin A and Floratheasaponin D were the main saponin components in Baiye No.1 tea flowers [20].

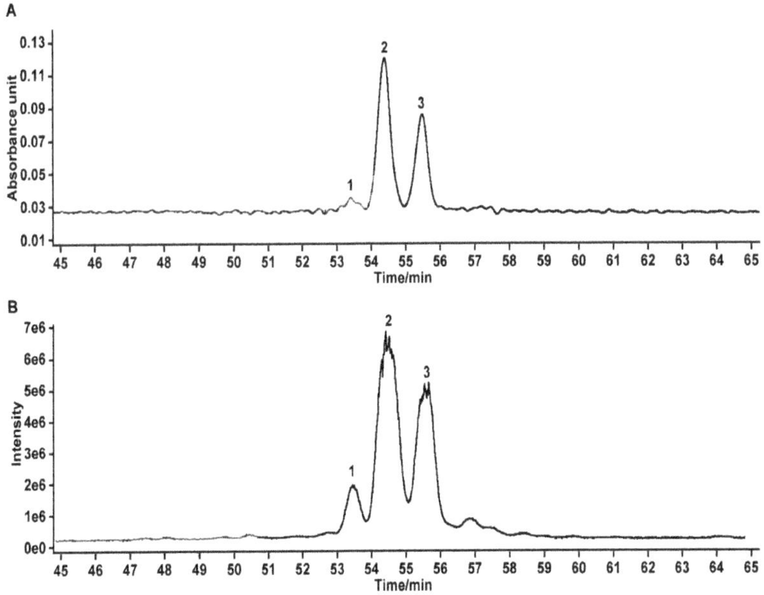

Figure 1. Typical chromatograms of BTFS. (**A**) Ultraviolet chromatograms. (**B**) Total ion chromatograms.

Table 1. MS data in negative mode of saponins extracted from tea flower.

Peak	Retention Time (min)	$[M-H]^-$	MS2	Formula	Peak Identity
1	53.40	1245.59	1083, 1065, 951, 915, 753, 709, 611	C60H94O27	Unknown [20]
2	54.45	1229.59	1083, 1067, 1049, 789, 611	C60H94O26	Floratheasaponin D [19,20]
3	55.57	1215.58	1083, 1035, 951, 933, 789, 611	C59H92O26	Floratheasaponin A [18,20]

2.2. BTFS Inhibits Ovarian Cancer Cell Proliferation

The effects of BTFS on cell viability were determined by CellTiter 96 Aqueous One Solution Cell Proliferation assay. BTFS reduced the cell viability of A2780/CP70 cells dose-dependently, while BTFS displayed less cytotoxicity to normal ovarian cell line IOSE-364 (Figure 2A). Colony formation assay is considered as an effective way to determine the long-term proliferation capacity of cancer cells. We then carried out this assay to further explore the inhibitory effect of BTFS on A2780/CP70 cells. The results found that the number of cell colonies was significantly lower for cells subjected to BTFS than for the control cell (Figure 2B,C). Besides, we also analyzed the protein expression of proliferating cell nuclear antigen (PCNA) by Western blot; the results showed that PCNA was downregulated in the BTFS-treated group, compared to the vehicle group. (Figure 2D,E, the original images for Figure 2D can be seen in Supplementary Materials). In summary, the results demonstrated that BTFS exhibited an antiproliferative effect and cytotoxicity on A2780/CP70 cells.

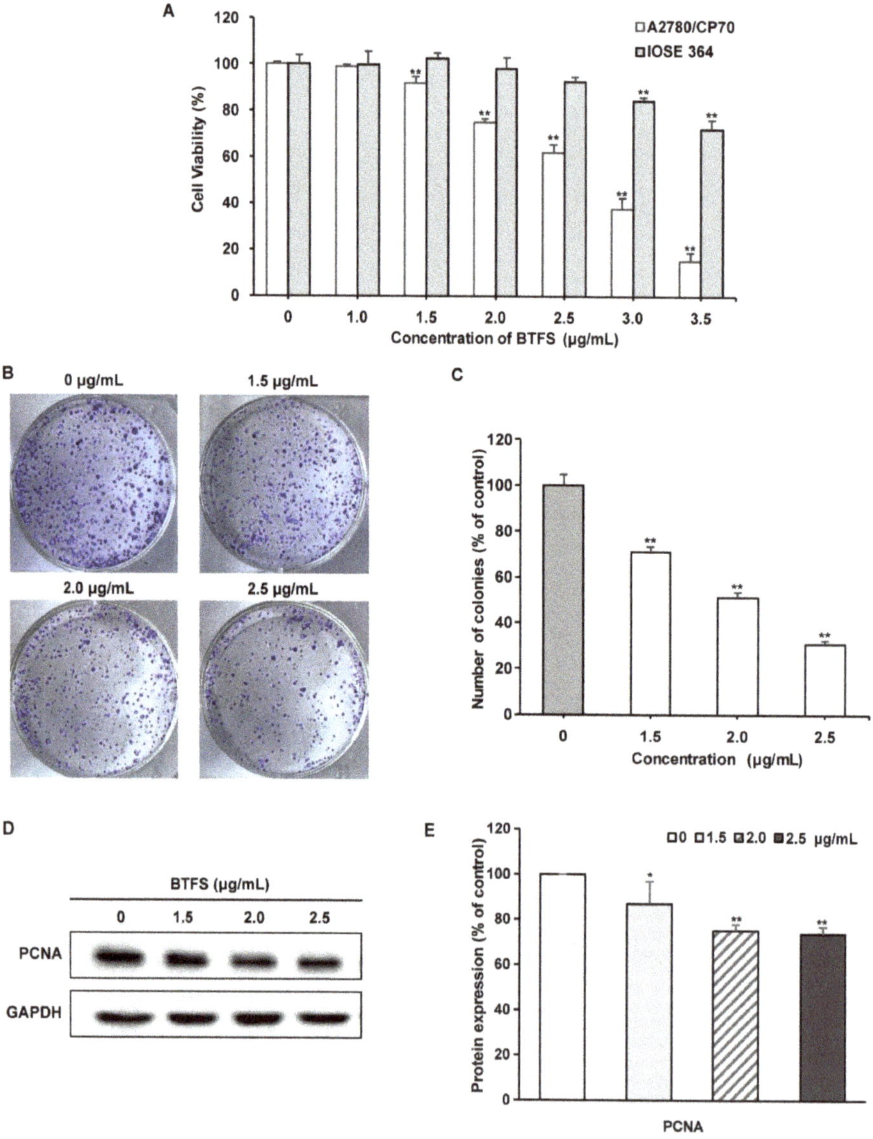

Figure 2. BTFS inhibits proliferation of A2780/CP70 cells. (**A**) BTFS inhibited the cell viability of A2780/CP70 and showed moderate effect on IOSE-364 cells. (**B**) The effect of BTFS on colony formation of A2780/CP70 cells. (**C**) Statistical histogram. $^*p < 0.05$; $^{**}p < 0.01$ versus control. (**D**)Effects of BTFS on protein expression of PNCA in A2780/CP70 cells. (**E**) Statistical histogram of protein quantization. * $p < 0.05$; ** $p < 0.01$ versus control.

2.3. BTFS Induces Cell Cycle Arrest in the S Phase in A2780/CP70 Cells

In order to elucidate the mechanism of BTFS inhibiting cell proliferation, flow cytometry was used to detect the cell cycle phase distribution of BTFS-treated human ovarian cells stained with propidium iodide (PI). The results showed that BTFS treatment induced a dose-dependent increase in the proportion of A2780/CP70 cells in the S phase. We also observed a reduction of cell proportion in the G0/G1 and G2/M phases (Figure 3A,B). When cells were treated with 1.5, 2.0, and 2.5 μg/mL BTFS for 24 h, the proportion of cells at the S phase were 29.04%, 35.60%, and 43.52%, respectively, compared with 20.30% in the vehicle-treated cells.

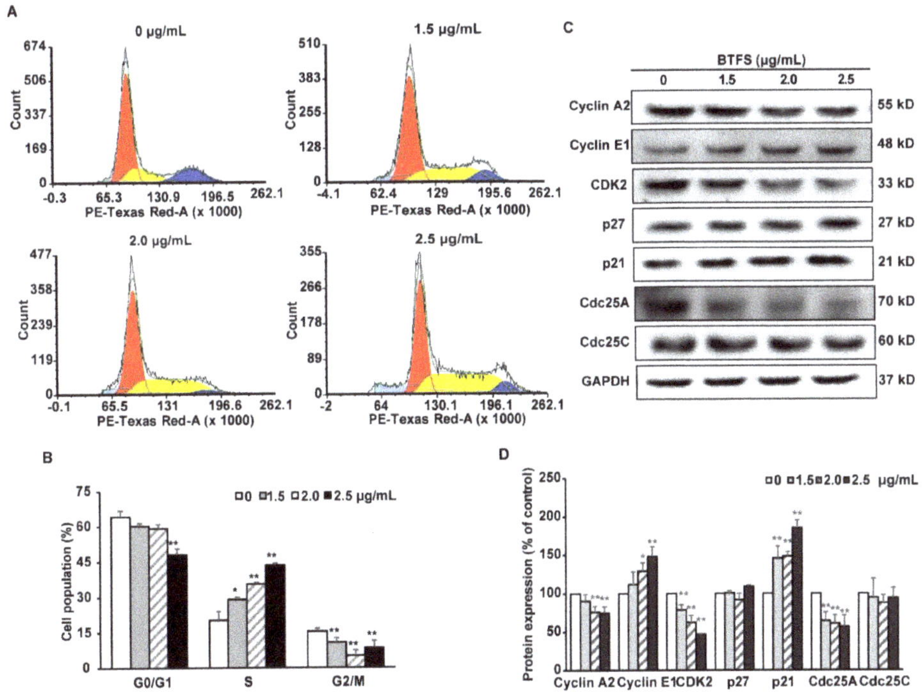

Figure 3. BTFS-induced cell cycle arrest at S phase in A2780/CP70 cells and regulated proteins expression related with S phase. (**A**,**B**) BTFS induced cell cycle arrest at S phase by flow cytometry. Statistical analysis bar chart, * $p < 0.05$ and ** $p < 0.01$ versus control. (**C**,**D**) Effects of BTFS on the expression of cell cycle-related proteins in A2780/CP70 cancer cells. Statistical histogram of protein quantization, * $p < 0.05$; ** $p < 0.01$ versus control.

2.4. The Effects of BTFS on Cell Cycle Regulatory Protein Expression

We then evaluated the expression of cell cycle regulatory proteins by western blot after BTFS treatment. Cyclin and Cyclin dependent kinase (CDK) form Cyclin/CDK complex to regulate cell cycle progression. Furthermore, p21 and p27 are CDK inhibitors (CDKI), which negatively regulate cell cycle; the Cdc25 phosphatase family have a positive regulation effect on cell cycle. We found that BTFS could effectively suppress the expression of CDK2, Cyclin A, and Cdc25A and increased the expression of Cyclin E1 and p21, while showing no effect on the protein levels of p27 and Cdc25C (Figure 3C,D). The results demonstrated that the down-regulation of Cdc25A, up-regulation of p21, and reduction of kinase activities of CyclinE1/CDK2 and CyclinA2/CDK2 complexes might be responsible for S phase arrest induced by BTFS in A2780/CP70 cells.

2.5. BTFS Activates Apoptosis in A2780/CP70 Cells

The increasing of sub-G1 phase population demonstrates that BTFS might cause cellular apoptosis in A2780/CP70 cells. Accordingly, we further explored whether BTFS caused apoptosis in A2780/CP70 cells. Hoechst 33342 staining was performed to observe the morphological changes of apoptosis. As shown in Figure 4A, after treating with BTFS, A2780/CP70 cells showed more apoptotic cells, which were brighter blue with condensed or fragmented nuclei than the untreated group. We then used quantitative fluorescence spectrophotometer to evaluate the mitochondrial membrane potential of A2780/CP70 cells. BTFS treatment resulted in a notable reduction in the red-green fluorescence ratio of JC-1 dye, which indicated that BTFS could induce apoptosis of A2780/CP70 cells (Figure 4B). Flow cytometric analysis was then conducted to further verify the pro-apoptotic effect of BTFS. As shown in Figure 4C,D, BTFS could significantly reduce the proportion of live cells and increase the proportion of apoptotic cells dose-dependently. Together, these results suggested that inducing apoptosis may be an important factor for the antiproliferative effect of BTFS on A2780/CP70 cells.

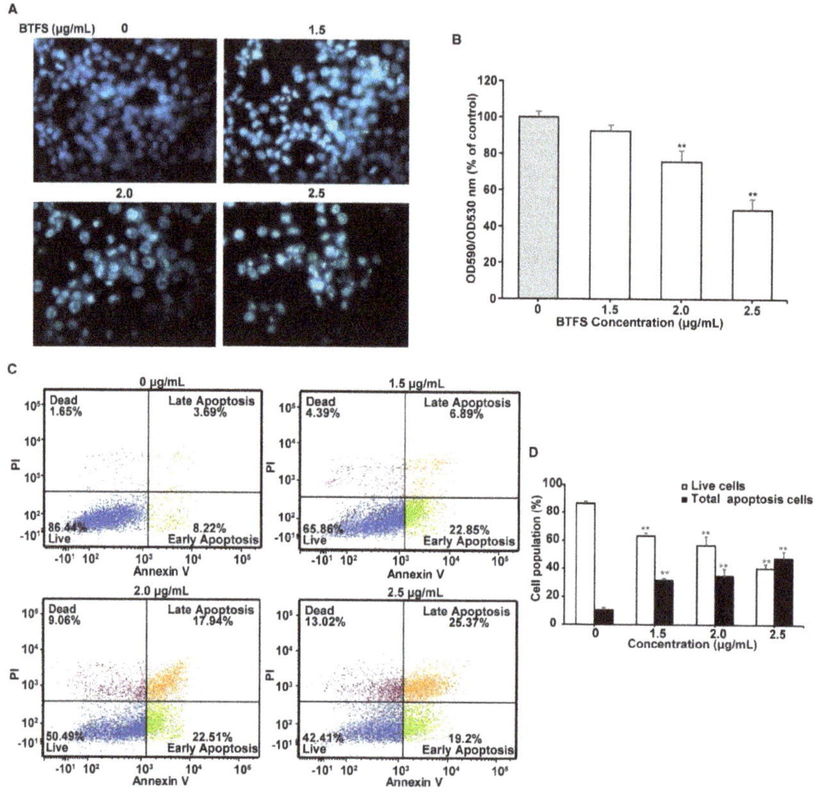

Figure 4. BTFS-induced apoptosis in A2780/CP70 cells. (**A**) Hoechst 33342 staining confirmed the apoptotic effect induced by BTFS in A2780/CP70 cells. (**B**) The effect of BTFS on mitochondrial membrane potential in A2780/CP70 cells was determined by JC-1 staining. ** $p < 0.01$ versus control. (**C**,**D**) BTFS-induced apoptosis in A2780/CP70 cells evidenced by flow cytometry. Statistical analysis bar chart, ** $p < 0.01$ versus control.

2.6. BTFS Mediates Apoptosis via Intrinsic and Extrinsic Apoptotic Pathways

Apoptosis could be classified into the intrinsic (mitochondrial mediated) pathway and the extrinsic (death receptor mediated) pathway. To investigate the specific pathway of BTFS in inducing apoptosis in A2780/CP70 cells, caspase-Glo assay was used to detected the caspase activation. As shown in Figure 5A, caspase-3/7, -8 and -9 activities in BTFS-treated cells were increased significantly compared with vehicle treated cells, which hinted that BTFS might trigger both the intrinsic and extrinsic apoptotic pathway. Furthermore, western blot assay was then conducted to examine the key proteins in both apoptotic pathways. After BTFS treatment, cleaved PARP protein, served as a marker of apoptosis, increased significantly, further confirming that BTFS could induce apoptosis in A2780/CP70 cells. Meanwhile, extrinsic pathway related proteins were investigated to confirm whether the extrinsic pathway was involved in BTFS-induced apoptosis. The results showed that BTFS could markedly up-regulate the expression of death receptors, Fas and DR5, and dose-dependently increased the cell death adaptor protein FADD (Figure 5B,C). With regard to the intrinsic apoptosis-related proteins, BTFS obviously decreased the protein expression of Bcl-2 and Bcl-xL, while Bax, Cytochrome C, and Apaf apoptotic protease activating factor-1(Apaf-1) were significantly upregulated and had no effect on Bad expression (Figure 5D,E). These results suggested that both intrinsic and extrinsic pathways were involved in BTFS-induced apoptosis in A2780/CP70 cells.

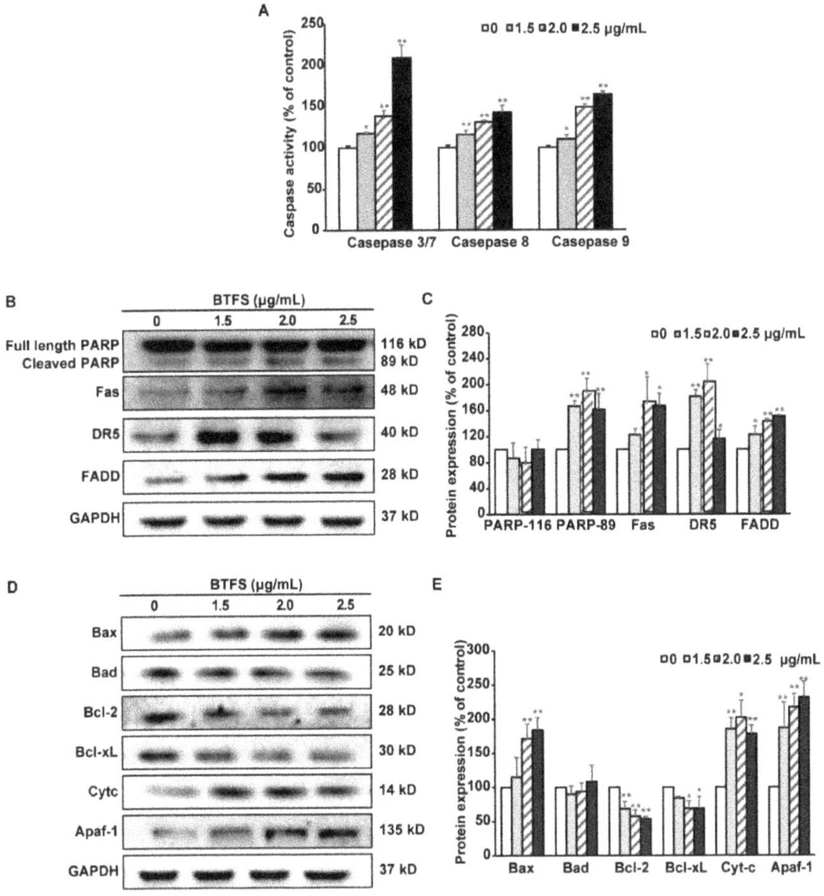

Figure 5. BTFS trigged both extrinsic and intrinsic pathways. (**A**) Effects of BTFS on the activity of caspase-3/7, 8 and 9. * $p < 0.05$ and ** $p < 0.01$ versus control. (**B**,**C**) Effects of BTFS on extrinsic apoptosis-related protein expression in A2780/CP70 cells. (**D**,**E**) Effect of BTFS on intrinsic apoptosis-related protein expression in A2780/CP70 cells.

2.7. BTFS Induces DNA Damage and Affects the Expression of Upstream Regulators AKT, MDM2, and P53

ROS and DNA damages could mediate cell cycle arrest and apoptosis [21,22]. Firstly, DCFH-DA fluorescence probe assay was conducted to assess the effect of BTFS on intracellular ROS production. ROS generation was obviously elevated when A2780/CP70 cells were exposed to BTFS, compared to the vehicle-treated group (Figure 6A). Next, western blot assay was then performed to investigate the effect of BTFS on DNA damage response. The phosphorylation of histone H2A.X at serine 139 is considered as a reliable marker of DNA damage [23]. BTFS dramatically increased the phosphorylation of histone H2A.X. ATM/Chk is one of the important signaling pathways mediating DNA damage. After exposure to BTFS, both the phosphorylation of ATM at Ser1981 as well as the phosphorylation of Chk2 at Thr68 were up-regulated (Figure 6B,C), suggesting that ATM-Chk2 pathway was activated. These results suggested that BTFS promoted ROS generation and DNA damage, which is responsible for the cytotoxicity of BTFS. Moreover, BTFS induced DNA damage may be mediated by ROS generation, the specific mechanism of which needs to be further elucidated.

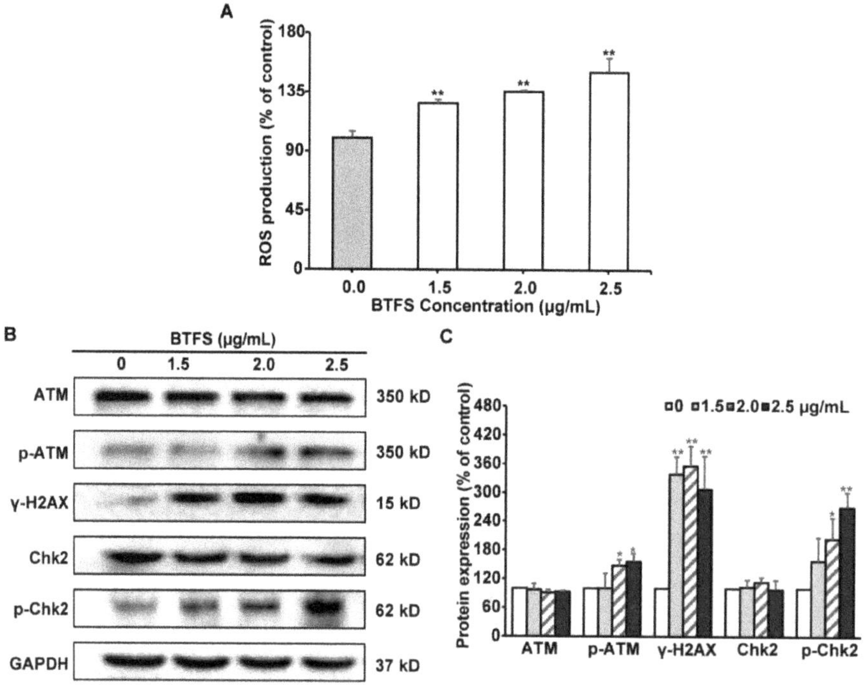

Figure 6. BTFS caused DNA damage in A2780/CP70 cells. (**A**) The effect of BTFS 3 on ROS production in A2780/CP70 cells. * $p < 0.05$; ** $p < 0.01$ versus control. (**B**,**C**) The effect of BTFS on the expression of DNA damage-related proteins in A2780/CP70 cells. * $p < 0.05$; ** $p < 0.01$ versus control.

AKT, MDM2, and p53 are upstream regulators of the cell cycle and apoptosis related proteins mentioned above. To further explore the mechanism underlying BTFS-induced S phase cell cycle arrest and apoptosis, we evaluated the protein expression levels of these upstream regulators in A2780/CP70 cells after BTFS exposure. Western blot analysis illustrated that p-AKT and MDM2 were dramatically decreased by BTFS, meanwhile p53 and p-p53 were increased compared with the controls (Figure 7A,B).

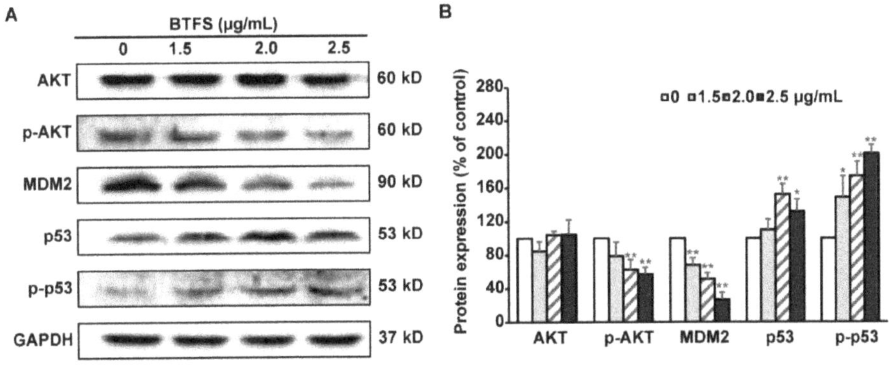

Figure 7. Effect of BTFS on AKT/MDM/P53 pathway related proteins. (**A**) Western blot image (**B**) Statistical histogram of protein quantization. * $p < 0.05$; ** $p < 0.01$ versus control.

3. Discussion

Ovarian cancer is considered to be one of the deadliest gynecological cancers in the world. Although platinum-based chemotherapy is the most broadly used treatment for this disease, chemoresistance and adverse side-effects still remain major obstacles to successful treatment [24]. Compounds derived from natural products have recently gained much attention in cancer therapy due to the higher biological activity and lower toxicity [25]. It has been proved that various triterpenoid saponins have extensive anticancer activity [14,15] and some triterpenoid saponins, such as Albizia gummifera saponins [26], ginsenoside 20(S)-Rg3 [27], ginsenoside Rh2 [28], Camellia oleifera Abel seed saponins [29], and *Camellia sinensis* seed saponins [30], exhibited obvious anti-proliferative effect against ovarian cancer cells. In this study, we extracted and isolated the characteristic saponin complex BTFS from Baiye No.1 tea flowers, which mainly contained Floratheasaponin A and Floratheasaponin D, and found that BTFS strongly inhibited cell proliferation of human ovarian cancer cells A2780/CP70 by induction of S phase cell cycle arrest and apoptosis.

This research measured the cytotoxic effect of BTFS on ovarian cells and found that BTFS significantly reduced the viability of A2780/CP70 cells, whereas it hardly affected the normal human immortalized ovarian surface epithelial IOSE 364 cells at indicated concentrations. Ovarian cancer cells have unlimited proliferation ability, while healthy cells normally proliferate. BTFS can inhibit cell proliferation by inducing apoptosis and S-phase cycle arrest in A2780/CP70. BTFS may not cause apoptosis and cycle arrest of normal cells. This may be why BTFS is selective towards ovarian cancer cells. The IC50 value of BTFS on A2780/CP70 cells was calculated to be 2.6 μg/mL, lower than theaflavin-3,3′-digallate (IC50 was about 20.7 μg/mL on A2780/CP70 cells) [31], and tea seed saponins (IC50 was about 5.9 μg/mL on OVCAR-3 and A2780/CP70 cells) [30]. Besides, the results obtained from colony formation assay and the Western blot of PCNA further demonstrated that BTFS had obvious inhibitory effects on A2780/CP70 cells.

The cell cycle disorder leading to the abnormal cell proliferation is one of the main mechanisms of tumorigenesis [32]. The S phase in the DNA synthesis phase is when DNA is replicated; thus, it is a pivotal part of the cell cycle [33]. The cell cycle is a sequential process and any phase of arrest will cause cell proliferation stagnation or death. Numerous chemotherapeutic agents exert anticancer properties by interfering with the cell cycle. In our research, analysis of the distribution of cell cycle showed that BTFS could cause S phase cell cycle arrest in A2780/CP70 cells. This result was consistent with studies that many saponins extracted from natural plants also inhibit cancer cell proliferation by arresting cells in S phase, such as Astragalus saponins [34], Albiziae Cortex total saponins [35], and ginsenoside Re [36]. Cell cycle progression is regulated by cyclins, CDKs, and other regulatory proteins [37]. Cyclin E/CDK2 complex actively participates in G1/S transition and plays important role in the initial stage of S phase. S phase progression is impacted by Cyclin A/CDK2 complex, and the S/G2 transition also requires Cyclin A/CDK2 complex [38,39]. Moreover, Cyclin/CDK complexes are modulated by Cyclin-dependent kinase inhibitors and the Cdc25 phosphatase family. The p21 protein is considered as a Cyclin dependent kinase inhibitor, which inhibits the formation of Cyclins/CDK2 complex, ultimately blocking cell cycle progression from S to G2/M phase [40,41]. CDC25A, a dual specificity phosphatase, activates the Cyclin/CDK complexes, which promotes cell cycle progression, and overexpression of CDC25A will lead to abnormal cell cycle regulation and lead to tumorigenesis [42,43]. In this study, after BTFS treatment, Cyclin A2, CDK2, and Cdc25A were downregulated significantly, while p21 and Cyclin E1 proteins were significantly upregulated. Thus, these data suggest that BTFS-induced S phase arrest might be due to changes in the S phase related proteins in A2780/CP70 cells.

Apoptosis is considered one of the most widespread forms of programmed cell death, playing a pivotal role in various physiological processes and pathological conditions [44]. Inducing apoptosis is regarded as one of the major mechanisms for cancer treatments with natural compounds. In this study, the results obtained from Hoechst 33342 staining, JC-1 fluorescent staining, and flow cytometry assay suggest that BTFS induced apoptosis in A2780/CP70 cells as evidenced by much brighter and more condensed nuclei within cells, notable reduction of mitochondrial membrane potential, and higher percentage of apoptotic cells. Two well-known pathways to trigger apoptosis are the extrinsic and intrinsic apoptotic pathways. Activation of caspase-8 and caspase-9 are regarded as essential markers of the extrinsic and intrinsic apoptotic pathways, respectively, and can further activate downstream effector caspase-3 and caspase-7, which are able to mediate the cleavage of PARP, and then regulate apoptosis [45,46]. In our research, BTFS obviously activated caspase-3/7, -8 and -9 and increased the level of cleaved PARP-1, indicating that BTFS triggered both the extrinsic and intrinsic apoptotic pathways in A2780/CP70 cells. For the extrinsic pathway, tumor necrosis factor-related apoptosis-inducing ligands (TRAIL), for instance, Apo2L/TRAIL and Fas ligand (FasL), bind with their respective death receptors, such as DR4/DR5 or Fas, and subsequently interact with the adaptor molecule, Fas-associated death domain (FADD) [47]. FADD combines with caspase-8, followed by initiating the caspase-3/7 cascade reaction and ultimately cell death [48]. The current research found that BTFS evidently up-regulated DR5, Fas, and FADD, suggesting activation of the extrinsic apoptotic pathway. Previous research reported that tea seeds saponins could also increase protein expression of DR5 and FADD and induced apoptosis in ovarian cancer cell, which are consistent with our results [30]. In the intrinsic pathway, the Bcl-2 family proteins, which include pro-apoptotic (Bax, Bad, and Bak) and anti-apoptotic (Bcl-2, Bcl-xL and Bcl-B) members, are key regulators by governing the mitochondrial outer membrane permeabilization (MOMP) [30]. After the decrease of mitochondrial membrane potential caused through the increase of MOMP, cytochrome c is released from the mitochondria into the cytosol, and then binds with Apaf-1 to form the apoptosome complex, which will activate pro-caspase 9 and trigger an enzymatic cascade leading to cell death [49,50]. In this case, BTFS increased the ratio of pro- versus anti-apoptotic Bcl-2 family protein and the release of cytochrome C and Apaf-1. A similar study reported that Paris saponin II induced apoptosis in ovarian cancer cell might also result from its effects on the expression of Bax, Bcl-2, and cytochrome c proteins [11]. These results demonstrate that induction of apoptosis through both extrinsic and intrinsic pathways might also account for the anti-proliferation activity of BTFS on A2780/CP70 cells. Previously we reported the anti-cancer effect of saponin extract, which contained 14 triterpenoid saponins [17]. In this paper, a higher-purity BTFS, which mainly contained Floratheasaponin D and Floratheasaponin A, was obtained and it showed strong antiproliferative effect against A2780/CP70 cells. Though BTFS could also induce apoptosis and cell cycle arrest, the specific contribution of Floratheasaponin D and Floratheasaponin A remains to be further elucidated. Moreover, structure-activity relationship may play a pivotal role in its anticancer effect. It has been reported that the differences of saponin type, position, and sugar moieties affect anticancer activity [51,52]. BTFS was classified as triterpenes saponins in our study; we obtained a mixture of three saponin monomers, which makes it complex to evaluate the anticancer effect and the chemical structures. However, the specific structure-activity relationship of tea flower saponins is worth investigation in future work after we obtain the monomers.

Inducing intracellular ROS generation is considered as an important mechanism of the anticancer effect of most drugs [53]. Excessive ROS generation could cause DNA double-strand break, DNA locus mutation, and other forms of DNA damage [54]; and elevated ROS levels have been regarded as a causative trigger for DNA damage [55]. Cell cycle checkpoints and effector kinases could be activated to regulate cellular decision among cell cycle arrest, apoptosis, or other cell death modalities in response to ROS-mediated DNA damage [56]. In our research, we demonstrated ROS generation and DNA damage after treatment with BTFS in A2780/CP70 cells. Ataxia telangiectasia mutated (ATM) kinase is an important DNA damage sensor for oxidative stress response. When responding to DNA damage, ATM is activated by autophosphorylation and further phosphorylates downstream substrates such as Chk1 and Chk2 [57,58]. Furthermore, activated Chk1 and Chk2 cause the phosphorylation of their downstream effectors, for instance Cdc25A, which could mediate the transformation of cell cycle S/G2 by regulating CDK2 activity [59]. Moreover, Chk2 could phosphorylate and activate p53 protein directly [60]. This experiment revealed that p-ATM and p-Chk2 were remarkably increased by BTFS in A2780/CP70 cells, suggesting that the ATM-Chk2 pathway was activated following DNA damage.

A serine/threonine kinase named AKT can be activated by autophosphorylation at Ser473 and Thr308, thereby inhibiting apoptosis and promoting cell survival. MDM2 is one of the downstream proteins of AKT, which can promote cell proliferation and growth, and is related to the development of a variety of tumors [61]. MDM2 is also a ubiquitin ligase of p53, which can be phosphorylated by p-AKT at Ser166 and Ser186 and enter the nucleus to form a complex with p53, thereby inhibiting p53 activity [62]. P53 is an important tumor suppressor, which plays an important role in cellular response. DNA damage can induce p53 phosphorylation at Ser15 and Ser20 sites, weakening the interaction between p53 and MDM2 and inducing apoptosis, cell cycle arrest, etc. [62,63]. P53 mainly induces apoptosis by activating the death receptor pathway and the mitochondrial pathway; meanwhile, p53 can promote apoptosis by activating death receptors such as Fas, DR4, and DR5 located on the cell membrane. On the other hand, Bcl-2 family proteins as well as mitochondria proteins are also associated with p53-dependent apoptosis [64]. It has been reported that triterpenoid saponin ginsenoside Rh2 can activate the p53 pathway to induce apoptosis in colorectal cancer cells [64], and can induce apoptosis in human epidermal cancer cells by inhibiting AKT activity [65]. Based on our study, we found that BTFS can significantly reduce p-AKT and MDM2 and increase p53 and p-p53 protein levels in A2780/CP70 cells, suggesting that BTFS can reduce the cross-linking of MDM2 and p53 by inhibiting AKT autophosphorylation, and thus effectively enhance p53 activity and promote cell apoptosis. Our finding is consistent with the study that the active tea component theaflavins can induce apoptosis of ovarian cancer cellA2780/CP70 through AKT-MDM2-p53 pathway [31].

4. Materials and Methods

4.1. Materials and Reagents

RPMI-1640 medium, Fetal bovine serum (FBS), and DMSO were purchased from Sigma (St. Louis, MO, USA). Caspase-Glo 3/7, Caspase-8, Caspase-9, and CellTiter 96 Aqueous kit were purchased from Promega (Madison, WI, USA). Propidium iodide (PI) and Alexa Fluor 488 Annexin V were purchased from Invitrogen (Waltham, MA, USA). Antibodies against PCNA, p21, p27, CDK2, Cdc25A, Cdc25C, CyclinA2, Cyclin E1, ATM, p-ATM (Ser1981), γ-H2AX (Ser139), PARP, Fas, DR5, FADD, Bax, Bcl-2, Bcl-xL, Apaf-1, Cytc, p53, p-p53 (Ser15), AKT, p-AKT (Ser473), and MDM2 were purchased from Cell Signaling Technology (Beverly, MA, USA). Antibodies against Chk2, p-Chk2 (Thr 68), Bad, and GAPDH were purchased from Santa Cruz Biotechnology (Dallas, TX, USA).

4.2. Extraction and Identification of Baiye No.1 Tea Flower Saponins (BTFS)

Dried tea flowers of tea Baiye No.1 variety were obtained from Zhe-jiang Yilongfang Co., Ltd. (Kaihua, Zhe-jiang, China). After smashing, the powder was distilled at 80 °C for 45 min. The aqueous extract was separated by AB-8 macroporous adsorption resin, followed by preparative HPLC to obtain BTFS. BTFS was then identified by UPLC-Q-TOF/MS/MS system with ultra-high performance chromatography (Agilent, Santa Clara, CA, USA) coupled with electro-spray ionization quadrupole time-of-flight mass spectrometry (AB SCIEX, Framingham, MA, USA) according to the methods we described previously, with certain modifications [20]. BTFS was dissolved in dimethyl sulfoxide (DMSO) to make a 20 mg/mL stock solution and stored at −20 °C before use.

4.3. Cell Lines and Cell Culture

Human ovarian cancer cell line A2780/CP70 was provided by Dr. Bing-Hua Jiang from Thomas Jefferson University, and the normal ovarian surface epithelial cell line IOSE-364 was provided by Dr Auersperg from the University of British Columbia. The cell lines were cultured in RPMI-1640 medium with 10% FBS, and incubated at 37 °C in a humidified incubator with 5% CO_2.

4.4. Cell Viability Assay

A2780/CP70 and IOSE-364 cells were seeded in 96-well plates at a density of 2×10^4 cells/well incubated overnight, and treated with BTFS (1.0, 1.5, 2.0, 2.5, 3.0, 3.5 μg/mL) or an equal concentration of DMSO (as vehicle) for 24 h. CellTiter 96 Aqueous kit was then used to assess the cell viability according to the manufacturer's protocol. Results were presented as percentage of control.

4.5. Colony Formation Assay

A2780/CP70 cells were seeded into 6-well plates at 6×10^5 cells/well incubated overnight and treated with BTFS (0, 1.5, 2.0, 2.5 μg/mL) for 24 h. The cells were then cultured for 7 days with drug-free medium at 2×10^3 cells/well. Colonies were fixed with ice-cold methanol for 10 min, then stained with 0.5% crystal violet solution in 25% methanol for another 10 min. The plates were rinsed with distilled water carefully several times and directly photographed. Image J software (Bethesda, MD, USA) was used to count the number of colonies; the results were adjusted to the percentage of control.

4.6. Cell Cycle Analysis by Flow Cytometry

After treating with BTFS (0, 1.5, 2.0, 2.5 μg/mL) for 24 h, the cells were washed with cold PBS twice and then fixed with ice-cold 70% ethanol at 4 °C overnight. Afterwards, the cells were washed twice with PBS and incubated with 180 μg/mL RNase (Invitrogen) for 15 min at 37 °C, then incubating with 50 μg/mL propidium iodide (PI) solution (Sigma) for 15 min in the dark at 37 °C. The cells were then analyzed by FACSCalibur flow cytometry (BD Biosciences, San Jose, CA, USA) and data were analyzed by FCS software (De Novo Software, CA, USA).

4.7. Hoechse 33342 Staining

The cells were seeded in 96 well plates at density of 2×10^4 cells/well and incubated overnight, after treating with BTFS (0, 1.5, 2.0, 2.5 μg/mL) for 24 h. The cells were stained with 10 μg/mL Hoechst 33342 (Sigma) in PBS for 15 min in the dark at 37 °C. Fluorescence microscope (ZEISS, Heidelberg, Germany) was used to examine the cellular morphology.

4.8. Evaluation of Mitochondrial Membrane Potential

The cells were seeded in black 96 well plates at density of 2×10^4 cells/well and incubated overnight, and treated with BTFS (0, 1.5, 2.0, 2.5 μg/mL) for 24 h. After washing twice, the cells were incubated with 10 μg/mL JC-1 solution for 30 min at 37 °C. The fluorescent intensity was measured using Synerg HT Multi Mode Microplate reader (BioTek, Winooski, VT, USA) at excitation: emission of 485/590 and 485/528 for red aggregates and green monomers, respectively.

4.9. Apoptosis Analysis by Flow Cytometry

The apoptotic cells were evaluated using an Alexa Fluor 488 Annexin V/Dead Cell Apoptosis Kit (Invitrogen, Waltham, MA, USA). After treating with BTFS (0, 1.5, 2.0, 2.5 μg/mL) for 24 h, the cells were harvested and centrifuged for 8 min at 1000 rpm; after washing twice with PBS, the cells were suspended in Annexin-binding buffer with Alexa Fluor 488 Annexin V and PI solution for in dark 15 min at room temperature. The stained cells were then analyzed by FACSCalibur flow cytometry (BD Biosciences) with fluorescence emission at 530 nm and excitation at 488 nm.

4.10. Cellular Caspase Activity Assay

The cells were seeded in 96 well plates at density of 2×10^4 cells/well and incubated overnight, after treating with BTFS (0, 1.5, 2.0, 2.5 μg/mL) for 24 h. Caspase Glo-3/7, -8 and -9 regents (Promega, Madison, WI, USA) were added to each well and incubated for 30 min at 37 °C. Luminescence was measured by Synerg HT Multi Mode Microplate reader (BioTek). Total protein levels were detected with a BCA assay kit to normalize the caspases activities. The results were presented as percentage of control.

4.11. Detection of Intracellular ROS Production

Intracellular ROS production was measured by peroxide-sensitive fluorescent probe DCFH-DA. The cells were treated with BTFS (0, 1.5, 2.0, 2.5 μg/mL) for 24 h, followed by treatment with 10 μM DCFH-DA for 30 min at 37 °C. The fluorescence intensity was measured with excitation at 485 nm and emission at 528 nm by Synergy HT Multi-Mode Microplate Reader (BioTek). Total protein levels were detected by BCA assay kit to normalize the ROS generation. The results were presented as percentage of control.

4.12. Western Blotting

Cells were treated with BTFS (0, 1.5, 2.0, 2.5 μg/mL) for 24 h and then harvested and extracted with Mammalian Protein Extraction Reagent (Pierce, Rockford, IL, USA) supplemented with Halt Protease and Phosphatase Inhibitor (Pierce). BCA protein assay kit (Pierce) was used to determine the total protein concentrations of cell lysates. Protein samples of cell lysates were mixed with equal amount of SDS loading buffer and denatured by heating for 8 min, then separated by SDS-polyacrylamide gel electrophoresis before transferring onto nitrocellulose membranes. The membranes were blocked with 5% non-fat milk in Tris-buffer saline, which contained 0.1% Tween 20 (TBST) for 1 h at room temperature. Specific primary antibodies were used and the membrane was incubated at 4 °C overnight. After washing with TBST, appropriate secondary antibodies conjugated with horseradish peroxidase were used. The antigen-antibody complex was visualized with the ECL Western blot detection kit (Bio-Rad) and ChemiDoc MP System (Bio Rad, Hercules, CA, USA). Image J software was used to quantitate the protein bands; the indicated protein was then normalized by GAPDH.

4.13. Statistical Analysis

Data were presented as mean ± standard deviation (SD) for at least three independent experiments. One-way ANOVA followed with Dunnett's test was performed by SPSS software (IBM, Version 22.0, Armonk, NY, USA). The criterion for statistical significance were $p < 0.05$ and $p < 0.01$.

5. Conclusions

The high-purity standardized saponin extract we obtained from Baiye No.1 tea flower, namely BTFS, shows a strong antiproliferative effect against A2780/CP70 cells at low concentrations, while causing less cytotoxicity to normal cells. BTFS caused cellular DNA damage in A2780/CP 70 cells and induced cell cycle arrest in the S phase via regulating ATM-Chk2 signaling pathway related proteins. BTFS also trigged both intrinsic and extrinsic apoptosis in A2780/CP70 cells through the AKT-MDM2-p53 signaling pathway. Based on our results, BTFS has the potential to serve as a nutraceutical for the prevention and treatment of ovarian cancer. The specific contribution of Floratheasaponins A and D to the antiproliferative activity of A2780/CP70 cells needs further investigation.

Supplementary Materials: The Supplementary Materials are available online.

Author Contributions: Conceptualization, L.C., Y.T. and Y.C.C; methodology, L.C. and Y.C.C.; formal analysis, L.C., N.R. and Y.W. (Yuanyuan Wu); resources, Y.T., Y.R. and G.O.R.; writing—original draft preparation, L.C., B.L. and Y.W. (Yaomin Wang); writing—review and editing, Y.W. (Yaomin Wang), Y.T. and Y.C.C.; funding acquisition, Y.T. and Y.C.C., Y.W. (Yaomin Wang); All authors have read and agreed to the published version of the manuscript.

Funding: This research was funded by Key Research and Development Projects in Zhejiang Province "Industrialization Model Projects on Exploring Functional Components and Related Products from Tea Flowers and Fruits" (2018C02012), the National Key Research and Development Plan "Processing of Tea Products, Key Technology of Quality Control during Storage and Equipment Development" (2017YFD0400803), the Natural Science Foundation of Hubei Province (Grant No: 2019CFB187). This research was also supported by NIH grants P20RR016477 from the National Center for Research Resources and P20GM103434 from the National Institute for General Medical Sciences (NIGMS) awarded to the West Virginia IDeA Network of Biomedical Research Excellence. This study was also supported by Grant Number P20GM104932 from NIGMS, a component of the National Institutes of Health (NIH) and its contents are solely the responsibility of the authors and do not necessarily represent the official view of NIGMS or NIH. This study was also supported by COBRE grant GM102488/RR032138, ARIA S10 grant RR020866, FORTESSA S10 grant OD016165, and INBRE grant GM103434.

Acknowledgments: We would like to thank Kathy Brundage from Flow Cytometry Core at West Virginia Excellence.

Conflicts of Interest: The authors declare no conflict of interest.

References

1. Momenimovahed, Z.; Tiznobaik, A.; Taheri, S.; Salehiniya, H. Ovarian cancer in the world: Epidemiology and risk factors. *Int. J. Womens Health* **2019**, *11*, 287–299. [CrossRef]
2. Chen, W.; Zheng, R.; Baade, P.D.; Zhang, S.; Zeng, H.; Bray, F.; Jemal, A.; Yu, X.Q.; He, J. Cancer statistics in China, 2015. *CA: Cancer J. Clin.* **2016**, *66*, 115–132. [CrossRef]
3. Siegel, R.L.; Miller, K.D.; Jemal, A. Cancer statistics, 2018. *CA: Cancer J. Clin.* **2018**, *68*, 7–30. [CrossRef]
4. Jayson, G.C.; Kohn, E.C.; Kitchener, H.C.; Ledermann, J.A. Ovarian cancer. *Lancet* **2014**, *384*, 1376–1388. [CrossRef]
5. Zhou, Q. Targeting Cyclin-Dependent Kinases in Ovarian Cancer. *Cancer Investig.* **2017**, *35*, 367–376. [CrossRef]
6. D'Andrilli, G.; Kumar, C.; Scambia, G.; Giordano, A. Cell Cycle Genes in Ovarian Cancer. *Clin. Cancer Res.* **2004**, *10*, 8132. [CrossRef]
7. Ghobrial, I.M.; Witzig, T.E.; Adjei, A.A. Targeting apoptosis pathways in cancer therapy. *CA: Cancer J. Clin.* **2005**, *55*, 178–194. [CrossRef]
8. Shi, Z.Y.; Zeng, J.Z.; Wong, A.S.T. Chemical Structures and Pharmacological Profiles of Ginseng Saponins. *Molecules* **2019**, *24*, 2443. [CrossRef]
9. Zhang, W.; Zhang, D.; Ma, X.; Liu, Z.; Li, F.; Wu, D. Paris saponin VII suppressed the growth of human cervical cancer Hela cells. *Eur. J. Med. Res.* **2014**, *19*, 41. [CrossRef]
10. Zong, J.; Wang, R.; Bao, G.; Ling, T.; Zhang, L.; Zhang, X.; Hou, R. Novel triterpenoid saponins from residual seed cake of Camellia oleifera Abel. show anti-proliferative activity against tumor cells. *Fitoterapia* **2015**, *104*, 7–13. [CrossRef]
11. Xiao, X.; Zou, J.; Bui-Nguyen, T.M.; Bai, P.; Gao, L.; Liu, J.; Liu, S.; Xiao, J.; Chen, X.; Zhang, X.; et al. Paris saponin II of Rhizoma Paridis—a novel inducer of apoptosis in human ovarian cancer cells. *Bioscience Trends* **2012**, *6*, 201–211. [CrossRef] [PubMed]
12. Yan, J.L.J.; He, K.; Pan, R.; Hu, Q.; Peng, B.; Liu, X. Apoptosisi induced by solanum lyratum on ovarian carcinoma cell SKOV3. *World Sci. Technol.* **2008**, 60–63.
13. Zhao, Y.Z.; Zhang, Y.Y.; Han, H.; Fan, R.P.; Hu, Y.; Zhong, L.; Kou, J.P.; Yu, B.Y. Advances in the antitumor activities and mechanisms of action of steroidal saponins. *Chin. J. Nat. Med.* **2018**, *16*, 732–748. [CrossRef]

14. Koczurkiewicz, P.; Czyż, J.; Podolak, I.; Wójcik, K.; Galanty, A.; Janeczko, Z.; Michalik, M. Multidirectional effects of triterpene saponins on cancer cells—mini-review of in vitro studies. *Acta Biochim. Pol.* **2015**, *62*, 383–393. [CrossRef]
15. Xu, X.H.; Li, T.; Fong, C.M.; Chen, X.; Chen, X.J.; Wang, Y.T.; Huang, M.Q.; Lu, J.J. Saponins from Chinese Medicines as Anticancer Agents. *Molecules* **2016**, *21*, 1326. [CrossRef]
16. Kitagawa, N.; Morikawa, T.; Motai, C.; Ninomiya, K.; Okugawa, S.; Nishida, A.; Yoshikawa, M.; Muraoka, O. The Antiproliferative Effect of Chakasaponins I and II, Floratheasaponin A, and Epigallocatechin 3-O-Gallate Isolated from Camellia sinensis on Human Digestive Tract Carcinoma Cell Lines. *Int. J. Mol. Sci.* **2016**, *17*, 1979. [CrossRef]
17. Wang, Y.; Ren, N.; Rankin, G.O.; Li, B.; Rojanasakul, Y.; Tu, Y.; Chen, Y.C. Anti-proliferative effect and cell cycle arrest induced by saponins extracted from tea (Camellia sinensis) flower in human ovarian cancer cells. *J. Funct. Foods* **2017**, *37*, 310–321. [CrossRef]
18. Yoshikawa, M.; Morikawa, T.; Yamamoto, K.; Kato, Y.; Nagatomo, A.; Matsuda, H. Floratheasaponins A-C, acylated oleanane-type triterpene oligoglycosides with anti-hyperlipidemic activities from flowers of the tea plant (Camellia sinensis). *J. Nat. Prod.* **2005**, *68*, 1360–1365. [CrossRef]
19. Yoshikawa, M.; Nakamura, S.; Kato, Y.; Matsuhira, K.; Matsuda, H. Medicinal flowers. XIV. New acylated oleanane-type triterpene oligoglycosides with antiallergic activity from flower buds of chinese tea plant (Camellia sinensis). *Chem. Pharm. Bull.* **2007**, *55*, 598–605. [CrossRef]
20. Shen, X.; Shi, L.Z.; Pan, H.B.; Li, B.; Wu, Y.Y.; Tu, Y.Y. Identification of triterpenoid saponins in flowers of four Camellia Sinensis cultivars from Zhejiang province: Differences between cultivars, developmental stages, and tissues. *Ind. Crop. Prod.* **2017**, *95*, 140–147. [CrossRef]
21. Greenshields, A.L.; Shepherd, T.G.; Hoskin, D.W. Contribution of reactive oxygen species to ovarian cancer cell growth arrest and killing by the anti-malarial drug artesunate. *Mol. Carcinog.* **2017**, *56*, 75–93. [CrossRef]
22. Jacobson, M.D. Reactive oxygen species and programmed cell death. *Trends Biochem. Sci.* **1996**, *21*, 83–86. [CrossRef]
23. Mah, L.J.; El-Osta, A.; Karagiannis, T.C. gammaH2AX: A sensitive molecular marker of DNA damage and repair. *Leukemia* **2010**, *24*, 679–686. [CrossRef]
24. Abedini, M.R.; Muller, E.J.; Bergeron, R.; Gray, D.A.; Tsang, B.K. Akt promotes chemoresistance in human ovarian cancer cells by modulating cisplatin-induced, p53-dependent ubiquitination of FLICE-like inhibitory protein. *Oncogene* **2010**, *29*, 11–25. [CrossRef]
25. Dutta, S.; Mahalanobish, S.; Saha, S.; Ghosh, S.; Sil, P.C. Natural products: An upcoming therapeutic approach to cancer. *Food Chem. Toxicol.* **2019**, *128*, 240–255. [CrossRef]
26. Cao, S.; Norris, A.; Miller, J.S.; Ratovoson, F.; Razafitsalama, J.; Andriantsiferana, R.; Rasamison, V.E.; TenDyke, K.; Suh, T.; Kingston, D.G. Cytotoxic triterpenoid saponins of Albizia gummifera from the Madagascar rain forest. *J. Nat. Prod.* **2007**, *70*, 361–366. [CrossRef]
27. Liu, T.; Zhao, L.; Zhang, Y.; Chen, W.; Liu, D.; Hou, H.; Ding, L.; Li, X. Ginsenoside 20(S)-Rg3 targets HIF-1α to block hypoxia-induced epithelial-mesenchymal transition in ovarian cancer cells. *PLoS ONE* **2014**, *9*, 103887. [CrossRef]
28. Nakata, H.; Kikuchi, Y.; Tode, T.; Hirata, J.; Kita, T.; Ishii, K.; Kudoh, K.; Nagata, I.; Shinomiya, N. Inhibitory effects of ginsenoside Rh2 on tumor growth in nude mice bearing human ovarian cancer cells. *Jpn. J. Cancer Res. Gann* **1998**, *89*, 733–740. [CrossRef]
29. Fu, H.Z.; Wan, K.H.; Yan, Q.W.; Zhou, G.P.; Feng, T.T.; Dai, M.; Zhong, R.J. Cytotoxic triterpenoid saponins from the defatted seeds of Camellia oleifera Abel. *J. Asian Nat. Prod. Res.* **2018**, *20*, 412–422. [CrossRef]
30. Jia, L.Y.; Wu, X.J.; Gao, Y.; Rankin, G.O.; Pigliacampi, A.; Bucur, H.; Li, B.; Tu, Y.Y.; Chen, Y.C. Inhibitory Effects of Total Triterpenoid Saponins Isolated from the Seeds of the Tea Plant (Camellia sinensis) on Human Ovarian Cancer Cells. *Molecules* **2017**, *22*, 1649. [CrossRef]
31. Tu, Y.; Kim, E.; Gao, Y.; Rankin, G.O.; Li, B.; Chen, Y.C. Theaflavin-3, 3′-digallate induces apoptosis and G2 cell cycle arrest through the Akt/MDM2/p53 pathway in cisplatin-resistant ovarian cancer A2780/CP70 cells. *Int. J. Oncol.* **2016**, *48*, 2657–2665. [CrossRef]
32. Blagosklonny, M.V. Cell immortality and hallmarks of cancer. *Cell Cycle* **2003**, *2*, 296–299. [CrossRef]
33. Yi, S.; Chen, Y.; Wen, L.; Yang, L.; Cui, G. Expression of connexin 32 and connexin 43 in acute myeloid leukemia and their roles in proliferation. *Oncol. Lett.* **2012**, *4*, 1003–1007. [CrossRef]

34. Tin, M.M.; Cho, C.H.; Chan, K.; James, A.E.; Ko, J.K. Astragalus saponins induce growth inhibition and apoptosis in human colon cancer cells and tumor xenograft. *Carcinogenesis* **2007**, *28*, 1347–1355. [CrossRef]
35. Qian, Y.; Han, Q.H.; Wang, L.C.; Guo, Q.; Wang, X.D.; Tu, P.F.; Zeng, K.W.; Liang, H. Total saponins of Albiziae Cortex show anti-hepatoma carcinoma effects by inducing S phase arrest and mitochondrial apoptosis pathway activation. *J. Ethnopharmacol.* **2018**, *221*, 20–29. [CrossRef]
36. Jang, H.J.; Han, I.H.; Kim, Y.J.; Yamabe, N.; Lee, D.; Hwang, G.S.; Oh, M.; Choi, K.C.; Kim, S.N.; Ham, J.; et al. Anticarcinogenic effects of products of heat-processed ginsenoside Re, a major constituent of ginseng berry, on human gastric cancer cells. *J. Agric. Food Chem.* **2014**, *62*, 2830–2836. [CrossRef]
37. Lim, S.; Kaldis, P. Cdks, cyclins and CKIs: Roles beyond cell cycle regulation. *Development* **2013**, *140*, 3079–3093. [CrossRef]
38. Schwartz, G.K.; Shah, M.A. Targeting the cell cycle: A new approach to cancer therapy. *J. Clin. Oncol.* **2005**, *23*, 9408–9421. [CrossRef]
39. Desdouets, C.; Sobczak-Thépot, J.; Murphy, M.; Bréchot, C. Cyclin A: Function and expression during cell proliferation. *Prog. Cell Cycle Res.* **1995**, *1*, 115–123. [CrossRef]
40. Karimian, A.; Ahmadi, Y.; Yousefi, B. Multiple functions of p21 in cell cycle, apoptosis and transcriptional regulation after DNA damage. *DNA Repair* **2016**, *42*, 63–71. [CrossRef]
41. You, L.; Yang, C.; Du, Y.; Liu, Y.; Chen, G.; Sai, N.; Dong, X.; Yin, X.; Ni, J. Matrine Exerts Hepatotoxic Effects via the ROS-Dependent Mitochondrial Apoptosis Pathway and Inhibition of Nrf2-Mediated Antioxidant Response. *Oxid. Med. Cell Longev.* **2019**, *2019*, 1045345. [CrossRef]
42. Sur, S.; Agrawal, D.K. Phosphatases and kinases regulating CDC25 activity in the cell cycle: Clinical implications of CDC25 overexpression and potential treatment strategies. *Mol. Cell. Biochem.* **2016**, *416*, 33–46. [CrossRef]
43. Dozier, C.; Mazzolini, L.; Cénac, C.; Froment, C.; Burlet-Schiltz, O.; Besson, A.; Manenti, S. CyclinD-CDK4/6 complexes phosphorylate CDC25A and regulate its stability. *Oncogene* **2017**, *36*, 3781–3788. [CrossRef]
44. Fulda, S. Targeting apoptosis for anticancer therapy. *Semin. Cancer Biol.* **2015**, *31*, 84–88. [CrossRef]
45. Riedl, S.J.; Shi, Y. Molecular mechanisms of caspase regulation during apoptosis. *Nat. Rev. Mol. Cell Biol.* **2004**, *5*, 897–907. [CrossRef]
46. Chaitanya, G.V.; Steven, A.J.; Babu, P.P. PARP-1 cleavage fragments: Signatures of cell-death proteases in neurodegeneration. *Cell Commun. Signal. CCS* **2010**, *8*, 31. [CrossRef]
47. Jia, L.T.; Chen, S.Y.; Yang, A.G. Cancer gene therapy targeting cellular apoptosis machinery. *Cancer Treat. Rev.* **2012**, *38*, 868–876. [CrossRef]
48. Lavrik, I.; Golks, A.; Krammer, P.H. Death receptor signaling. *J. Cell Sci.* **2005**, *118*, 265–267. [CrossRef]
49. Brown, G.C.; Borutaite, V. Regulation of apoptosis by the redox state of cytochrome c. *Biochim. Biophys. Acta* **2008**, *1777*, 877–881. [CrossRef]
50. Shakeri, R.; Kheirollahi, A.; Davoodi, J. Apaf-1: Regulation and function in cell death. *Biochimie* **2017**, *135*, 111–125. [CrossRef]
51. Jiang, Y.L.; Liu, Z.P. Natural products as anti-invasive and anti-metastatic agents. *Curr. Med. Chem.* **2011**, *18*, 808–829. [CrossRef]
52. Man, S.; Gao, W.; Zhang, Y.; Huang, L.; Liu, C. Chemical study and medical application of saponins as anti-cancer agents. *Fitoterapia* **2010**, *81*, 703–714. [CrossRef]
53. Verrax, J.; Pedrosa, R.C.; Beck, R.; Dejeans, N.; Taper, H.; Calderon, P.B. In situ modulation of oxidative stress: A novel and efficient strategy to kill cancer cells. *Curr. Med. Chem.* **2009**, *16*, 1821–1830. [CrossRef]
54. Yang, L.; Yuan, Y.; Fu, C.; Xu, X.; Zhou, J.; Wang, S.; Kong, L.; Li, Z.; Guo, Q.; Wei, L. LZ-106, a novel analog of enoxacin, inducing apoptosis via activation of ROS-dependent DNA damage response in NSCLCs. *Free Radic. Biol. Med.* **2016**, *95*, 155–168. [CrossRef]
55. Liu, H.; Zhou, L.; Shi, S.; Wang, Y.; Ni, X.; Xiao, F.; Wang, S.; Li, P.; Ding, K. Oligosaccharide G19 inhibits U-87 MG human glioma cells growth in vitro and in vivo by targeting epidermal growth factor (EGF) and activating p53/p21 signaling. *Glycobiology* **2014**, *24*, 748–765. [CrossRef]
56. Guachalla, L.M.; Rudolph, K.L. ROS induced DNA damage and checkpoint responses: Influences on aging? *Cell Cycle* **2010**, *9*, 4058–4060. [CrossRef]
57. Maréchal, A.; Zou, L. DNA damage sensing by the ATM and ATR kinases. *Cold Spring Harb. Perspect. Biol.* **2013**, *5*. [CrossRef]

58. Zhao, J.; Liao, Y.; Chen, J.; Dong, X.; Gao, Z.; Zhang, H.; Wu, X.; Liu, Z.; Wu, Y. Aberrant Buildup of All-Trans-Retinal Dimer, a Nonpyridinium Bisretinoid Lipofuscin Fluorophore, Contributes to the Degeneration of the Retinal Pigment Epithelium. *Investig. Ophthalmol Vis. Sci.* **2017**, *58*, 1063–1075. [CrossRef]
59. Puente, X.S.; Jares, P.; Campo, E. Chronic lymphocytic leukemia and mantle cell lymphoma: Crossroads of genetic and microenvironment interactions. *Blood* **2018**, *131*, 2283–2296. [CrossRef]
60. Liu, Y.; Wang, L.; Wang, B.; Yue, M.; Cheng, Y. Pathway Analysis Based on Attractor and Cross Talk in Colon Cancer. *Dis. Markers* **2016**, *2016*, 2619828. [CrossRef]
61. Urso, L.; Calabrese, F.; Favaretto, A.; Conte, P.; Pasello, G. Critical review about MDM2 in cancer: Possible role in malignant mesothelioma and implications for treatment. *Crit. Rev. Oncol. Hematol.* **2016**, *97*, 220–230. [CrossRef] [PubMed]
62. Shieh, S.Y.; Ikeda, M.; Taya, Y.; Prives, C. DNA damage-induced phosphorylation of p53 alleviates inhibition by MDM2. *Cell* **1997**, *91*, 325–334. [CrossRef]
63. Zhang, J.; Wu, D.; Xing, Z.; Liang, S.; Han, H.; Shi, H.; Zhang, Y.; Yang, Y.; Li, Q. N-Isopropylacrylamide-modified polyethylenimine-mediated p53 gene delivery to prevent the proliferation of cancer cells. *Colloids Surf. B Biointerfaces* **2015**, *129*, 54–62. [CrossRef] [PubMed]
64. Li, B.; Zhao, J.; Wang, C.Z.; Searle, J.; He, T.C.; Yuan, C.S.; Du, W. Ginsenoside Rh2 induces apoptosis and paraptosis-like cell death in colorectal cancer cells through activation of p53. *Cancer Lett.* **2011**, *301*, 185–192. [CrossRef]
65. Park, E.K.; Lee, E.J.; Lee, S.H.; Koo, K.H.; Sung, J.Y.; Hwang, E.H.; Park, J.H.; Kim, C.W.; Jeong, K.C.; Park, B.K.; et al. Induction of apoptosis by the ginsenoside Rh2 by internalization of lipid rafts and caveolae and inactivation of Akt. *Br. J. Pharm.* **2010**, *160*, 1212–1223. [CrossRef]

Sample Availability: Samples of the compounds BTFS are not available from the authors.

molecules MDPI

Review

Targeting Toxins toward Tumors

Henrik Franzyk and **Søren Brøgger Christensen** *

Department of Drug Design and Pharmacology, University of Copenhagen, Universitetsparken 2, DK-2100 Copenhagen Ø, Denmark; henrik.franzyk@sund.ku.dk
* Correspondence: soren.christensen@sund.ku.dk

Abstract: Many cancer diseases, e.g., prostate cancer and lung cancer, develop very slowly. Common chemotherapeutics like vincristine, vinblastine and taxol target cancer cells in their proliferating states. In slowly developing cancer diseases only a minor part of the malignant cells will be in a proliferative state, and consequently these drugs will exert a concomitant damage on rapidly proliferating benign tissue as well. A number of toxins possess an ability to kill cells in all states independently of whether they are benign or malignant. Such toxins can only be used as chemotherapeutics if they can be targeted selectively against the tumors. Examples of such toxins are mertansine, calicheamicins and thapsigargins, which all kill cells at low micromolar or nanomolar concentrations. Advanced prodrug concepts enabling targeting of these toxins to cancer tissue comprise antibody-directed enzyme prodrug therapy (ADEPT), gene-directed enzyme prodrug therapy (GDEPT), lectin-directed enzyme-activated prodrug therapy (LEAPT), and antibody-drug conjugated therapy (ADC), which will be discussed in the present review. The review also includes recent examples of protease-targeting chimera (PROTAC) for knockdown of receptors essential for development of tumors. In addition, targeting of toxins relying on tumor-overexpressed enzymes with unique substrate specificity will be mentioned.

Keywords: chemotherapy; prodrug; drug targeting; overexpressed enzymes; ADC; ADEPT; GDEPT; LEAPT; PROTAC

Citation: Franzyk, H.; Christensen, S.B. Targeting Toxins toward Tumors. *Molecules* **2021**, *26*, 1292. https://doi.org/10.3390/molecules26051292

Academic Editors: Marialuigia Fantacuzzi and Alessandra Ammazzalorso

Received: 9 January 2021
Accepted: 22 February 2021
Published: 27 February 2021

1. Introduction

According to the International Union of Pure and Applied Chemistry (IUPAC), prodrugs are defined as chemically modified drugs that undergo biological and/or chemical transformation(s) before eliciting pharmacological responses [1]. Drugs may be converted into prodrugs in order to: (i) increase their bioavailability, (ii) target the drugs toward tissues such as tumors, (iii) decrease toxicity, (iv) increase chemical stability, (v) increase solubility, or (vi) mask unpleasant taste [2,3]. Prodrugs are formed by covalent attachment of the drug to a carrier, also often termed as the promoiety, which is subjected to cleavage within the body to release the active drugs. Promoieties and their degradation products should be nontoxic and nonimmunogenic [2]. Pharmacologically inactive compounds, which in the organism are modified into active drugs, are known as bio-precursor prodrugs. Examples of such prodrugs are proguanil that in the liver is converted into the antimalarial drug cycloguanil [4], salicin that is converted into salicylic acid [5], and acetanilide that is converted into acetaminophen [3]. Both salicylic acid and acetaminophen are antipyretics and analgesics. Another class of prodrugs is the co-drugs that consist of two drugs covalently attached to each other—either directly or via a linker in a way so that they act as promoieties for each other [2,6]. Examples of co-drugs comprise sulfasalazine, which in the body is degraded to 5-aminosalicylic acid and sulfapyridine [6,7], and benorylate, which is an ester of acetylsalicylic acid with paracetamol [6].

A review focused on the prodrug approach revealed the state of the art in 2017 [8]. In the present review new developments in the fields of boronic acids as prodrugs, of anthracyclines, and of antibody–drug conjugates, targeting of paclitaxel and refined use of prostate-specific membrane antigen (PSMA) for delivery of payloads are described. The problem of targeting oncogenes for neoplastic tissue in gene-directed enzyme prodrug therapy is discussed (which often has been omitted in previous reviews). Finally, a new group of prodrugs, which link two pharmacophores, i.e., PROtease Targeting Chimeras (PROTACs; [9,10]) and lectin-directed enxym activated prodrugs, are discussed. One of these pharmacophores has a high affinity for an E3 ubiquitin ligase (an enzyme that, with assistance of an E2 ubiquitin-conjugating enzyme, transfers ubiquitin to its protein substrate), while the other has an affinity for the targeted protein e.g., a receptor or ion channel. After binding of the protein and the ubiquitin ligase, the biomolecule will be modified with ubiquitin and subsequently cleaved by a 26S proteasome, which degrades ubiquitinated proteins [9,10].

Thus, the present review comprises the following: (i) prodrugs cleaved in the acidic microenvironment of cancer cells (Section 2.1.1), (ii) prodrugs cleaved by reactive oxygen species (ROS) in cancer cells (Section 2.1.2), (iii) prodrugs cleaved by glutathione (Section 2.1.3), (iv) prodrugs cleaved by enzymes overexpressed in cancer cells (Section 2.1.4), (v) prodrugs cleaved by glucuronidase (Section 2.1.5), (vi) prodrugs cleaved by prostate-specific antigen (PSA) or PSMA (Section 2.1.6), (vii) antibody–drug conjugates (Section 2.2), (viii) antibody-directed enzyme prodrug therapy (Section 2.3), (ix) gene-directed enzyme prodrug therapy (Section 2.4), (x) lectin-directed enzyme-activated prodrug therapy (Section 2.5), and (xi) protease-targeting chimeras (Section 3).

2. Prodrugs

2.1. *Targeting by Selective Cleavage of Prodrugs in the Microenvironment of Cancer Cells*

The metabolism in cancer cells involves a high rate of anaerobic glycolysis resulting in an overproduction of lactic acid and carbonic acid. Since the acid protons of these acids are exported into the extracellular medium, intracellular pH of cancer cells typically is higher (pH 7.4 versus 7.2 in normal cells). [8,11,12]. As a consequence of the proton transport the microenvironment surrounding cancer cells has a pH of 6.8 in contrast to the is estimated pH of blood 7.4 [13]. A high rate of glycolysis without oxygen supply causes hypoxia inside cancer cells [8,11,14,15]. The ensuing rise in the intracellular level of reactive oxygen species (ROS), such as hydrogen peroxide, formed during hypoxia conditions may be employed as a mode of targeting drugs toward cancer cells. Cancer cells also have an increased level of glutathione [16], β-glucuronidase [17], and some specific proteolytic enzymes [17–19].

2.1.1. Prodrugs Cleaved in Acidic Media

Salts of dithiocarbamates (e.g., **1**) are stable at physiological pH, but they will after protonation in the acidic microenvironment surrounding cells undergo cleavage to release the free amine (**2**) and carbondisulfide (Scheme 1). In a similar way the emitine monoamide (**3**) with 2-methylmaleic acid was used to simultaneously increase the solubility of emitine in water and enable its release from the prodrug in slightly acidic media [20].

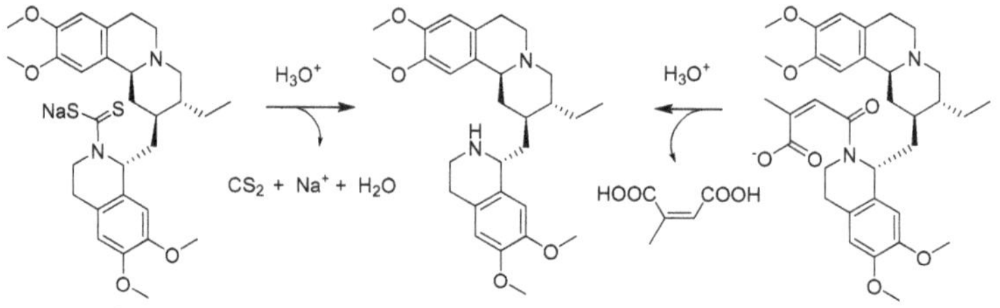

Scheme 1. Dithiocarbamates and methylmaleic amides cleaved at low pH [20].

A prodrug of doxorubicin (DOXO-EMCH, **4**) is linked via a hydrazone promoiety to a maleimide *N*-substituted with a 6-aminohexanoic spacer. This prodrug is designed to enable reaction with Cys-34 of serum albumin (to give **5**), present as the most abundant protein in blood. The resulting albumin-linked drug (**5**) cannot penetrate into cells until the hydrazone is hydrolyzed in the acidic environment around cancer cells to provide the free doxorubicin (**6**; Scheme 2). The clinical phase III trial, however, did not enable registration of the compound as a drug [14,21,22]. Despite these preliminary results, attempts to overcome the cardiotoxicity of DOX-EMCH continue.

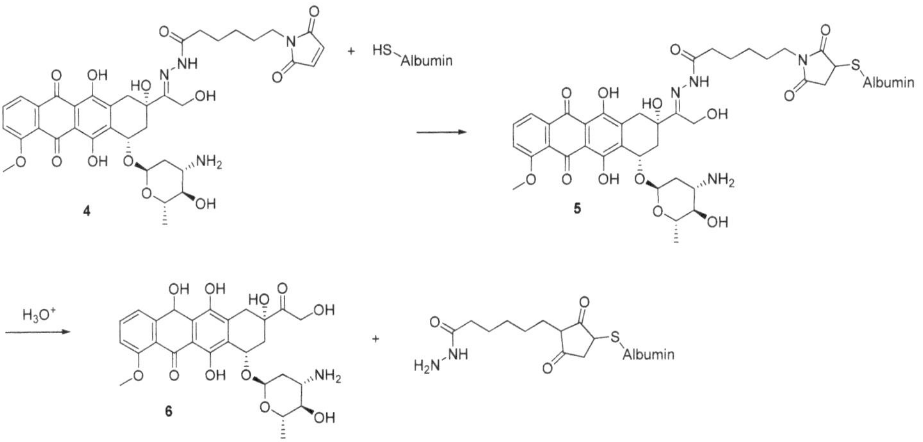

Scheme 2. Linkage of doxorubicin to serum albumin to prevent its penetration into benign cells; only in the acidic microenvironment of cancer cells is doxorubicin released [14,21,22].

Polyethylene glycol-coated liposomes encapsulating doxoxrubicin (Caelyx) show less cardiotoxicity than doxorubicin itself. The drug is used for treatment of breast cancer and ovarian cancer [23].

Paclitaxel is widely used for treatment of various cancers; however, poor solubility limits its use. The formulation vehicle Cremophor EL (CrEL; macrogolglycerol ricinoleate; polyethylene glycol (PEG)-35 castor oil) and ethanol are used to increase its solubility, but unfortunately CrEL causes side effects like hypersensitivity, neurotoxicity and nephrotoxicity [24]. These side effects have been overcome by a new formulation of lyophilized paclitaxel with serum albumin (i.e., Abraxane®) that provides nanoparticles (average size: 130 nm). This drug formulation has been approved by the U. S. Food and Drug Administration (FDA) for treatment of pancreatic cancer and non-small cell lung cancer (NSCLC) [25]. Moreover, paclitaxel (**7**) has been attached to nanoparticles via acetal linkages (**8**). Acetals are cleaved in the acidic environment of cancer cells (Scheme 3) [26]. This method is also used for conjugation of paclitaxel to nanoparticles prepared from polyethylene glycols (PEGs) [13].

2.1.2. Prodrugs Cleaved by ROS

In normal cells, ATP is primarily produced by oxidative phosphorylation, whereas in cancer cells ATP primarily is produced by anaerobic glycolysis (the Warburg effect) [27,28]. The anaerobic pathway stimulates generation of ROS such as hydrogen peroxide [28]. The presence of hydrogen peroxide under certain physiological conditions can be used to facilitate cleavage of arylboronic acids, or esters thereof, to give phenols and boric acid [15]. The concentration of hydrogen peroxide in benign cells is estimated to approx. 1 μM, but in cancer cells it may reach even 10 μM [15]. Some boronic acids are oxidized by cytochrome P450 [15]. Boronic acids may also be oxidized by peroxynitrite [15]. It may be questioned whether arylboronic functionalities act as true promoieties, since the oxidation provides boric acid and the corresponding phenol. As an example, camptothecin-10-boronic (**9**) acid is oxidatively cleaved by hydrogen peroxide to give 10-hydroxycamptothecin (**10**; Scheme 4) [29]. The resulting 10-hydroxycamptothecin (**10**) proved to be a more potent topoisomerase inhibitor, and to be more cytotoxic in a number of cell systems than the original drug. Furthermore, this hydroxylated derivative exhibited tumor growth inhibition in xenograft models [29].

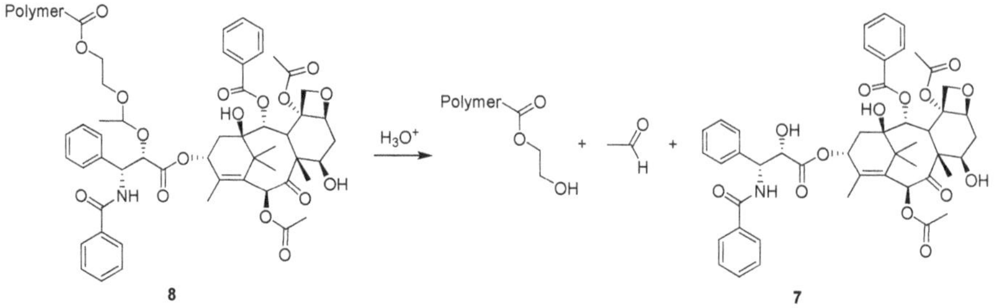

Scheme 3. Conjugation of paclitaxel (**7**) to polymers that increase solubility [26].

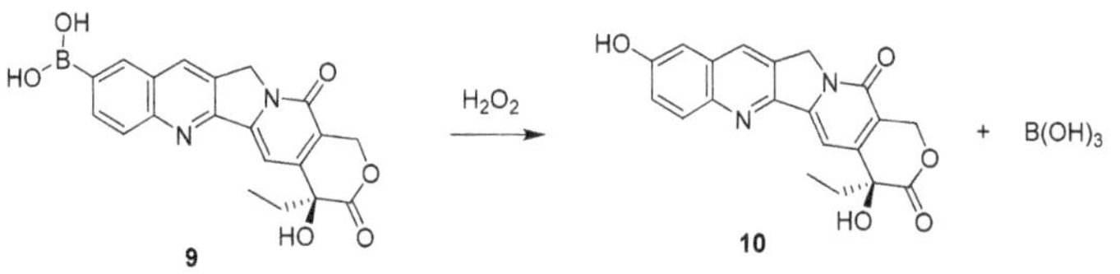

Scheme 4. Oxidation of camptothecin-10-boronic acid (**9**) to give 10-hydroxycamptothecin (**10**) [15].

Arylboronic acid prodrugs of doxorubicin (e.g., **11**) have also been reported. Oxidative cleavage of the boronic acid moiety releases a phenol that spontaneously cleaves itself from the self-immolative spacer 4-hydroxybenzyl carbamate (**12**; Scheme 5) [15]. Doxorubicin (**6**) very efficiently kills cancer cells, however, a severe cardiotoxicity limits its use as a chemotherapeutic drug [30]. Targeting of the drug may reduce this side effect. The prodrug was found to induce regression of pancreatic tumors in mice, and further analysis revealed that the prodrug was cleaved to doxorubicin inside tumors (Scheme 5) [31].

Similarly, an aryl boronic acid prodrug (**13**) of paclitaxel (**7**), also containing a self-immolative linker, has been reported (Scheme 6) [15]. The size of the PEG moiety was adjusted so that the prodrug self-assembles into micelles with a size of ca. 50 nm. Native paclitaxel (**7**) was only released in the acidic microenvironment of the cells containing a high level of ROS. Consequently, reduced toxicity of the prodrug as compared to treatment with paclitaxel was observed in mice while retaining similar tumor regression [32]. At present no boronic acid prodrugs have been approved, despite intensive research being performed in the field [15].

2.1.3. Prodrugs Cleaved by Glutathione

Glutathione (H-γGlu-Cys-Gly-OH) is present in almost all mammalian tissues, but usually it is overexpressed in cancer cells [33]. The active functionality of glutathione is the thiol, which enables the molecule to participate in redox reactions, and may thus protect the cell from a high level of ROS [33]. The molecule is able to cleave disulfides including linkages within prodrugs. Hence, this feature has been utilized in the construction of prodrugs attached to a promoiety via a disulfide linkage, and e.g., camptothecin (**14**) has been linked to a near-infrared (NIR) dicyanomethylenebenzopyran fluorophore (**15**; Scheme 7). An in vivo experiment using a mouse BCap-37 tumor xenograft model showed a significantly improved regression of tumors on mice treated with the prodrug as compared to that found for those treated with camptothecin or another prodrug in which the linkage consisted of a stable carbon–carbon bond instead of the disulfide bond [16].

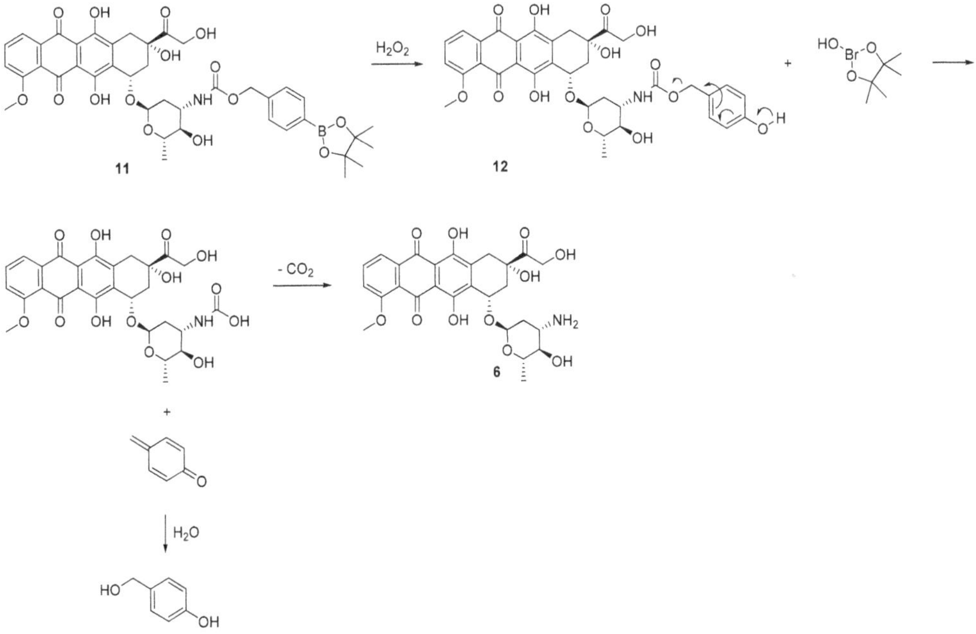

Scheme 5. Prodrug of doxorubicin (**6**) cleaved by ROS [15].

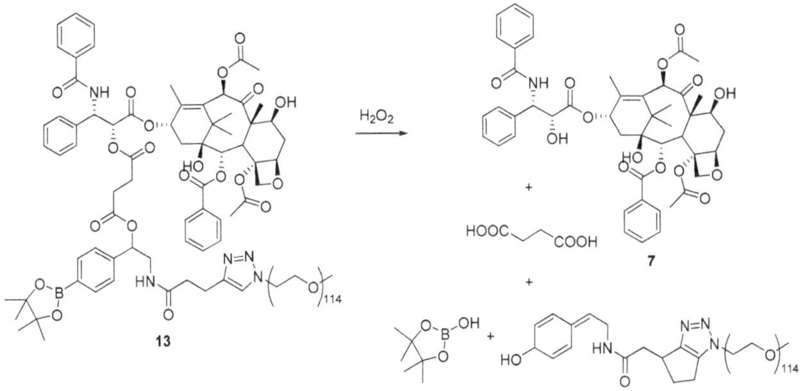

Scheme 6. Polyethylene glycol (PEG)-containing prodrug (**13**) of paclitaxel (**7**) that is cleaved by reactive oxygen species (ROS) [13].

2.1.4. Prodrugs Cleaved by Expressed Enzymes

A number of enzymes are overexpressed in cancer cells. These enzymes include oxidoreductases, hydrolases, and matrix metalloproteinases (MMPs) [8]. A prodrug based on the overexpression of MMPs was designed for doxorubicin (Scheme 8) [34]. The peptide promoiety conjugated to the amine in doxorubicin prevents entry into cells, and consequently the compound is harmless to benign cells. By contrast, in the microenvironment of cancer cells the peptide is cleaved at the Gly-hPhe position. Proteases subsequently remove the remaining amino acids. In a HT1080 xenograft mouse preclinical model, the prodrug was more efficient in reducing tumor growth than doxorubicin itself, and less undesired toxicity was observed [34].

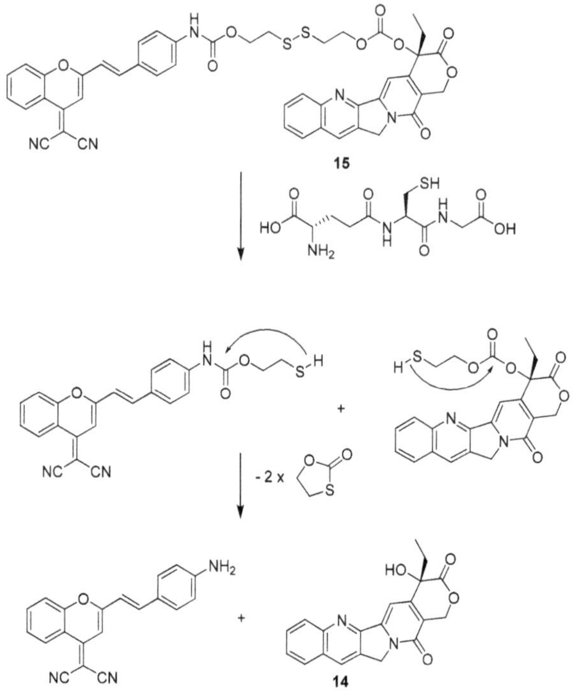

Scheme 7. Prodrug (i.e., **15**) of camptothecin (**14**) that is cleaved by glutathione [16].

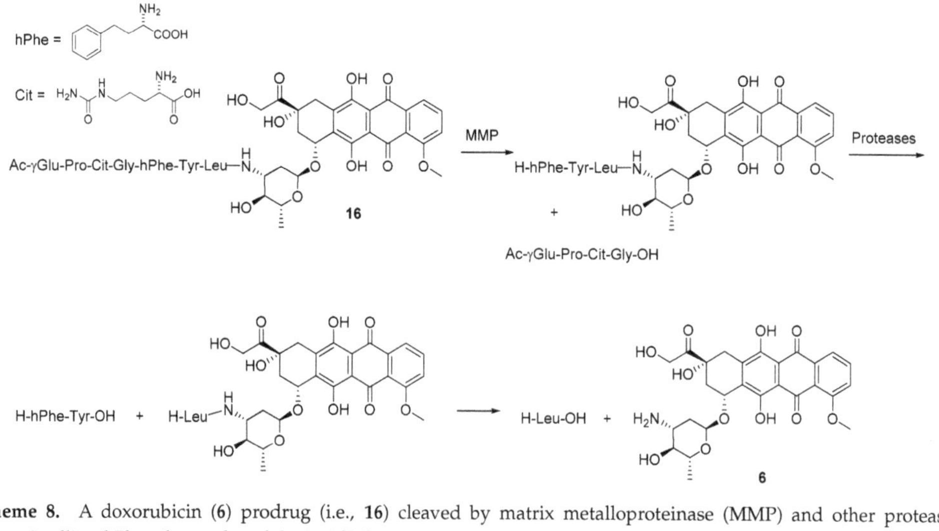

Scheme 8. A doxorubicin (**6**) prodrug (i.e., **16**) cleaved by matrix metalloproteinase (MMP) and other proteases (Cit = citrulline; hPhe = homophenylalanine) [34].

Cathepsin B is involved in cancer invasion and metastasis, and it is overexpressed in cancer tissue [35]. A prodrug (**17**) consisting of doxorubicin conjugated via the self-immolative linker 4-aminobenzyl alcohol to a dipeptide fragment (Ac-Phe-Lys-OH), which is a substrate for cathepsin B, has been designed (Scheme 9). In a mouse model this prodrug inhibited development of peritoneal carcinomatosis as well as its progression more efficiently and with fewer side effects than doxorubicin itself [35].

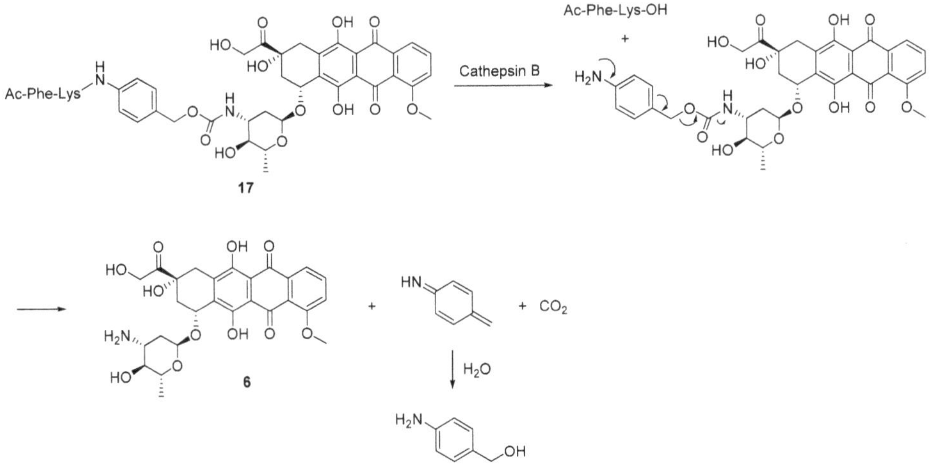

Scheme 9. Prodrug of doxorubicin (i.e., **17**) that is cleaved by cathepsin B [35].

2.1.5. Prodrugs Cleaved by β-glucuronidase

Glucuronides are formed as a phase II metabolism of drugs. β-Glucuronidases are expressed excessively in a number of tumors such as breast, lung and gastrointestinal tract carcinomas as well as in melanomas, where they are particularly abundant in necrotic areas [17,36,37]. Prodrugs based on this selective enzyme distribution include glucuronides of doxorubicin (**6**) and 4′-epi-doxorubicin (**19**) [17]. A self-immolative linker was introduced, since the β-glucuronide (i.e., **18**) conjugated directly to the sugar part of doxorubicin was not a substrate for β-glucuronidase (Scheme 10) [17].

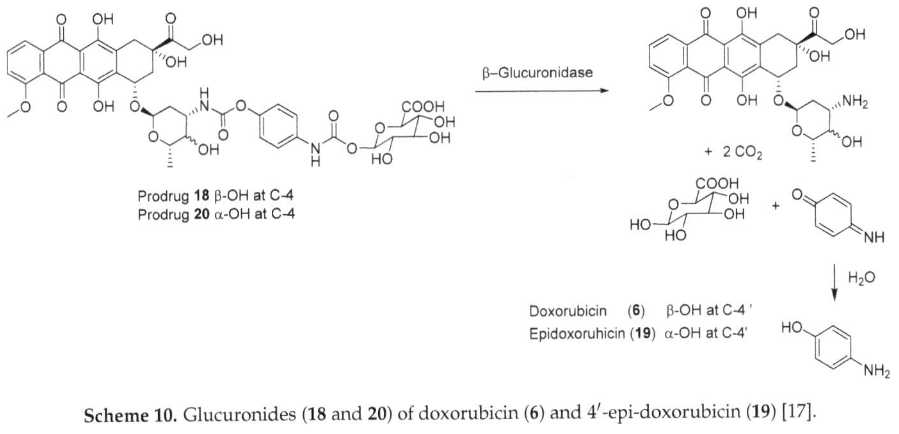

Scheme 10. Glucuronides (**18** and **20**) of doxorubicin (**6**) and 4′-epi-doxorubicin (**19**) [17].

In an attempt to circumvent the poor solubility of paclitaxel (**7**) in water a glucuronide (i.e., **21**) was made. The resulting glucuronide (**21**) proved indeed to be soluble in water, and it was rapidly converted into paclitaxel (**7**) in the presence of high concentrations of β-glucuronidase (Scheme 11) [38].

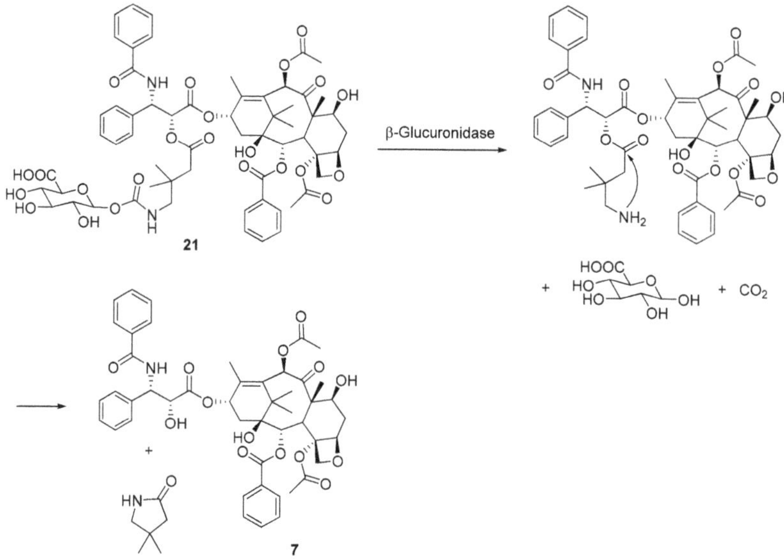

Scheme 11. Water-soluble glucuronide-based prodrug (**21**) of paclitaxel (**7**) [38].

Likewise, 7-Aminocamptothecin was conjugated to glucuronic acid via another self-immolative linker (Scheme 12).

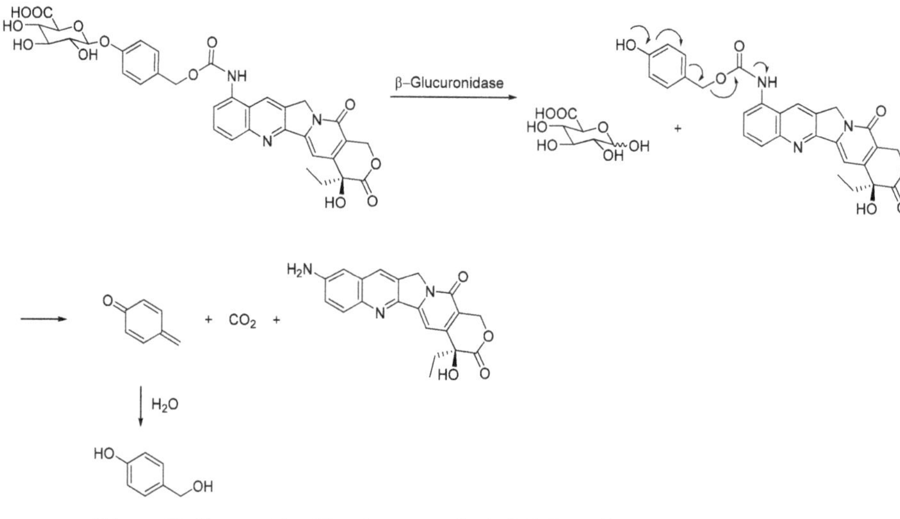

Scheme 12. Glucuronide of 7-aminocamptothecin (**23**) cleaved by β-glucuronidase [39].

2.1.6. Prodrugs Cleaved by PSA or PSMA

Prostate cancer is a slowly developing cancer disease. In high-income countries it is the cancer disease that causes second-most deaths among men. In its initial stages the disease can be treated with androgen ablation therapy. However, if progression of disease occurs during treatment with anti-androgens, resulting in development of distant metastasis, the prostate cancer is defined as metastatic Castration-Resistant Prostate Cancer (mCRPC) which is not sensitive to hormone ablation [40]. All tumors of mCRPCs secrete the enzyme prostate-specific antigen (PSA) into their microenvironment. PSA is a chymotrypsin-like protease with a unique substrate specificity [18]. PSA also diffuses into the bloodstream, but PSA in the blood is inactivated by complexing with blood proteins like serum albumin [40]. Conjugation of cytotoxins with different selectively labile peptides has been used for targeting of mCRPCs. Thus, *O*-desacetylvinblastine (**24**) has been targeted to mCRPCs by conjugation to a PSA-specific peptide substrate to give a prodrug (i.e., **25**) (Scheme 13) [19].

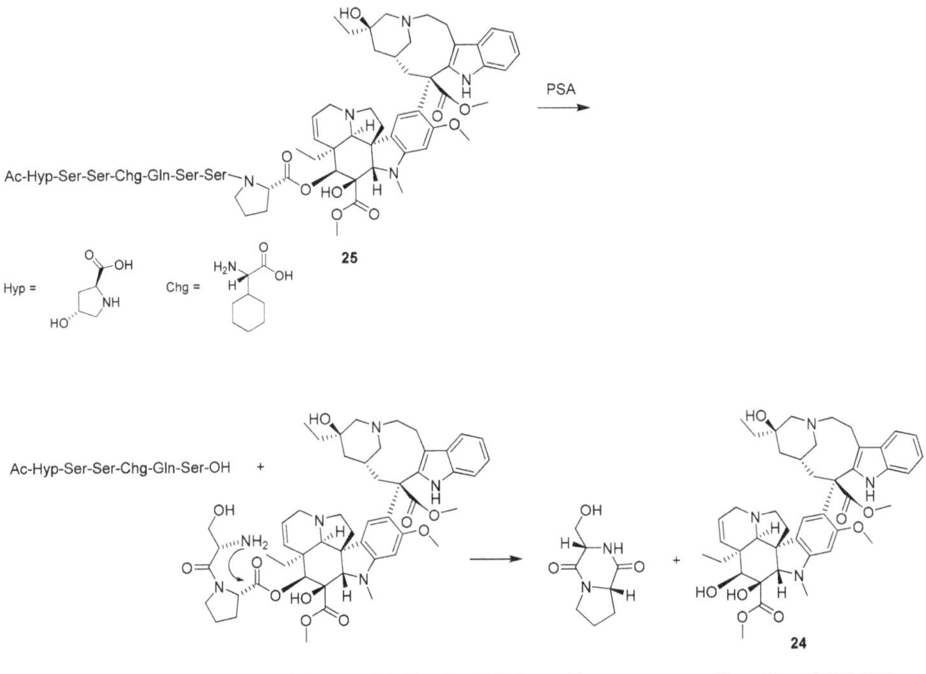

Scheme 13. Prodrug (i.e., **25**) of desacetylvinblastine (**24**) cleaved by prostate-specific antigen (PSA) [19].

PSA cleaves the peptide between the two Ser residues adjacent to the C-terminal Pro residue, whereupon a spontaneous intramolecular attack of the amino group of the terminal Ser on the Pro carboxylate affords desacetylvinblastine (**24**) and a diketopiperazine. This intramolecular diketopiperazine formation appeared to depend on the presence of the Pro residue, as it did not occur when Leu was incorporated instead. Desacetylvinblastine (**24**) proved equally efficient in inducing mitotic arrest as the original vinblastine (Scheme 13) [19].

A number of peptides have been conjugated to doxorubicin (**6**) [41]. Among these different promoities the peptide H_2N-Glu-Hyp-Ala-Ser-Chg-Ser-Leu-OH was found to afford a prodrug that was efficiently cleaved by PSA, and it showed a dramatically increased activity in reducing LNCaP xenografts in mice as compared to that of native doxorubicin (**6**). The released active drug consists of a mixture of doxorubicin and H-Leu-doxorubicin (Scheme 14) [41].

A drawback of using vinblastine or doxorubicin (**6**) as drugs for treatment of prostate cancer is that both compounds cause mitotic arrest, and consequently they primarily target proliferating cells. A more pronounced cell death is expected when toxins capable of killing cells in all stages are used. Thapsigargin (**27**) is a cytotoxic compound that kills cells in all states by blocking the sarco/endoplasmic reticulum Ca^{2+} ATPase (SERCA), thereby inducing the unfolded protein response leading to apoptosis [42]. The general toxicity of the compound requires targeting via a prodrug in order to avoid general systemic toxicity [43]. No obvious anchoring point for conjugation to a peptide exists in native thapsigargin, but replacement of the butanoyl moiety with a 12-aminododecanoic acid spacer (to give **28**) allows for introduction of an amine functionality that may serve as attachment point for a peptide promoiety (Scheme 15).

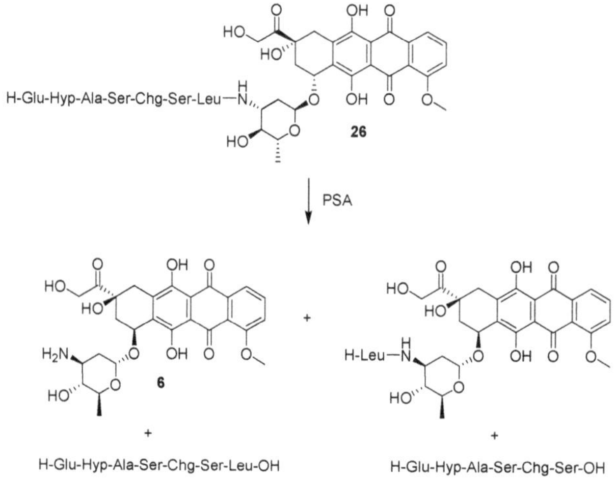

Scheme 14. Doxorubicin prodrug (**26**) cleaved by PSA [41].

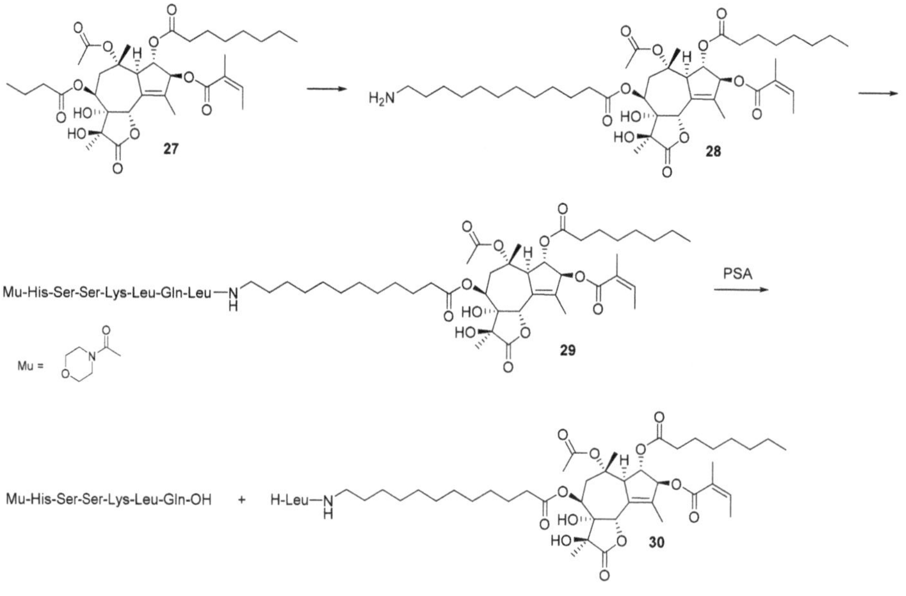

Scheme 15. Prodrug of ω-aminododecanolydesbutanoylthapsigargin (**28**) cleaved by PSA [43].

Conjugation of a thapsigargin analogue to a polar peptide was expected to inhibit diffusion into cells, thereby preventing the prodrug from reaching the intracellular SERCA pump. The hexapeptide H-His-Ser-Ser-Lys-Leu-Gln-OH is very efficiently released from the prodrug by PSA, but only to a limited extent by any other proteases in the human body [18]. The C-terminal Leu residue was introduced in order to make the prodrug a substrate for PSA. In vivo experiments in mice confirmed that the prodrug was only cleaved in the blood to a limited extent, but very efficiently cleaved by PSA to release the active Leu derivative within tumors. Thus, this prodrug prevented growth of tumors in mice [44].

KLK2 is another enzyme (previously named human kallikrein 2, hK2) that may be used for targeting drugs toward prostate cancers [45,46]. Similarly to PSA, KLK2 is also secreted from the prostate and prostate cancer cells. The level of KLK2 in blood can be used as a biomarker for prostate cancer, and KLK2 is inactivated upon entering the bloodstream by binding to blood proteins [47].

An alternative enzyme, characteristic for the prostate glandule, is prostate-specific membrane antigen (PSMA). The catalytic site of this enzyme extends outwards into the extracellular environment. The enzyme is not only expressed in the prostate glandule, but also in human prostatic carcinoma and in neovascular tissue of a number of tumors [48,49]. In a healthy individual the enzyme is exclusively expressed in the prostate, ensuring that cleavage of the peptide conjugated to its payload solely occurs in the prostata glandula [49–53]. As the only enzyme outside the central nervous system PSMA cleaves the amide linkage in the γ-Glu tetramer [54]. Taking advantage of this feature, a prodrug of the 12-aminododeanoate of desbutanoylthapsigargin (**28**), (i.e., mipsagargin, **31**) was made (Scheme 16). The C-terminal βAsp residue was introduced in order to make the prodrug a substrate for PSMA [49]. This prodrug, which has been prepared by solid-phase synthesis [55], was cleaved rapidly in tumors to release the βAsp derivative, which slowly was cleaved to provide the free mipsagargin. A solid-phase synthesis of these guaianolide prodrugs were developed [55].

In the clinical phase II trial this prodrug conferred a prolonged stabilization of the disease in patients with hepatocellular carcinoma [56]. Hepatocellular cancer also expresses PSMA in neovascular tissue, which thus should be sensitive to mipsagargin [57]. However, the results obtained in clinical phase II trial did not meet the expectations, and hence the drug was not marketed [58]. A major problem might be that the prodrug, despite its five negative charges on its peptide side chains, has been found to be able to penetrate cell membranes in benign cells, thereby causing unspecific toxicity [59].

2.2. *Antibody–Drug Conjugates (ADCs)*

An antibody–drug conjugate (ADC) is a prodrug consisting of a monoclonal antibody conjugated to a cytotoxin (i.e., the payload) via a linker. The prodrug is designed based on the hypothesis that appropriate antibodies that preferentially bind to cancer-specific antigens (located on the surface of cancer cells) can be obtained. Indeed, the two first ADCs, Adcetris® (brentuximab vedotin) for Hodgkin lymphoma and Kadcyla® (trastuzumab emtansine) for breast cancer, were approved by the FDA in 2011 and in 2013, respectively. Since then six additional ADCs have been approved by the FDA (i.e., Besponsa® (inotuzumab ozogamicin), Mylotarg® (gemtuzumab ozogamicin), Polivy®, Enhertu®, Padcev®, and Trodelvy®) [61]. More than 60 ADC prodrugs are under clinical development [62–64].

The linker should be stable in circulation to avoid release of free cytotoxin causing systemic toxicity, as is often seen with conventional chemotherapeutics (Figure 1).

Monoclonal antibodies of rodent origin may cause severe immunogenic reactions in humans. The use of chimeric humanized antibodies has to some extent solved this problem [65].

The ideal cytotoxin should be very toxic since only a limited number of antigens are present on the surface of malignant cells, and consequently only a limited number of ADCs can be internalized to exert the cytotoxic effect [66]. A number of toxins have been used as payloads, e.g., the peptide monomethyl auristatin E, the polyketide macrolides ansamitocin (as a mixture of aliphatic alkyl esters) and maytansins (= maitansins) as well as doxorubicin

(**6**), duocarmycin (**32**), and enediynes like calicheamicin γ_1^{I} (**33**) have been converted into ADCs (Figure 2) [61,63].

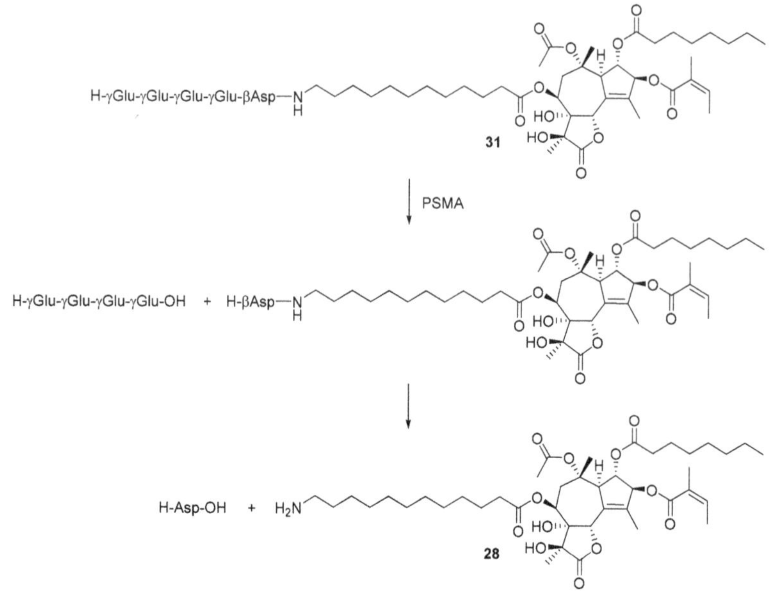

Scheme 16. The PSMA-sensitive prodrug mipsagargin (**31**) [56,60].

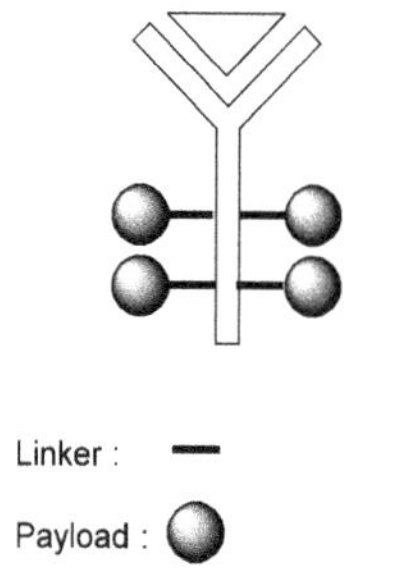

Figure 1. Cartoon illustrating the structure of an antibody–drug conjugate (ADC) drug.

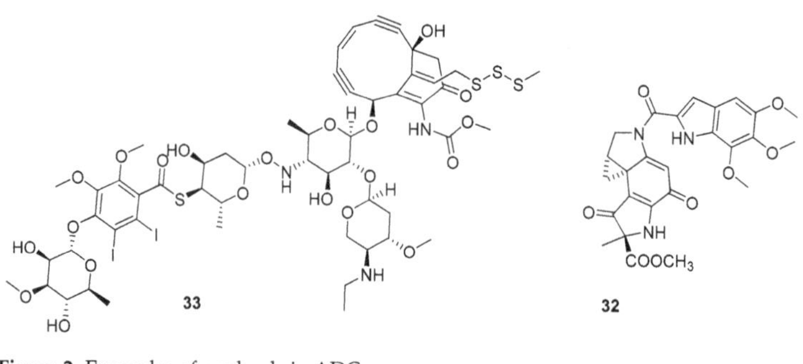

Figure 2. Examples of payloads in ADCs.

The calicheamycins is a group of extremely potent cytotoxins. Originally the compounds were tested as antibiotics, and their minimum inhibitory cancentration (MIC) values were found to be from 0.5 µg/mL toward *Eschericia coli* to less than 0.2 ng/mL against *Bacillus subtilis* [67]. Antitumor activity was tested against P388 leukemia and B16 melanoma in mice by intraperitoneal injection. The optimum dose was found to be 5 µg/kg as compared to 1.6 mg/kg for cisplatin against P388 cells, and 1.25 µg/kg as compared to 300 mg/kg for cisplatin against B16 cells [67]. All mice died, indicating a high general toxicity. Calicheamicin $\gamma_1{}^{I}$ is an interesting payload because of its extreme cytotoxicity [66]. This molecule represents an extraordinary example of natural bioengineering that has occurred during evolution. The sugar part including the iodinated aromatic residue confers affinity for DNA. After complexing with DNA, a nucleophilic attack, e.g., by glutathione on the central sulfur in the trisulfide, leads to the cleavage of this linkage, thereby releasing the free thiol, which undergoes an intramolecular thiol Michael addition to the α,β-unsaturated ketone. By changing the trigonal bridgehead β-carbon to a tetragonal carbon, sufficient tension is induced in the 10-membered ring to initiate a Bergman cyclization. The resulting intermediate diradical finally cleaves the DNA [66] (Scheme 17).

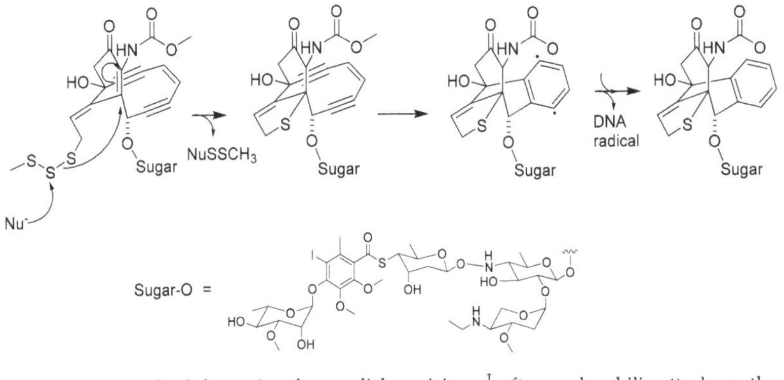

Scheme 17. Diradical formation from calicheamicin $\gamma_1{}^{I}$ after nucleophilic attack on the α,β-unsaturated ketone [66].

In particular two functional groups are used for conjugation of drugs via a linker to the antibody, namely the thiol group of cysteine and/or the amino groups of lysine residues [61]. Traut's reagent or carbodiimides with or without hydroxysuccinimide have been used for coupling of a carboxylic acid to lysine side chains [63]. As an example, Scheme 18 depicts how calicheamicin $\gamma_1{}^{I}$ (**33**) has been coupled to an antibody in Mylotarg (gemtuzumab ozogamicin) [63].

After internalization of the antibody–antigen complex, enzymes within the cell facilitate hydrolysis of the hydrazone moiety [63]. The disulfide will be cleaved by glutathione, enabling Bergman cyclization. Other linkers have been designed to be cleaved by intracellular proteases like cathepsin B (e.g., Adcetris). After internalization of the ADC Kadcyla, in which mertansine (**34**) is linked to an antibody, the linker including the lysine residue remains attached to the payload after decomposition of the antibody (Scheme 19). This extended linker moiety appears not to compromise the effect of the drug. Other examples of ADCs have been reported by Nicolaou and Rigol [63].

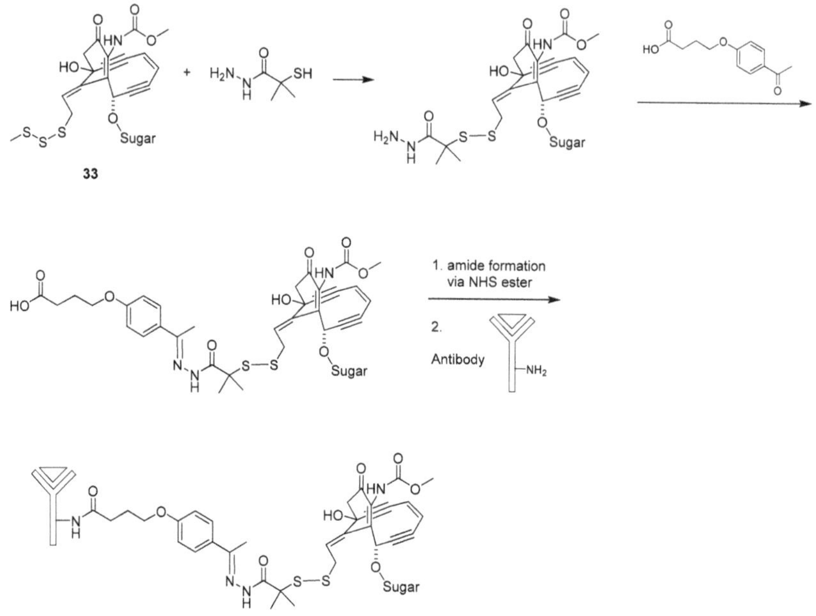

Scheme 18. Coupling of a calicheamicin to antibodies via lysine residues (the O-Sugar moiety is defined in Scheme 17) [63].

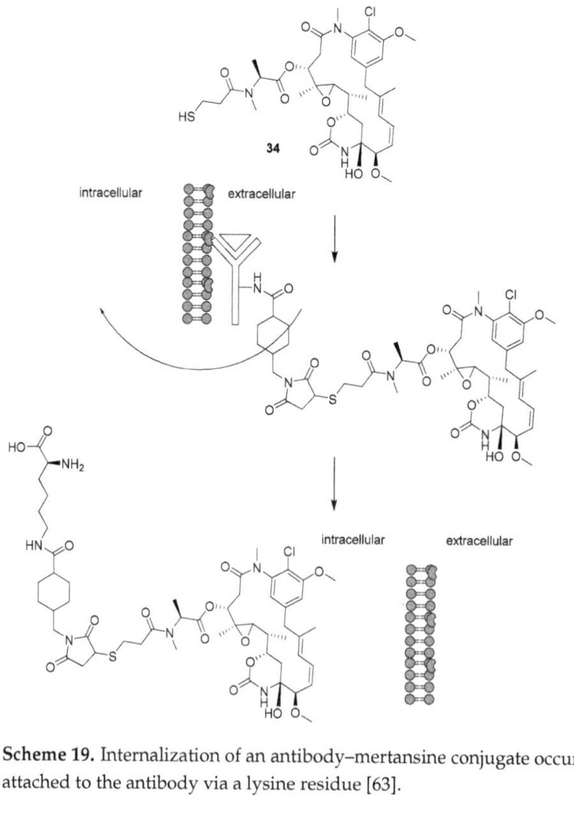

Scheme 19. Internalization of an antibody–mertansine conjugate occurs while the payload remains attached to the antibody via a lysine residue [63].

2.3. *Antibody-Directed Enzyme Prodrug Therapy*

Similarly to ADCs, the concept of antibody-directed prodrug therapy (ADEPT) is based on the ability of antibodies to selectively target antigens expressed abundantly on the surface of cancer cells [68,69]. The principle involves a preferential binding of a non-human enzyme to the surface of cancer cells via an antibody–antigen complex. The choice of a non-human enzyme makes it possible to choose a linker which solely is cleaved by this enzyme and not by any endogenous enzymes. On the other hand, a potential drawback of using a non-human enzyme may be a strong allergic reaction due to unforeseen immunogenicity. In contrast to the ADC approach, non-internalizing antigens can be targeted. The enzyme is linked to the antibody by using a bisfunctional linker, where one functionality can be linked to the lysine side chains present on the enzyme, while the other functionality can be linked to thiols of cysteines on the antibody (Figure 3) [68–70]. After administration to the patient the antibody binds to the surface of the cancer cell. When the excess free antibody–enzyme conjugate is completely cleared from the body the prodrug is administered.

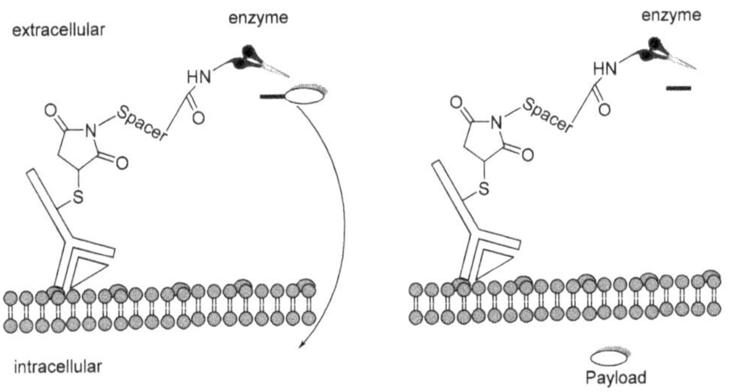

Figure 3. Antibody–enzyme conjugate bound to antigens on the surface of malignant cells.

As mentioned above, a prerequisite for the use of enzymes not present in the human body is that they are non-immunogenic [70]. Enzymes belonging to the families of alkaline phosphatases (cleaving phosphate from prodrugs), peptidases, sulfatases (for cleavage of sulfate monoesters), carboxylesterases and carboxypeptidases (for cleavage of e.g., glutamic amides), have been investigated in this respect [70].

Some antibodies themselves possess catalytic properties, e.g., the antibody 38C2 catalyzes retroaldol and retro-Mannich reactions; for example, a prodrug of doxoxrubicin is cleaved by 38C2 (Scheme 20). [70,71].

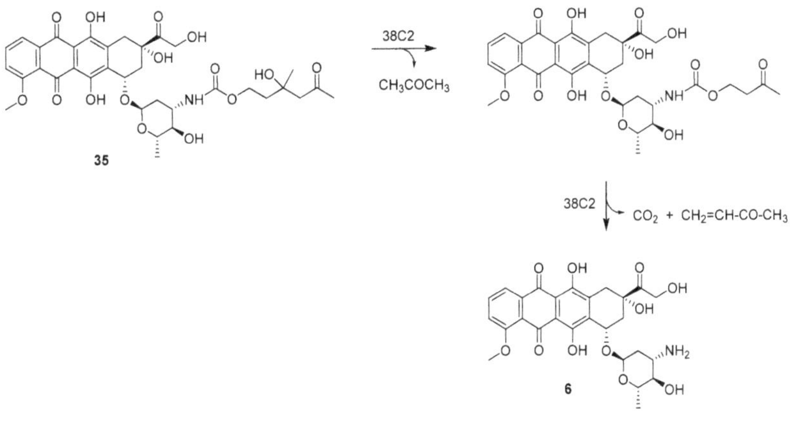

35

6

Scheme 20. Doxorubicin prodrug (**35**) cleaved by 38C2 [70,71].

Even though some promising clinical results have been obtained, no drugs based on ADEPT are in clinical use at present [68,69].

2.4. Gene-Directed Enzyme Prodrug Therapy (GEPDT)

In gene-directed enzyme prodrug therapy (GEPDT), a gene encoding for a unique enzyme is introduced into the tumor cells by using a vector. The technique was already introduced in 1986, and the gene introduced into cells is called a suicide gene [72]. Upon expression of the enzyme on the cancer cell surface, the enzyme enables cleavage of the linkage between the payload and the promoiety, after which the payload may diffuse into the cancer cell (Figure 4) [69,70]. A major drawback in GDEPT is the prerequisite of achieving selective transfer of a gene into malign cells. Retroviruses, adenoviruses and herpes viruses have been studied as potential vectors [73]. Retroviral vectors have some selectivity, since they are only incorporated into the genome of actively dividing cells [73]. Attachment of tissue-specific promoters may allow for transgenic expression only in neoplastic cells. The use of receptor-specific vectors has also been proposed [73]. Mesenchymal stem cells, exhibiting strong tropism toward tumors and metastases expressing receptors on their surface, can efficiently be transduced with vectors [72]. Virus-like particles have also been used to internalize the gene into cells [74]. No drugs based on the principle of GDEPT have been approved so far.

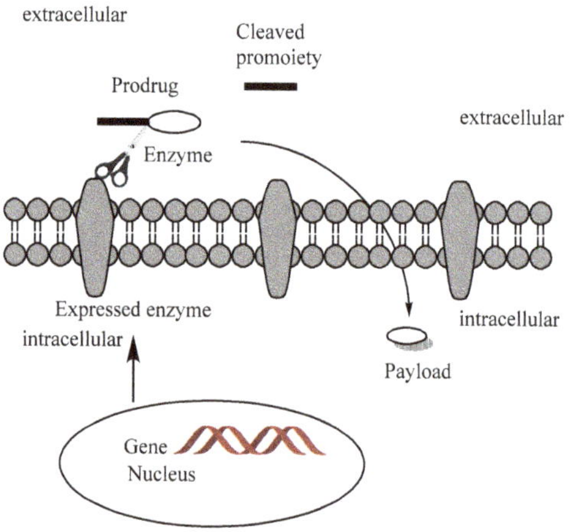

Figure 4. Cartoon illustrating the principle of gene-directed enzyme prodrug therapy (GEPDT) [69,70].

2.5. Lectin-Directed Enzyme-Activated Prodrug Therapy (LEAPT)

In lectin-directed enzyme-activated prodrug therapy (LEAPT), a drug or an enzyme is targeted toward cancer cells by using sugar–protein recognition, whereas antigen–antibody recognition is used for targeting in ADEPT and GDEPT. Lectins are proteins involved in biological carbohydrate recognition comprising cellular processes such as growth, differentiation, proliferation or apoptosis [75]. In order to improve the selectivity of doxorubicin, a galacturonamide derivative (i.e., **36**) was prepared (Figure 5) [76]. Here, the expression of asialoglycoprotein receptors (ASGPRs) 1 and 2 on the surface of hepatocytes with a high affinity for D-galactose and L-rhamnose was exploited. After binding to the receptor, the appropriate carbohydrate-containing ligand is internalized. The ASGPRs are expressed on the surface of HT-29, MCF-7 and A549 cells to a much higher extent than in normal liver cells [76]. The Gal-Dox derivative proved to exhibit higher selectivity toward cancer cell lines than doxorubicin (**6**) itself. In S180 tumor-bearing mice, the Gal-Dox-treated group had a higher accumulation of the drug in the malignant tissue than the doxorubicin-treated group as well as an improved survival rate [76]. However, in this case the doxorubicin derivative may in fact not be a true prodrug, since probably the Gal derivative may also interact with the topoisomerase target.

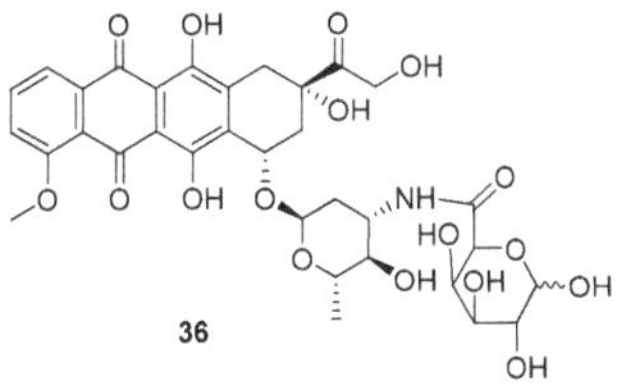

36

Figure 5. Galacturonamide of doxorubicin (**36**) for lectin-directed enzyme-activated prodrug therapy (LEAPT) [76].

Another approach utilizes the overexpression of glucose transporters (GLUT) in cancer tissue. By preparing glucose or glucuronic acid derivatives of paclitaxel, two advantages are obtained: (i) the compounds become more soluble in water, and (ii) increased uptake through the GLUT into the cancer tissue (Figure 6) [77].

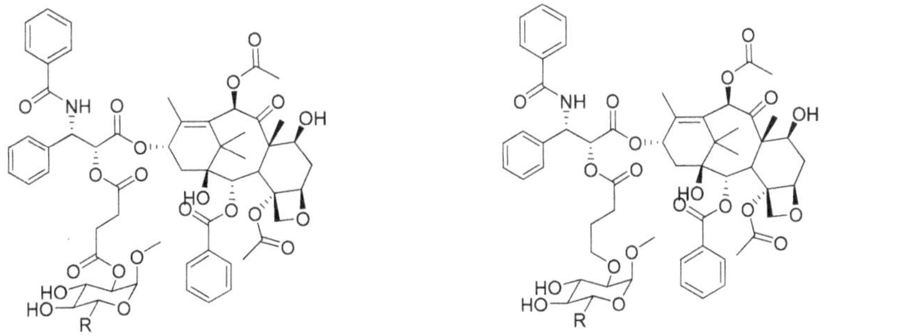

R = CH_2OH (**37**)
R = COOH (**38**)

R = CH_2OH (**39**)
R = COOH (**40**)

Figure 6. Glucose and glucuronic acid derivatives (i.e., **37** and **38**) of paclitaxel (**7**) displaying improved selectivity via LEAPT [77].

The glucose and glucuronic acid derivatives (**37** and **38**) were found to exert a low cytotoxicity on benign cells, but an activity similar to that of paclitaxel (**7**) itself on cell lines expressing GLUT. It is assumed that the prodrug is cleaved by intracellular β-glucosidases. A mechanism involving cleavage of the methyl glucoside followed by self-immolative cleavage to give paclitaxel (**7**) has been proposed [77]. However, the glucose derivative reported was an α-glycoside.

A two-phase LEAPT mechanism overcoming the requirement for intracellular cleavage of the prodrug has been suggested. In the first phase a glycosylated enzyme interacts with a carbohydrate-recognizing lectin on the surface of the cells in the targeted tissue. After similar interactions, a glycosylated prodrug, which is a substrate for the glycosylated enzyme, becomes internalized as well. Inside the cells, the internalized enzyme cleaves the glycosylated prodrug to liberate the active drug (Scheme 21).

A procedure for pergalactosylation of a naringinase produced by *Penicillium decumbens* has been developed to give a pergalactosylated enzyme, which showed high affinity for ASGPRs on the surface of hepatocytes. Binding to ASPGR triggers internalization of the bound ligand. The naringinase possesses α-rhamnosidase and β-glucosidase activities. Thus, a rhamnose derivative of doxorubicin (**6**) was prepared, and the stability of this derivative was tested [78]. At present, no drugs based on the LEAPT principle have been approved.

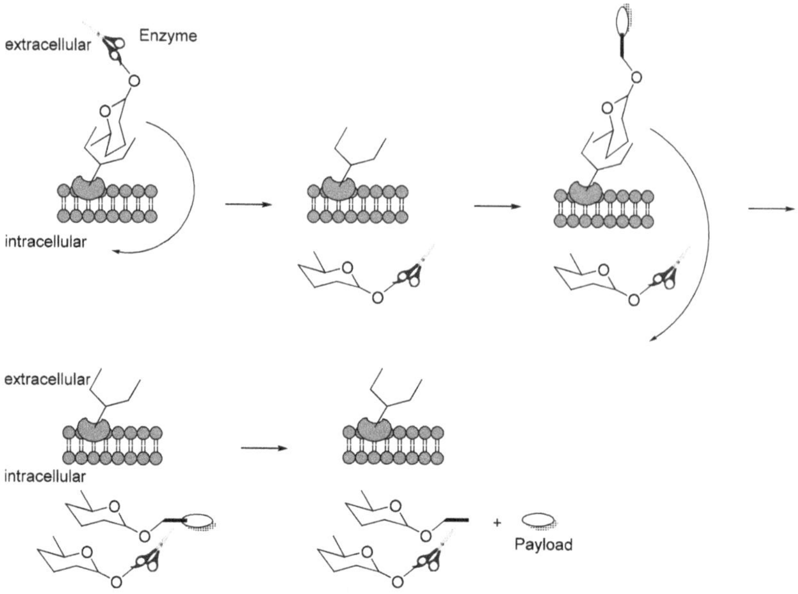

Scheme 21. Two-phase LEAPT. First a glycosylated enzyme binds to the cell surface and becomes internalized. Secondly, a glycosylated prodrug binds to the surface, and is then internalized whereafter it is cleaved by the internalized enzyme [78].

3. Protease-Targeting Chimeras (PROTAC)

In living cells, misfolded, damaged or mutated proteins are removed from the cells by natural processes, in which the protein first becomes covalently bound to one of a number of ubiquitins, which are highly conserved 76-residue peptides [79]. This conjugation process involves ubiquitin-activating enzymes E1, which transfer ubiquitin to E2 from where ubiquitin is transferred to a von Hippel–Lindau(VHL)-cullin-RING ligase complex including E3 that conjugates ubiquitin to the target protein mainly via lysine residues [9,10]. Subsequently, the ubiquitin-modified protein is degraded by a 26S proteasome to give a number of small peptides and a number of lysine-modified ubiquitins [9,10,80]. Other proteases finally cleave the oligopeptides into free amino acids [81].

Advantages of this system are that drugs may be developed to selectively remove intracellular proteins. A chimera consisting of a residue with high affinity for the VHL complex was via a linker attached to a moiety with high affinity for the estrogen-related receptor α (ERRα). After complexing with VHL, knockdown of the ERRα level was observed. The first experiment was performed in MCF7 cells after incubation with the chimeras to knock down ERRα [9]. Moreover, a serine-threonine kinase (RIPK2) was knocked down after incubation of MCF7 cells with a chimera consisting of a moiety with high affinity for the VHL complex (Figure 7) [9].

The effect of small-molecule drugs as ligands for biomolecules in treatment of cancer diseases can be limited by mutations in the gene encoding the biomolecule, thereby making the modified target insensitive to the agent. Such mutations are observed for the epidermal growth factor receptors and androgen receptors [82]. PROTAC has been used to enable knockdown of steroid receptors and for non-small lung cancer by knockdown of epidermal growth factor. In addition, the anaphylactic lymphoma kinase can similarly be removed as a possible treatment of different types of human cancers [82]. The PROTAC technique is still at an early stage, and at present no such drugs are currently in clinical use.

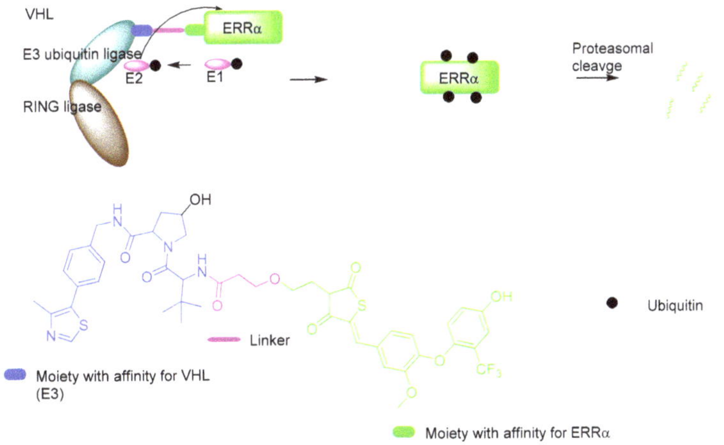

Figure 7. Cartoon illustrating the principle of protease-targeting chimera (PROTAC) [9,10,80]. A compound with affinity for the Hippel–Lincau-cullin-Ring (VHL) complex and the target protein (e.g., estrogen-related receptor α (ERRα)) is used to attach the protein to the E3 ligase in the VHL complex. After complexation the E3 conjugates ubiquitin to the protein making it a target for proteasomal degradation.

4. Conclusions

In recent decades, several diverse methods have been developed for the targeting of toxins to cancer tissue to avoid their general systemic toxicity. In the present review, the initial sections concern new attempts developed for prodrugs to be cleaved predominantly in the microenvironment of cancer cells and tumors. Thus, the lower pH characterizing cancer tissue has been explored for selective cleavage of prodrugs based on amides of a substituted maleic acid [20], a hydrazone promoiety [14,21,22], and labile acetal linkage to polymers [26]. A prodrug of doxorubicin (Aldoxorubicin) designed to prevent cardiotoxicity expected to be cleaved by the acidic microenvironment of cancer cells failed in clinical trial III [22]. Moreover, proof-of-concept studies of prodrugs relying on selective cleavage due to the increased ROS production in cancer cells comprise examples of arylboronic acid derivatives [13,15,29]. An example of glutathione-promoted cleavage of a disulfide-based prodrug has also appeared [16].

Next, enzymes, overexpressed by cancer cells or neovascular tissue in tumors, capable of selective cleavage of prodrugs carrying a peptide substrate moiety, offer several examples: e.g., MMP [34], cathepsin B [35], β-glucuronidase [17,38,39], and PSA [19,41,43] and PSMA [56,60]. One prodrug, mipsagargin, actually went into clinical phase III trials but, despite the polarity of the γGlu-γGlu-γGlu-γGlu-βAsp peptide moiety, the compound appeared to be able to penetrate cell membranes of benign cells also, and thus cause general toxicity [58].

In addition, the progress within the field of ADCs (with an anticancer drug as payload) comprise >60 entities in clinical development [62–64]. In total eight ADCs have been approved by the FDA as new and improved cancer therapies, albeit not in the period 2014 to 2019 [83–88]. Calicheamicin and maytansine have been used as the payload in many of these drugs [63].

Another approach also involving antibodies is ADEPT [70,71]; however, even though promising clinical results have been reported, no drugs based on ADEPT are currently approved for clinical use [68,69].

In addition, an advanced approach requiring selective introduction of a gene, coding for an enzyme capable of cleaving a prodrug, into cancer cells (i.e., GDEPT) [69,70] is considered a promising approach, but so far no drugs based on this concept have been approved. Similarly, targeting to cancer cells via sugar–protein recognition processes involving lectins present on the surface of cancer cells (i.e., LEAPT) have been explored [76–78]. Nevertheless, no drugs based on these principles have been approved as yet.

Finally, recent examples of protease-targeting chimeras (PROTACs) involve ubiquitination enzyme complexes that undergo proteolytic degradation to release the drug [9,10,80], however, this technique is at an early stage, and no examples of its clinical use have appeared.

Even though the described techniques have been utilized to improve the solubility of paclitaxel and selectivity of doxorubicin, the associated prodrugs have not as yet shown sufficiently improved properties to convince medical agencies that they can be approved as drugs. In conclusion, the new approaches reviewed here may indeed lead to future new anticancer drugs that are urgently needed for treatment of cancer diseases for which no cure exists. Nevertheless, most of these recently developed targeting principles remain to result in approved drugs, which emphasizes the need for further research to unleash the full potential of these concepts currently considered for experimental therapies.

Author Contributions: Both authors have contributed to the manuscript. Both authors have read and agreed to the published version of the manuscript.

Funding: This research received no external funding.

Institutional Review Board Statement: Not applicable.

Informed Consent Statement: Not applicable.

Data Availability Statement: No supporting information for this work.

Conflicts of Interest: The authors declare no conflict of interest.

References

1. Mishra, A.P.; Chandra, S.; Tiwari, R.; Srivastava, A.; Tiwari, G. Therapeutic potential of prodrugs towards targeted drug delivery. *Open Med. Chem. J.* **2018**, *12*, 111–123. [CrossRef]
2. Elsharif, N.A. Review: Prodrug concept in drug design. *Res. Rev. J. Pharm. Sci.* **2018**, *9*, 22–28.
3. Zawilska, J.B.; Wojcieszak, J.; Olejniczak, A.B. Prodrugs: A challenge for the drug development. *Pharm. Rep.* **2013**, *65*, 1–14. [CrossRef]
4. McKeage, K.; Scott, L.J. Atovaquone/proguanil: A review of its use for the prophylaxis of *Plasmodium falciparum malaria*. *Drugs* **2003**, *63*, 597–623. [CrossRef]
5. Oketch-Rabah, H.A.; Marles, R.J.; Jordan, S.A.; Low Dog, T. United States pharmacopeia safety review of willow bark. *Planta Med.* **2019**, *85*, 1192–1202. [CrossRef]
6. Das, N.; Dhanawat, M.; Dash, B.; Nagarwal, R.C.; Shrivastava, S.K. Codrug: An efficient approach for drug optimization. *Eur. J. Pharm. Sci.* **2010**, *41*, 571–588. [CrossRef] [PubMed]
7. Greenstein, R.J.; Su, L.; Shahidi, A.; Brown, S.T. On the action of 5-amino-salicylic acid and sulfapyridine on *M. avium* including subspecies paratuberculosis. *PLoS ONE* **2007**, *2*, e516.
8. Zhang, X.; Li, X.; You, Q.; Zhang, X. Prodrug strategy for cancer cell-specific targeting: A recent overview. *Eur. J. Med. Chem.* **2017**, *139*, 542–563. [CrossRef] [PubMed]
9. Bondeson, D.P.; Mares, A.; Smith, I.E.D.; Ko, E.; Campos, S.; Miah, A.H.; Mulholland, K.E.; Routly, N.; Buckley, D.L.; Gustafson, J.L.; et al. Catalytic in vivo protein knockdown by small-molecule PROTACs. *Nat. Chem. Biol.* **2015**, *11*, 611–617. [CrossRef] [PubMed]
10. Paiva, S.-L.; Crews, C.M. Targeted protein degradation: Elements of PROTAC design. *Curr. Opin. Chem. Biol.* **2019**, *50*, 111–119. [CrossRef]
11. Weber, C.E.; Kuo, P.C. The tumor microenvironment. *Surg. Oncol.* **2012**, *21*, 172–177. [CrossRef] [PubMed]
12. Corbet, C.; Feron, O. Tumour acidosis: From the passenger to the driver's seat. *Nat. Rev. Cancer* **2017**, *17*, 577–593. [CrossRef] [PubMed]
13. Mu, J.; Zhong, H.; Zou, H.; Liu, T.; Yu, N.; Zhang, X.; Xu, Z.; Chen, Z.; Guo, S. Acid-sensitive PEGylated paclitaxel prodrug nanoparticles for cancer therapy: Effect of PEG length on antitumor efficacy. *J. Control. Release* **2020**, *326*, 265–275. [CrossRef] [PubMed]
14. Souza, C.; Pellosi, D.S.; Tedesco, A.C. Prodrugs for targeted cancer therapy. *Expert Rev. Anticancer* **2019**, *19*, 483–502. [CrossRef] [PubMed]
15. Maslah, H.; Skarbek, C.; Pethe, S.; Labruere, R. Anticancer boron-containing prodrugs responsive to oxidative stress from the tumor microenvironment. *Eur. J. Med. Chem.* **2020**, *207*, 112670. [CrossRef] [PubMed]
16. Wu, X.; Sun, X.; Guo, Z.; Tang, J.; Shen, Y.; James, T.D.; Tian, H.; Zhu, W. In Vivo and In Situ tracking cancer chemotherapy by highly photostable NIR fluorescent theranostic prodrug. *J. Am. Chem. Soc.* **2014**, *136*, 3579–3588. [CrossRef]

17. De Graaf, M.; Boven, E.; Scheeren, H.W.; Haisma, H.J.; Pinedo, H.M. Beta-glucuronidase-mediated drug release. *Curr. Pharm. Des.* **2002**, *8*, 1391–1403. [CrossRef]
18. Denmeade, S.R.; Lou, W.; Lovgren, J.; Malm, J.; Lilja, H.; Isaacs, J.T. Specific and efficient peptide substrates for assaying the proteolytic activity of prostate-specific antigen. *Cancer Res.* **1997**, *57*, 4924–4930. [PubMed]
19. Brady, S.F.; Pawluczyk, J.M.; Lumma, P.K.; Feng, D.M.; Wai, J.M.; Jones, R.; Feo-Jones, D.; Wong, B.K.; Miller-Stein, C.; Lin, J.H.; et al. Design and synthesis of a pro-drug of vinblastine targeted at treatment of prostate cancer with enhanced efficacy and reduced systemic toxicity. *J. Med. Chem.* **2002**, *45*, 4706–4715. [CrossRef]
20. Akinboye, E.S.; Rosen, M.D.; Denmeade, S.R.; Kwabi-Addo, B.; Bakare, O. Design, synthesis, and evaluation of pH-dependent hydrolyzable emetine analogues as treatment for prostate cancer. *J. Med. Chem.* **2012**, *55*, 7450–7459. [CrossRef]
21. Kratz, F. Doxo-emch (INNO-206): The first albumin-binding prodrug of doxorubicin to enter clinical trials. *Expert Opin. Investig. Drugs* **2007**, *16*, 855–866. [CrossRef] [PubMed]
22. Cranmer, L.D. Spotlight on aldoxorubicin (INNO-206) and its potential in the treatment of soft tissue sarcomas: Evidence to date. *OncoTargets Ther.* **2019**, *12*, 2047–2062. [CrossRef] [PubMed]
23. O'Brien, M.E.R.; Wigler, N.; Inbar, M.; Rosso, R.; Grischke, E.; Santoro, A.; Catane, R.; Kieback, D.G.; Tomczak, P.; Ackland, S.P.; et al. Reduced cardiotoxicity and comparable efficacy in a phase III trial of pegylated liposomal doxorubicin HCl (CAELYX/Doxil) versus conventional doxorubicin for first-line treatment of metastatic breast cancer. *Ann. Oncol.* **2004**, *15*, 440–449. [CrossRef]
24. Gelderblom, H.; Verwij, J.; Nooter, K.; Sparreboom, A. Cremophor EL: The drawbacks and advantages of vehicle selection for drug formulation. *Eur. J. Cancer* **2001**, *37*, 1590–1598. [CrossRef]
25. Miele, E.; Spinelli, G.P.; Miele, E.; Tomao, F.; Tomao, S. Albumin-bound formulation of paclitaxel (Abraxane®ABI-007) in the treatment of breast cancer. *Int. J. Nanomed.* **2009**, *4*, 99–105.
26. Gu, Y.; Zhong, Y.; Meng, F.; Cheng, R.; Deng, C.; Zhong, Z. Acetal-linked paclitaxel prodrug micellar nanoparticles as a versatile and potent platform for cancer therapy. *Biomacromolecules* **2013**, *14*, 2772–2780. [CrossRef]
27. Björkling, F.; Moreira, J.; Stenvang, J. Anticancer Agents. In *Textbook of Drug Design and Discovery*, 5th ed.; Strømgaard, K., Krogsgaard-Larsen, P., Madsen, U., Eds.; CRC Press: Boca Raton, FL, USA, 2017; pp. 369–386.
28. Pascale, R.M.; Calvisi, D.F.; Simile, M.M.; Feo, C.F.; Feo, F. The warburg effect 97 years after its discovery. *Cancers* **2020**, *12*, 2819. [CrossRef]
29. Wang, L.; Xie, S.; Ma, L.; Chen, Y.; Lu, W. 10-Boronic acid substituted camptothecin as prodrug of SN-38. *Eur. J. Med. Chem.* **2016**, *116*, 84–89. [CrossRef]
30. Octavia, Y.; Tocchetti, C.G.; Gabrielson, K.L.; Janssens, S.; Crijns, H.J.; Moens, A.L. Doxorubicin-induced cardiomyopathy: From molecular mechanisms to therapeutic strategies. *J. Mol. Cell. Cardiol.* **2012**, *52*, 1213–1225. [CrossRef]
31. Skarbek, C.; Serra, S.; Maslah, H.; Rascol, E.; Labruere, R. Arylboronate prodrugs of doxorubicin as promising chemotherapy for pancreatic cancer. *Bioorg. Chem.* **2019**, *91*, 103158. [CrossRef] [PubMed]
32. Dong, C.; Zhou, Q.; Xiang, J.; Liu, F.; Zhou, Z.; Shen, Y. Self-assembly of oxidation-responsive polyethylene glycol-paclitaxel prodrug for cancer chemotherapy. *J. Control. Release* **2020**, *321*, 529–539. [CrossRef] [PubMed]
33. Gamcsik, M.P.; Kasibhatla, M.S.; Teeter, S.D.; Colvin, O.M. Glutathione levels in human tumors. *Biomarkers* **2012**, *17*, 671–691. [CrossRef]
34. Albright, C.F.; Graciani, N.; Han, W.; Yue, E.; Stein, R.; Lai, Z.; Diamond, M.; Dowling, R.; Grimminger, L.; Zhang, S.-Y.; et al. Matrix metalloproteinase-activated doxorubicin prodrugs inhibit HT1080 xenograft growth better than doxorubicin with less toxicity. *Mol. Cancer* **2005**, *4*, 751–760. [CrossRef]
35. Shao, L.-H.; Liu, S.-P.; Hou, J.-X.; Zhang, Y.-H.; Peng, C.-W.; Zhong, Y.-J.; Liu, X.; Liu, X.-L.; Hong, Y.-P.; Firestone, R.A.; et al. Cathepsin B cleavable novel prodrug Ac-Phe-Lys-PABC-ADM enhances efficacy at reduced toxicity in treating gastric cancer peritoneal carcinomatosis An experimental study. *Cancer* **2012**, *118*, 2986–2996. [CrossRef] [PubMed]
36. Fujita, M.; Taniguchi, N.; Makita, A.; Oikawa, K. Cancer-associated alteration of β-glucuronidase in human lung cancer: Elevated activity and increased phosphorylation. *GANN Jpn. J. Cancer Res.* **1984**, *75*, 508–517.
37. Sperker, B.; Werner, U.; Murdter, T.E.; Tekkaya, C.; Fritz, P.; Wacke, R.; Adam, U.; Gerken, M.; Drewelow, B.; Kroemer, H.K.; et al. Expression and function of β-glucuronidase in pancreatic cancer: Potential role in drug targeting. *Naunyn Schmiedeberg's Arch. Pharm.* **2000**, *362*, 110–115. [CrossRef]
38. De Bont, D.B.A.; Leenders, R.G.G.; Haisma, H.J.; van der Meulen-Muileman, I.; Scheeren, H.W. Synthesis and biological activity of β-glucuronyl carbamate-based prodrugs of paclitaxel as potential candidates for ADEPT. *Bioorg. Med. Chem.* **1997**, *5*, 405–414. [CrossRef]
39. Leu, Y.-L.; Roffler, S.R.; Chern, J.-W. Design and synthesis of water-soluble glucuronide derivatives of camptothecin for cancer prodrug monotherapy and antibody-directed enzyme prodrug therapy (ADEPT). *J. Med. Chem.* **1999**, *42*, 3623–3628. [CrossRef] [PubMed]
40. Akinboye, E.S.; Brennen, W.N.; Denmeade, S.R.; Isaacs, J.T. Albumin-linked prostate-specific antigen-activated thapsigargin- and niclosamide-based molecular grenades targeting the microenvironment in metastatic castration-resistant prostate cancer. *Asian J. Urol.* **2019**, *6*, 99–108. [CrossRef]
41. Garsky, V.M.; Lumma, P.K.; Feng, D.-M.; Wai, J.; Ramjit, H.G.; Sardana, M.K.; Oliff, A.; Jones, R.E.; DeFeo-Jones, D.; Freidinger, R.M.; et al. The synthesis of a prodrug of doxorubicin designed to provide reduced systemic toxicity and greater target efficacy. *J. Med. Chem.* **2001**, *44*, 4216–4224. [CrossRef]

42. Lindner, P.; Christensen, S.B.; Nissen, P.; Møller, J.V.; Engedal, N. Cell death induced by the ER stressor thapsigargin involves death receptor 5, anon-autophagic function of MAP1LC3B, anddistinct contributions from unfoldedprotein response components. *Cell. Commun. Signal.* **2020**, *18*, 12. [CrossRef]
43. Denmeade, S.R.; Isaacs, J.T. The SERCA pump as a therapeutic target: Making a "Smart bomb" for prostate cancer. *Cancer Biol.* **2005**, *4*, 14–22. [CrossRef]
44. Denmeade, S.R.; Jakobsen, C.M.; Janssen, S.; Khan, S.R.; Garrett, E.S.; Lilja, H.; Christensen, S.B.; Isaacs, J.T. Prostate-specific antigen-activated thapsigargin prodrug as targeted therapy for prostate cancer. *J. Natl. Cancer Inst.* **2003**, *95*, 990–1000. [CrossRef]
45. Darson, M.F.; Pacelli, A.; Roche, P.; Rittenhouse, H.G.; Wolfert, R.L.; Young, C.Y.; Klee, G.G.; Tindall, D.J.; Bostwick, D.G. Human glandular kallikrein 2 (hK2) expression in prostatic intraepithelial neoplasia and adenocarcinoma: A novel prostate cancer marker. *Urology* **1997**, *49*, 857–862. [CrossRef]
46. Darson, M.F.; Pacelli, A.; Roche, P.; Rittenhouse, H.G.; Wolfert, R.L.; Saeid, M.S.; Young, C.Y.; Klee, G.G.; Tindall, D.J.; Bostwick, D.G. Human glandular kallikrein 2 expression in prostate adenocarcinoma and lymph node metastases. *Urology* **1999**, *53*, 939–944. [CrossRef]
47. Janssen, S.; Rosen, D.M.; Ricklis, R.M.; Dionne, C.A.; Lilja, H.; Christensen, S.B.; Isaacs, J.T.; Denmeade, S.R. Pharmacokinetics, biodistribution, and antitumor efficacy of a human glandular kallikrein 2 (hK2)-activated thapsigargin prodrug. *Prostate* **2006**, *66*, 358–368. [CrossRef] [PubMed]
48. Pinto, J.; Suffoletto, B.; Berzin, T.; Qiao, C.; Lin, S.; Tong, W.; Heston, W. Identification of a membrane-bound pteroyl poly gamma-glutamyl carboxypeptidase (folate hydrolase) that is highly expressed in human prostatic carcinoma cells. *FASEB J.* **1996**, *10*, A496.
49. Denmeade, S.R.; Mhaka, A.M.; Rosen, D.M.; Brennen, W.N.; Dalrymple, S.; Dach, I.; Olesen, C.; Gurel, B.; DeMarzo, A.M.; Wilding, G.; et al. Engineering a prostate-specific membrane antigen-activated tumor endothelial cell prodrug for cancer therapy. *Sci. Transl. Med.* **2012**, *4*. [CrossRef] [PubMed]
50. Wang, H.-L.; Wang, S.-S.; Song, W.-H.; Pan, Y.; Yu, H.-P.; Si, T.-G.; Liu, Y.; Cui, X.-N.; Guo, Z. Expression of prostate-specific membrane antigen in lung cancer cells and tumor neovasculature endothelial cells and its clinical significance. *PLoS ONE* **2015**, *10*. [CrossRef]
51. Nomura, N.; Pastorino, S.; Jiang, P.; Lambert, G.; Crawford, J.R.; Gymnopoulos, M.; Piccioni, D.; Juarez, T.; Pingle, S.C.; Makale, M.; et al. Prostate specific membrane antigen (PSMA) expression in primary gliomas and breast cancer brain metastases. *Cancer Cell Int.* **2014**, *14*, 1–9. [CrossRef]
52. Kasoha, M.; Unger, C.; Solomayer, E.-F.; Bohle, R.M.; Zaharia, C.; Khreich, F.; Wagenpfeil, S.; Juhasz-Boess, I. Prostate-specific membrane antigen (PSMA) expression in breast cancer and its metastases. *Clin. Exp. Metastasis* **2017**, *34*, 479–490. [CrossRef] [PubMed]
53. Nimmagadda, S.; Pullambhatla, M.; Chen, Y.; Parsana, P.; Lisok, A.; Chatterjee, S.; Mease, R.; Rowe, S.P.; Lupold, S.; Pienta, K.J.; et al. Low-level endogenous PSMA expression in nonprostatic tumor xenografts is sufficient for In Vivo tumor targeting and imaging. *J. Nucl. Med.* **2018**, *59*, 486–493. [CrossRef]
54. Pinto, J.T.; Suffoletto, B.P.; Berzin, T.M.; Qiao, C.H.; Lin, S.; Tong, W.P.; May, F.; Mukherjee, B.; Heston, W.D.W. Prostate-specific membrane antigen: A novel folate hydrolase in human prostatic carcinoma cells. *Clin. Cancer Res.* **1996**, *2*, 1445–1451.
55. Zimmermann, T.; Christensen, S.B.; Franzyk, H. Preparation of enzyme-activated thapsigargin prodrugs by solid-phase synthesis. *Molecules* **2018**, *23*, 1463. [CrossRef] [PubMed]
56. Mahalingam, D.; Tubb, B.; Nemunaitis, J.J.; Cen, P.; Rowe, J.H.; Sarantopoulos, J.; Kurman, M.R.; Allgood, V.; Campos, L.T. Clinical activity and correlative DCE-MRI imaging of G-202, a thapsigargin-based prostate-specific membrane antigen-activated prodrug, in progressive hepatocellular cancer. *J. Clin. Oncol.* **2015**, *33*, 301. [CrossRef]
57. Denmeade, S.R.; Isaacs, J.T. Engineering enzymatically activated "molecular grenades" for cancer. *Oncotarget* **2012**, *3*, 666–667. [CrossRef]
58. Mahalingam, D.; Mahalingam, D.; Arora, S.P.; Sarantopoulos, J.; Peguero, J.; Campos, L.; Cen, P.; Rowe, J.; Allgood, V.; Tubb, B.; et al. A phase ii, multicenter, single-arm study of mipsagargin (G-202) as a second-line therapy following sorafenib for adult patients with progressive advanced hepatocellular carcinoma. *Cancers* **2019**, *11*, 833. [CrossRef]
59. Tarvainen, I.; Zimmermann, T.; Heinonen, P.; Jantti, M.H.; Yli-Kauhaluoma, J.; Talman, V.; Franzyk, H.; Tuominen, R.K.; Christensen, S.B. Missing selectivity of targeted 4β-phorbol prodrugs expected to be potential chemotherapeutics. *ACS Med. Chem. Lett.* **2020**, *11*, 671–677. [CrossRef]
60. Jakobsen, C.M.; Denmeade, S.R.; Isaacs, J.T.; Gady, A.; Olsen, C.E.; Christensen, S.B. Design, synthesis, and pharmacological evaluation of thapsigargin analogues for targeting apoptosis to prostatic cancer cells. *J. Med. Chem.* **2001**, *44*, 4696–4703. [CrossRef] [PubMed]
61. Dan, N.; Setua, S.; Kashyap, V.K.; Khan, S.; Jaggi, M.; Yallapu, M.M.; Chauhan, S.C. Antibody-drug conjugates for cancer therapy: Chemistry to clinical implications. *Pharmaceuticals* **2018**, *11*, 1–22.
62. Poudel, Y.B.; Chowdari, N.S.; Cheng, H.; Iwuagwu, C.I.; King, H.D.; Kotapati, S.; Passmore, D.; Rampulla, R.; Mathur, A.; Vite, G.; et al. Chemical modification of linkers provide stable linker-payloads for the generation of antibody-drug conjugates. *ACS Med. Chem. Lett.* **2020**, *11*, 2190–2194. [CrossRef] [PubMed]
63. Nicolaou, K.C.; Rigol, S. The role of organic synthesis in the emergence and development of antibody-drug conjugates as targeted cancer therapies. *Angew. Chem. Int. Ed.* **2019**, *58*, 11206–11241. [CrossRef]

64. Tumey, L.N. Thinking Small and Dreaming Big: Medicinal Chemistry Strategies for Designing Optimal Antibody-Drug Conjugates (ADC's). In *2017-Medicinal Chemistry Reviews*; American Chemical Society: Washington, DC, USA, 2017; Volume 52, pp. 363–381.
65. Morrison, S.L.; Johnson, M.J.; Herzenberg, L.D.; Oi, V.T. Chimeric human antibody molecules: Mouse antigen-binding domains with human constant region domains. *Proc. Natl. Acad. Sci. USA* **1984**, *81*, 6851–6855. [CrossRef] [PubMed]
66. Nicolaou, K.C.; Smith, A.L.; Yue, E.W. Chemistry and biology of natural and designed enediynes. *Proc. Natl. Acad. Sci. USA* **1993**, *90*, 5881–5888. [CrossRef]
67. Maiese, W.M.; Lechevalier, M.P.; Lechevalier, H.A.; Korshalla, J.; Kuck, N.; Fantini, A.; Wildey, M.J.; Thomas, J.; Greenstein, M. Calicheamicins, a novel family of antitumor antibiotics: Taxonomy, fermentation and biological properties. *J. Antibiot.* **1989**, *42*, 558–563. [CrossRef]
68. Sharma, S.K.; Bagshawe, K.D. Antibody directed enzyme prodrug therapy (ADEPT): Trials and tribulations. *Advan. Drug Deliv. Rev.* **2017**, *118*, 2–7. [CrossRef]
69. Aloysius, H.; Hu, L. Targeted prodrug approaches for hormone refractory prostate cancer. *Med. Res. Rev.* **2015**, *35*, 554–585. [CrossRef]
70. Jung, M. Antibody directed enzyme prodrug therapy (ADEPT) and related approaches for anticancer therapy. *Mini-Rev. Med. Chem.* **2001**, *1*, 399–407. [CrossRef] [PubMed]
71. Tranoy-Opalinski, I.; Fernandes, A.; Thomas, M.; Gesson, J.P.; Papot, S. Design of self-immolative linkers for tumour-activated prodrug therapy. *Anticancer Agents Med. Chem.* **2008**, *8*, 618–637. [CrossRef] [PubMed]
72. Moradian Tehrani, R.; Verdi, J.; Noureddini, M.; Salehi, R.; Salarinia, R.; Mosalaei, M.; Simonian, M.; Alani, B.; Ghiasi, M.R.; Jaafari, M.R.; et al. Mesenchymal stem cells: A new platform for targeting suicide genes in cancer. *J. Cell. Physiol.* **2018**, *233*, 3831–3845. [CrossRef] [PubMed]
73. Singhal, S.; Kaiser, L.R. Cancer chemotherapy using suicide genes. *Surg. Oncol. Clin. N. Am.* **1998**, *7*, 505–536. [CrossRef]
74. Sanchez-Sanchez, L.; Tapia-Moreno, A.; Juarez-Moreno, K.; Patterson, D.P.; Cadena-Nava, R.D.; Douglas, T.; Vazquez-Duhalt, R. Design of a VLP-nanovehicle for CYP450 enzymatic activity delivery. *J. Nanobiotechnol.* **2015**, *13*, 1–10. [CrossRef] [PubMed]
75. Sharon, N.; Lis, H. History of lectins: From hemagglutinins to biological recognition molecules. *Glycobiology* **2004**, *14*, 53R–62R. [CrossRef]
76. Ma, Y.; Chen, H.; Su, S.; Wang, T.; Zhang, C.; Fida, G.; Cui, S.; Zhao, J.; Gu, Y. Galactose as broad ligand for multiple tumor imaging and therapy. *J. Cancer* **2015**, *6*, 658–670. [CrossRef] [PubMed]
77. Lin, Y.-S.; Tungpradit, R.; Sinchaikul, S.; An, F.-M.; Liu, D.-Z.; Phutrakul, S.; Chen, S.-T. Targeting the delivery of glycan-based paclitaxel prodrugs to cancer cells via glucose transporters. *J. Med. Chem.* **2008**, *51*, 7428–7441. [CrossRef]
78. Garnier, P.; Wang, X.-T.; Robinson, M.A.; van Kasteren, S.; Perkins, A.C.; Frier, M.; Fairbanks, A.J.; Davis, B.G. Lectin-directed enzyme activated prodrug therapy (LEAPT): Synthesis and evaluation of rhamnose-capped prodrugs. *J. Drug Target.* **2010**, *18*, 794–802. [CrossRef]
79. Mukhopadhyay, D.; Riezman, H. Proteasome-independent functions of ubiquitin in endocytosis and signaling. *Science* **2007**, *315*, 201–205. [CrossRef]
80. Teicher, B.A.; Tomaszewski, J.E. Proteasome inhibitors. *Biochem. Pharm.* **2015**, *96*, 1–9. [CrossRef]
81. Ciechanover, A. The unravelling of the ubiquitin system. *Nat. Rev. Mol. Cell Biol.* **2015**, *16*, 322–324. [CrossRef] [PubMed]
82. Bashraheel, S.S.; Domling, A.; Goda, S.K. Update on targeted cancer therapies, single or in combination, and their fine tuning for precision medicine. *Biomed. Pharm.* **2020**, *125*, 110009. [CrossRef]
83. Bronson, J.J.; Peese, K.M.; Black, A.; Dhar, M.; Pashine, A.; Ellsworth, B.A.; Merritt, J.R. To Market, To Market. In *2015 Medicinal Chemistry Reviews*; Desai, M.J.C., Ed.; American Chemcal Society: Washington, DC, USA, 2015; Volume 50, pp. 461–576.
84. Bronson, J.J.; Peese, K.M.; Dhar, M.; Pashine, A.; Duclos, F.J.; Ellsworth, B.A.; Garcia, R.; Merritt, J.R. To Market, To Market. In *2016 Medicinal Chemistry Reviews*; Desai, M.C., Ed.; Amercian Chemical Society: Washington, DC, USA, 2016; Volume 51, pp. 439–540.
85. Bolger, C.A.; Dhar, T.G.M.; Pashine, A.; Dragovich, P.S.; Mallet, W.; Robert, M.J.; Peese, K.M. To Market, To Market. In *2017 Medicinal Chemistry Review*; Bronson, J.J., Ed.; American Chemical Society: Washington, DC, USA, 2017; Volume 52, pp. 537–601.
86. Bolger, C.A.; Carpenter, J.E.; Dhar, T.G.M.; Pashine, A.; Dragovich, P.S.; Cook, J.H.; Gillis, E.P.; Peese, K.M.; Merritt, J.R. To Market, To Market. In *2018 Medicinal Chemistry Reviews*; Bonson, J., Ed.; American Chemical Society: Washington, DC, USA, 2018; Volume 53, pp. 587–696.
87. Bolger, C.A.; Kahn, S.A.; Lipovšek, D.; Mallet, W.; Wieler, J. To Market, To Market. In *2019 Medicinal Chemistry Reviews*; Bonson, J.J., Ed.; American Chemical Society: Washington, DC, USA, 2019; Volume 54, pp. 601–639.
88. Araujo, E.; Braun, M.-G.; Dragovich, P.S.; Converso, A.; Nantermet, P.G.; Roecker, A.J.; Dhar, T.G.M.; Haile, P.; Hurtley, A.; Merritt, J.R. To Market, To Market-2018: Small Molecules. In *2019 Medicinal Chemistry Reviews-2019*; Bonson, J.J., Ed.; American Chemical Society: Washington, DC, USA, 2019; Volume 54, pp. 469–596.

MDPI
St. Alban-Anlage 66
4052 Basel
Switzerland
Tel. +41 61 683 77 34
Fax +41 61 302 89 18
www.mdpi.com

Molecules Editorial Office
E-mail: molecules@mdpi.com
www.mdpi.com/journal/molecules

www.ingramcontent.com/pod-product-compliance
Lightning Source LLC
LaVergne TN
LVHW070748100526
838202LV00013B/1327
* 9 7 8 3 0 3 6 5 4 9 2 0 0 *